DATE DUE

MAR 1 0 2003

BRODART   Cat. No. 23-221

AFFECT REGULATION AND THE DEVELOPMENT OF PSYCHOPATHOLOGY

Affect Regulation and the Development of Psychopathology

SUSAN J. BRADLEY

THE GUILFORD PRESS
New York   London

© 2000 Susan J. Bradley
Published by The Guilford Press
A Division of Guilford Publications, Inc.
72 Spring Street, New York, NY 10012
www.guilford.com

Printed in the United States of America

This book is printed on acid-free paper.

Last digit is print number: 9   8   7   6   5   4   3   2   1

Library of Congress Cataloging-in-Publication Data
is available from the Publisher.

ISBN 1-57230-548-7

About the Author

Susan J. Bradley, MD, FRCP(C), is Professor in the Department of Psychiatry, University of Toronto, and formerly Head of the Division of Child Psychiatry and Psychiatrist-in-Chief at the Hospital for Sick Children, Toronto, Ontario, Canada. She is also consultant psychiatrist to the Child and Adolescent Gender Identity Clinic at the Centre for Addiction and Mental Health, Clarke Division, and has coauthored the book *Gender Identity Disorder and Psychosexual Problems in Children and Adolescents* with Kenneth J. Zucker (The Guilford Press, 1995). In addition to her research and theoretical interests in gender identity disorder and in affect regulation, Dr. Bradley has had a longstanding interest in parenting and evaluation of parenting programs. Currently, she engages in teaching, research, and some clinical work.

Preface

Psychiatry and related theories of psychopathology have been encumbered by the polarization of the biological versus the psychosocial, despite a widespread stated belief in a biopsychosocial model. I believe that one factor maintaining this dualistic approach is the lack of a theory that integrates the biological with the psychosocial without doing an injustice to the main tenets of either side. I propose that affect regulation affords us a way of reducing this dualism by providing a common ground understandable and relevant to both biological and psychosocial approaches.

My thesis is that emotional arousal and the failure to regulate this arousal constitute a general factor in the development, recurrence, and maintenance of various forms of psychopathology. In the so-called "internalizing" disorders, such dysregulation occurs most typically when an individual with heightened stress reactivity becomes stressed. In the "externalizing" disorders, stress reactivity may be less central to the affect dysregulation; a genetic vulnerability to anger and aggressive behavior may instead play the pivotal role. Other, more specific factors give each disorder its unique quality. As we advance our investigations and treatments of various disorders, I believe it is important to distinguish the aspects of each disorder that are related to affect regulation or general arousal difficulties from other, disorder-specific factors that may reflect different approaches to coping.

This theory is an attempt to integrate many factors that have been shown to relate independently to the development, onset, or maintenance of psychopathology. It has arisen out of the frustration expressed by students grappling with a multiplicity of views and theoretical approaches to psychopathology. It also attempts to address clinicians' need for a framework within which to integrate recent developments from the many empirical foundations that contribute to the understanding of psychopathology.

In Part I (Chapter 1), I first briefly outline the evidence for a general arousal factor in psychopathology. I then present an overview of the model and illustrate how it can be used to understand several disorders.

In Part II, I describe in detail the developmental literature as well as the neurological basis for the model. Chapter 2 is a brief introduction to the concept of affect regulation and its development. In Chapter 3, I present the evidence from studies of inhibited children, possibly best understood as contributing to a genetic basis for difficulties with affect regulation. Studies of reactivity or defensiveness in animals are described to illustrate the presumed common biological basis for this trait. The role of perinatal insults in inducing stress reactivity is considered as part of the review of constitutional factors. In Chapter 4, I review the attachment literature to demonstrate how insecure attachment contributes to difficulties with affect regulation. I also examine how exposure to parental and parent–child conflict may sensitize a child to subsequent situations of conflict, potentially interfering with the child's development of skills to manage both the experience and expression of affect.

In Chapter 5, I discuss the evidence that stress produces arousal and, if prolonged, may induce failure in the individual's capacity to modulate that arousal. Studies that point to the importance of the corticosteroid receptors in limbic areas in regulating the stress response are described. The effects of two particularly severe forms of stress—trauma and abuse—are then examined. Chapter 6 shows how an individual's attempts to cope with arousal are affected by many factors, including temperament, caregiver behaviors, and experience.

In Chapter 7, I discuss the various brain areas that have been implicated in the development of psychopathology. I focus on the limbic system and show how specific areas such as the amygdala may play a crucial role in the development of defensiveness. Some of the recent theorizing about neural networks that relate to specific aspects of psychopathology, such as cognitive deficits and thought disorder, is also described. The purposes of this chapter are to orient readers to the most recent developments in neurobiology, and to give some idea of the exciting potential for integrating theories of the mind with those of the body. Both nonspecialist and specialist readers are encouraged to consult additional sources for further information as they feel the need.

Moving from brain to mind, in Chapter 8, I present an analysis of how the various schools of psychotherapy deal with affect and its regulation. Common aspects of the psychotherapies, particularly as they may relate to improving the individual's capacity to manage affect, are outlined. Resistance to change, a common dilemma in psychotherapy, is addressed in the context of the patient's capacity to develop strategies for affect regulation.

In Part III, the model is illustrated by applying it to several syndromes. Chapter 9 covers disorders generally referred to as "internalizing" (primarily the anxiety and mood disorders); Chapter 10 discusses disruptive behavior disorders (the "externalizing" disorders); and Chapter 11 covers psychotic disorders. In each chapter, efforts are made to distinguish the general factors from the disorder-specific factors in psychopathology; to show how various factors may change with development; and to suggest how research and intervention strategies should attempt to distinguish between general and disorder-specific factors.

I conclude the book in Part IV (Chapter 12) with suggestions for future research regarding the development of affect regulation, its relationship to other aspects of development, and its potential for change through various interventions.

In undertaking this work, I have relied on a number of excellent reviews and monographs, particularly to cover areas outside psychiatry proper. Because I have attempted both to extract information from several different and large literatures, and to purposely focus only on areas relevant to affect regulation and the development of psychopathology, some readers may feel that I have not done justice to the richness of their particular literature. To build an integrated theory, I had to tease out common principles and may have forsaken richness in the service of selectivity. I have tried to create a framework that explicates many of the facts we now have, but that can be expanded with the development of new knowledge. Undoubtedly, with the growth of knowledge it will be possible to refine aspects of the model, especially in the area of brain development and functioning. It is also possible that the integration of various components will be modified. I look forward to extending and elaborating the model as new data become available and as my readers provide feedback.

Acknowledgments

In writing this book, I have been aided by many colleagues who have spent long hours reading and offering suggestions for improvement. I am indebted to them, as without this input I would not have had the courage to expose this work to more public scrutiny. First, I want to thank Susan Goldberg, who was my main resource on the attachment literature. J. Rodney Wachsmuth, Pier Bryden, and Wendy Moore read early drafts of specific chapters and provided valuable feedback. Paul Steinhauer has been an enthusiastic supporter of many of my ideas, and through our discussions has helped inform my thinking and writing. Mary Seeman, who read my first paper on affect regulation and who encouraged me to put these ideas into a book, has been a mentor in this as she has in other ways. Linda Miland, a member of the editorial services staff at the Hospital for Sick Children, was the initial editor of Chapter 1; she helped me examine my writing style and, I hope, improve it. The many students who have been exposed to my teaching in this area have, through their critical analysis and questioning, forced me to rewrite and rethink many sections. I also want to thank my former secretary, Wilma Aranha, who patiently typed and retyped headings for diagrams and who helped me become more computer-literate. My present secretary, Pat Follett, also deserves thanks for so graciously spending hours photocopying and mailing revisions to The Guilford Press.

Kitty Moore, senior editor at The Guilford Press, has been invaluable in providing critical but judicious feedback about my writing style and the organization of the manuscript. Jack Bates went beyond the bounds of his initial job as an endorser and provided a complete re-view of the book, with important suggestions about references and or-ganization. Graeme Taylor, Saul Levine, and Elaine Walker agreed to do quick reviews at very short notice. Guilford's copy editor, Marie Sprayberry, transformed my halting prose into coherent and flowing writing; Paul Gordon, art director, provided a thoroughly attractive cover; and Anna Nelson brought everything together in the produc-tion of the book. Without this support, I would still be struggling with whether these ideas were worth expressing.

Finally, I want to thank my immediate and extended family for their constant forbearance as I have removed myself from other activi-ties to pursue completion of this work. My husband, Michael, has been continually supportive; my children, Sarah and Lynne, have entered many of the references; and Sarah's partner, Brad Heys, has bailed me out when my computer skills have failed me (an invaluable and affect-regulating experience for writing a book). Lastly, my parents have given me the confidence to do the risk taking that has been necessary for me to believe I could offer new ideas to the world.

Lewis Hyde (1983), in his book *The Gift: Imagination and the Erotic Life of Property*, describes any creative undertaking as a "gift." It is in this spirit that I offer these ideas.

Contents

PART III. Clinical Syndromes

PART IV. Final Remarks

PART I

Overview

Chapter 1

The Model and Its Rationale

This chapter provides an overview of my model of affect dys-regulation as a core factor in various types of psychopathology. I begin by describing briefly how I use the key terms *affects, emotional feelings*, and *arousal* in this book. Next, I provide evidence for a general arousal factor in psychopathology by examining a number of risk factors for psychopathology, as well as what appears to be the common element in various pharmacological and psychotherapeutic interventions for mental disorders. This is followed by brief discussions of the various brain factors (anatomical structures and neurochemical pathways) and mind factors (internal psychological structures) involved in the regulation of affect. I then provide a description and a diagram of the model itself, which integrates these brain and mind factors. Finally, I illustrate how the model can be applied to explanations of various disorders, permitting both general distress and more disorder-specific features to be teased out. All of these topics are, of course, covered in more detail in subsequent chapters of the book; my intent here is simply to provide an orientation.

AFFECTS AND EMOTIONAL FEELINGS: DEFINITIONS

I believe that negative affective states are generally more important than are positive affective states in the development of psychopathology. Negative affect states tend to produce greater physiological arousal (involving variously the hypothalmic pituitary-adrenal axis, the reti-

3

cular activating system and the sympathetic nervous system) than do positive affect states. Arousal generally refers to activation of a system above a basal or resting level. I also believe that the individual's interpretation of negative affect is what leads to a specific negative emotion and to the amount of arousal experienced. For this reason, I have found Frijda's (1993) theorizing about affects and emotional feelings helpful. In contrast to investigators who argue for a set of basic, unanalyzable *emotional feelings*, such as happiness, sadness, fear, anger, disgust, and joy (Izard, 1971; Magai & McFadden, 1995; Tomkins, 1962, 1963), Frijda (1993) argues that "only *affect* proper—that is, the experience of *pleasantness or unpleasantness*—is both unanalyzable and specific for affective experience" (p. 382; italics added). He describes emotional feelings as having four components and one corollary. The components are (1) affect; (2) awareness of situational meaning structure, or felt appraisal of events; (3) felt state of action readiness; and (4) felt bodily change. The corollary is the emotion's "significance" (p. 383).

This notion of two basic affective states—positive and negative affect, which may be elaborated into emotional feelings through experience and cognition—allows for the clinical observation that much emotional distress appears to be unelaborated. This is consistent with findings of a general "negative affect" factor in the tripartite model of Clark and Watson (1991b), and with Eysenck's (1967) "neuroticism" dimension. (See also Malcarne & Ingram, 1994, and Gjone & Stevenson, 1997, regarding negative affectivity and child psychopathology.) Stearns (1993) sees no real distinction between the emotional feelings of sadness and anger except in the response options to act or to withdraw, which are dependent on the social situation in which the affect is elicited and on the individual's learning history. What Stearns regards as basic is distress. With respect to the development of psychopathology, Rapee, Mattick, and Murrell (1986) have argued that *unexplained arousal* is what is particularly effective in prompting negatively valenced emotional experience.

Because of the general tendency to regard negative affect and arousal as relevant to the development of distress, and because I believe that psychopathology develops as a consequence of difficulties with regulation of affect or arousal, I will use the terms *affect regulation* and *arousal regulation* interchangeably. I view affects, emotions, and arousal as dictated by neural circuitry (particularly circuits connected to the amygdala) and regulated by a complex interaction of this circuitry with neurotransmitters (LeDoux, 1993; Panksepp, 1993). For a more complete discussion, see Chapter 2.

EVIDENCE FOR A GENERAL AROUSAL FACTOR IN PSYCHOPATHOLOGY: RISK FACTS AND THERAPEUTIC EFFECTS

Studies of the development of psychopathology suggest risk factors common to many disorders. These include loss, trauma, and abuse; temperamental or stress reactivity; brain insult; attachment difficulties; and sensitivity to expressed emotion or familial conflict. I believe that these risk factors share a tendency to produce high levels of arousal or to interfere with the development of strategies for regulating arousal. Recently, studies examining the relatively high prevalence of anxiety across mental disorders have suggested a common factor in psychopathology, heightened stress reactivity (Garvey, Noyes, Anderson, & Cook, 1991), as have studies of the heritability of anxiety and depression (Kendler, Neale, Kessler, Heath, & Eaves, 1992a). Furthermore, the relatively nonspecific effects of many therapeutic interventions also suggest that the common element may be an anxiety- or distress-relieving mechanism, which over time may reduce stress reactivity. This reduction in stress reactivity may be more salient in the internalizing disorders; however, given the comorbid presence of internalizing psychopathology in the externalizing disorders, stress reactivity may play a role here as well. In the externalizing disorders genetic vulnerability to managing anger or aggression may be more etiologically important (Schmitz, Fulker, & Mrazek, 1995).

Risk Factors for Psychopathology

Trauma, Abuse, and Loss

A history of trauma, abuse, or loss is a feature common to many disorders, including anxiety and mood disorders, eating disorders, conduct disorder, and many personality disorders (Kessler, Davis, & Kendler, 1997). The impact of trauma and abuse in producing prolonged states of hyperarousal has become more evident from recent physiological studies of affected individuals (see van der Kolk, 1996, for an overview). The impact of loss has been well articulated by Bowlby (1969, 1973, 1980), who described the sequence of protest, despair, and detachment in children separated from their mothers for long periods. Extended to other loss experiences, this sequence is now generally accepted as a normative reaction. In nonhuman primates, loss of maternal caretakers early in life produces prolonged states of hyperarousal in reactive animals (Suomi, 1991b), and caretaker loss can impair physiological regulation in other mammals as well (Hofer, 1995). Studies of human children have shown that even brief separations from caretakers (e.g., a mother's hospitalization for a second child's birth or a business trip) can produce significant changes in infants' affect, play behavior, activity level, heart rate, and sleep and eating patterns (Field, 1994). The return of these functions to a normal pattern is partially dependent on the emotional availability of caretakers on their return (Field, 1994).

Temperamental or Stress Reactivity

General temperamental or emotional reactivity has been identified as a risk factor in many theories of personality development and psychopathology (Eysenck, 1967; Strelau, 1994; Gray, 1991; Cloninger, 1987). This notion has been pursued in studies of inhibited infants and young children. Inhibition is a trait that correlates highly with family histories of anxiety and mood disorders (Rosenbaum et al., 1988). Individuals with this trait exhibit higher levels of arousal to stressful stimuli than do noninhibited controls, and a pattern of withdrawal or avoidance when confronted with new or challenging situations (Garcia-Coll, Kagan, & Reznick, 1984; Kagan, Reznick, & Snidman, 1987; Gersten, 1989; Reznick, Gibbons, Johnson, & McDonough, 1989). Kagan (1989), who pioneered studies with inhibited children, reports that inhibition, which is a relatively stable trait (Broberg, Lamb, & Hwang, 1990) but can be modified by early experience, appears more resistant to change after age 7. Kagan theorizes that inhibition is the result of a nervous system that becomes sympathetically activated more readily than is the case for noninhibited individuals. Studies of primates show that this factor is heritable, with affected animals displaying more intense reactions to stress than nonaffected animals and showing behaviors mimicking human psychopathology when under prolonged or severe stress (Higley & Suomi, 1989; Suomi, 1991a, 1991b). Individuals with this trait are described as highly sensitive to a variety of sensory and affective stimuli (Bradley, 1985; Zucker & Bradley, 1995; see also Rothbart & Bates, 1998). Physiological studies suggest that inhibition produces more intense arousal and greater prolongation of arousal once it is initiated (Kagan et al., 1987).

Brain Dysfunction

Brain dysfunction, in the form of either developmental anomaly or perinatal trauma, has been implicated in the development of psychopathology—most systematically in schizophrenia (Hultman, Öhman,

Cnattingius, Wieselgren, & Lindstrom, 1997; Kendell, Juszczak, & Cole, 1996), and to lesser degrees in other forms of psychopathology (Gillberg, Gillberg, & Groth, 1989). Neurological "soft signs," felt to reflect brain dysfunction, have been connected with both internalizing and externalizing types of psychopathology (Neumann & Walker, 1996; Raine, Brennan, Mednick, & Mednick, 1996). Although arousal has not been studied systematically in subjects who have sustained brain insult, studies of low-birthweight and premature infants suggests that these infants have greater difficulties in regulating arousal than normal-birthweight infants do (Schraeder, Heverly, & O'Brien, 1996). Such infants present their parents with greater challenges in terms of reading their signals and responding to their needs, which contributes to increased vulnerability to difficulties in attachment (see below). Frank brain damage such as cerebral infarction produces affective intensification or diminution, depending on the site (Borod, 1992). Left-sided cerebral damage generally produces a depressive reaction (suggesting overregulation of affect), in contrast to right-sided damage, which produces a lack of emotional concern and sometimes a euphoric reaction (suggesting an underregulation of affect).

Attachment Difficulties

The literature on infant–caretaker attachment has begun to focus more systematically on variables of specific interest to psychopathology, such as affect regulation. Insecurely attached infants, especially those who are *avoidantly* attached, exhibit elevated arousal levels despite the appearance of lack of distress (Grossmann, Grossmann, & Schwann, 1986; Spangler & Grossmann, 1993). Although these infants appear to have learned to cope by avoidance, their arousal, especially in interactions with caregivers, suggests a state of inner distress. Studies of adolescents and young adults with dismissing attachment patterns (the adult equivalent of avoidant attachment in infants) also suggest difficulty modulating affect, as manifested by elevations of skin conductance when attention is directed to attachment themes (Dozier & Kobak, 1992), and by peer ratings of more anxiety and hostility (Kobak & Seery, 1988). Increased arousal and hostility in a young child will lead to a more conflicted pattern of interaction with the caregiver, producing more oppositional behavior and negativity—a common pattern found in many disorders of childhood (Kendziora & O'Leary, 1993; Malcarne & Ingram, 1994). The *resistant* or *ambivalent* pattern of insecure attachment, being somewhat less common than the avoidant pattern, has been less studied; theoretically, however, resistant infants' overt displays of intensely negative affect may be presumed to be problematic for some caregivers. The *disorganized/disoriented* pattern of insecure attachment has been found to occur commonly in abused children and suggests a lack of a pattern or strategy for regulation of affect. (See Magai & McFadden, 1995, for an overview.)

All three types of insecure attachment may be presumed to interfere with a child's capacity for developing adaptive affect regulation strategies, as well as to produce behaviors that have a negative impact on the interaction with the caregiver, thus intensifying the child's state of insecurity or arousal. Follow-up of children from the New York Longitudinal Study (Tubman & Lerner, 1994) confirms the enduring negative impact of early emotional negativity has on later parent–child relationships and on emotional and social functioning in adolescence and early adulthood (See also Estrada, Arsenio, Hess, & Holloway, 1987, for the impact of a mother–child negative affective relationship on later cognitive functioning).

Sensitivity to Expressed Emotion and Familial Conflict

Reactivity to *expressed emotion* (a term that refers specifically to the expression of hostile and critical feelings) has been studied predominantly in relationship to the impact that high expressed emotion can have on relapse in schizophrenia (Bebbington & Kuipers, 1994). More recently, the impact of high expressed emotion on other disorders has begun to be examined, including disorders in children. There is a well-documented literature attesting to the negative impact of parental conflict on children (Cummings & Davies, 1994; Henning, Leitenberg, Coffey, Bennett, & Jankowski, 1997), as well as the effects of parent–child conflict in producing arousal in parents (Bugental, 1992) and presumably in children. Elsewhere, I (Manassis & Bradley, 1994) have argued that parent–child conflict, particularly in sensitive children, is an important factor in contributing to the development of anxiety disorders. Others have noted the presence of high expressed emotion in families of children with both internalizing and externalizing disorders (Hibbs et al., 1991; Vostanis, Nicholls, & Harrington, 1994). It is a reasonable assumption that conflict within important relationships, especially in sensitive individuals, can produce prolonged states of inner tension or distress.

Effects of Pharmacological and Psychotherapeutic Interventions

Earlier biochemical theories of depression and schizophrenia focused on single neurotransmitters, such as dopamine in schizophrenia or norepinephrine in depression. This thinking was partly the result of early pharmacological studies in which the main neurotransmitter affected was presumed to be causally related to the disease process. As our understanding of the interactive complexity of neurotransmission has grown, these unitary theories, and with them simple notions of drug effects, have been replaced by the realization that drugs affect many systems, producing both short- and long-term effects (Hyman & Nestler, 1996). Although most psychotropic drugs have some specificity for disorders, many psychotropics have an anxiety-relieving function, some more powerful than others. The major tranquilizers are effective in the most intense and disorganizing anxiety (which produces a psychotic reaction), whereas the minor tranquilizers, as well as many of the antidepressants, have an anxiolytic effect in the less disorganizing types of anxiety (LeDoux, 1996). Although there may be an element of specificity with some medications, it would seem that what makes many of the psychotropic medications effective across disorders is a general effect of reducing distress or arousal.

Psychotherapy also appears to have general effects of reducing distress or arousal. This presumption arises in part from the finding that there is little difference in outcome across different psychotherapies (Messer & Warren, 1995; Roth & Fonagy, 1996). Despite different emphases, it can be argued that all effective psychotherapies appear to provide their recipients with improved capacity to regulate affect. Dynamically oriented therapies, which focus on insight or understanding (Messer & Warren, 1995); cognitive-behavioral therapies, emphasizing self-talk, attributional shifts, and problem solving (Beck, 1971; Safran & Segal, 1990); and experiential therapy, which promotes discovery of new meaning (Greenberg, Rice, & Elliott, 1993), can all be conceptualized as giving individuals improved understanding, motivation, and/or strategies to manage their affects more comfortably. In many behavioral approaches to the anxiety disorders, exposure to the feared situation until the anxiety diminishes is considered of central importance to achieving change. Expressing painful feelings in therapy and trying out insights in the real world—normal aspects of dynamic psychotherapies—can be thought of as a form of "exposure" that gradually leads to a sense of greater comfort with and control of affect. In a recent study of the various components of cognitive-behavioral therapy, none of the theory-specific components (e.g., exploring attributions, correcting cognitive distortions) were more effective with respect to the outcome than the more general strategies of encouraging the client to face the avoided issues and to be active (Jacobson et al., 1996). Recent versions of the three main schools of psychotherapy (psychodynamic, cognitive, and experiential) share a common theoretical belief with respect to central factors in psychopathology—namely, that maladaptive internal representations cause the individual to enact maladaptive emotional responses to stressful situations (Messer & Warren, 1995; Safran & Segal, 1990; Greenberg et al., 1993). They differ in their focus on how to help individuals change these responses.

Combining these sources of evidence suggests that there is a general vulnerability to high arousal (which can be genetic in origin and/or that can arise from experience), and that this vulnerability, in concert with stresses, gives rise to psychopathology. The nonspecific anxiolytic effect of psychotropic medication, and the common effect that the psychotherapies appear to have on affect regulation, imply that many interventions have an impact in reducing general distress or in providing the individual with ways of managing distress. If, as I propose, distress is a factor common to all mental disorders, distinguishing "general distress" or "arousal" aspects of disorders from those specific aspects that differentiate disorders from one another becomes very important.

BRAIN FACTORS RELATED
TO THE CONTROL OF AFFECT

Since the pioneering work of Papez (1937) in identifying the structures in the center of the brain that have become known as the *limbic system*, these structures have been thought to constitute the main area for the experience and control of feelings. MacLean (1993) provides a model of brain function in which the limbic system plays an intermediary role between the basal ganglia or striatal complex (the *reptilian brain*) and the prefrontal cortex (the *neomammalian brain*). He conceptualizes the role of the reptilian brain as carrying out the "daily master routine" (including displays used in social communication), and he describes the neomammalian brain as necessary for anticipation and planning. Requisite to anticipation and planning is the individual's capacity to maintain a perspective on his or her situation, balancing the perceptions arising from inner and outer experience. The limbic system plays a central role in affect-related activities, such as finding and searching for food, angry and defensive behavior, and procreative behavior; in doing this, it relies closely on intimate connections with the other two areas. Despite different definitions of what constitutes the limbic system (see Chapter 7 for one such definition), there is general agreement that the structures in this area play a central role in the affective control of experience (Mesulam, 1985).

LeDoux (1993, 1996) has focused attention on the role of one component of the limbic system, the amygdala, in evaluating the emotional significance of input from a variety of channels and in controlling the *emotional response* to these inputs. Of particular interest to the development of psychopathology is the amygdala's role in defensive and attack behavior. Work in cats by Adamec and Stark-Adamec (1989) suggests that seizure induction or *kindling* in the amygdala can induce a "defensive personality." Furthermore, these authors have demonstrated that experience can change both level of defensiveness and strength of neurotransmission between the basomedial nucleus of the amygdala and the ventromedial nucleus of the hypothalamus; thus this work has begun to delineate some of the pathways important to learning or regulating fear. LeDoux (1996) argues that because the amygdala is central to fear conditioning and because it appears to store emotional memories at an unconscious level (the level of *implicit* or *procedural* memory), it plays an important role in the development of anxiety disorders, such as phobias, panic disorder, and posttraumatic stress disorder. Although this implicit memory storage of emotional situations becomes dysfunctional in anxiety disorders, he views it as having a survival function, as it allows the individual to react quickly to threat or danger. He contrasts the amygdala's role in storage of implicit memory with the role of the hippocampus, which is more critical to the storage of *explicit* or *declarative* memories. Explicit memories are more available to conscious processing. He postulates that the medial prefrontal cortex plays a role in modulating the arousal related to amygdala activation. Damage to or dysfunction of this cortex may make it difficult for individuals to use strategies to regulate their arousal.

Hemispheric differences also play a role in affect regulation. Fox and Davidson (1987) provide evidence that negative affects elicit right anterior activation and withdrawal behavior, whereas positive affects elicit left anterior activation and approach behavior. Deficit states resulting from damage to these areas decrease withdrawal or approach, respectively. Fox (1994) has extended these findings by showing that infants who at 4 months show high motor and high cry behaviors are more likely to display a pattern of right frontal electroencephalographic (EEG) activation. Moreover, those infants with high motor and high cry behavior and right frontal activation at 4 months are most likely to be rated as inhibited at 14 months. These infants, when presented with novel stimuli or stressful situations, display negative affect and withdrawal. Henriques and Davidson (1990) have argued that differences in right frontal activation reflect threshold effects, with low thresholds (more right frontal activation) producing a greater readiness to react negatively to stress. Fox (1994) has proposed a model in which right frontal activation is associated with control over negative affect and left frontal activation is linked with control over positive affect. In contrast to the qualitative differences noted with asymmetrical patterns of activation of the frontal areas, Dawson (1994) has shown that intensity of affective distress is related to overall frontal activation. She speculates "that the pattern of generalized frontal lobe activation that accompanies the experience of intense emotions may reflect, in part, the relatively diffuse influence of subcortical structures on the cortex and may serve to increase the infant's general readiness to receive and respond to significant external stimuli" (p. 151). (See Dawson et al., 1999, for a recent overview.)

Neurochemical modulators are numerous and interactively complex. Simplistically, there is evidence that glutamate has a general excitatory function that gamma-aminobutyric acid (GABA) has a general inhibitory function, that norepinephrine increases the signal-to-noise ratio in the cortex, that dopamine mediates anticipatory eagerness and positive emotionality, that serotonin provides general inhibitory control over many emotional processes, and that acetylcholine mediates arousal and attentional processes (Panksepp, 1993). Clark, Geffen, and Geffen (1987a, 1987b) have provided a more elaborated model for the regulation of attention, which, because of its central role in mental functioning, is of interest in affect regulation. They propose that the noradrenergic system, which activates the sensory cortex, is an input regulator, while the dopaminergic system, connected with the association and motor cortices, acts as an output regulator. These main transmitters are affected by and affect a host of other more specific neuropeptides whose functions are gradually being elucidated. (See Chapter 7 for a more complete discussion of where and how these neurochemical modulators may work.)

These anatomical structures and neurochemical modulators appear to be central in regulation of mood states, in drives such as hunger and sex, and in modulation of general arousal, exemplified in the balance between defensive and attack propensities. Many of these functions can also be understood to be influenced by learning and experience (Kraemer, Ebert, Schmidt, & McKinney, 1989). Although some of our psychological theories have lacked a firm empirical base, they comprise and describe what we refer to as *mind*. Our challenge is to integrate the mind and brain in our models of psychopathology.

MIND FACTORS RELATED
TO REGULATION OF AFFECT

As noted above, all the major psychological theories—including psychoanalysis and its derivatives (self psychology and attachment theory), as well as the more recent cognitive-behavioral and interpersonal approaches—conceive of internal structures that influence our perception of the world and, more importantly, our relationship with others (for overviews, see Messer & Warren, 1995; Safran & Segal, 1990; Greenberg et al., 1993). Variously labeled *transferences, self-objects, internal working models,* and *schemata,* these hypothesized structures create expectations based on past experience about how others will relate to us. These structures are organized around affective issues and provide the basis for our affective interpretation of experience. In most of these theories, schemata or internal working models operate at a largely unconscious level. However, information can be retrieved through therapy or other forms of self-reflection. Consistent with all theories is the understanding that as the individual matures, he or she gradually elaborates action tendencies, which have been described as *defenses, attributions,* or *cognitive strategies.* These mechanisms are presumed to provide a way of regulating affects and relationships. Depending on the individual's experience, the responses of caretakers, learning, and involvement with other emotionally important figures, these mechanisms/strategies may be needed more or less frequently and may produce inflexible or flexible aspects of personality structure (Main, 1995). All theories assume some dependence on cognitive maturation for the development of these mechanisms and the more advanced strategies require reliance on intact language function (Crittenden, 1995; Kopp, 1989).

Other psychological factors deemed important in mood regulation include self-esteem, self-efficacy, and insight. *Self-esteem* can be conceived of as a general factor that allows the individual to cope with stresses and insults by being able to maintain a positive perspective on the self in a particular situation. Individuals with self-esteem deficits or negative views of themselves may find their capacity to maintain a realistic perspective on their world easily disrupted. *Self-efficacy* (particularly as it relates to dealing with specific stresses), according to Bandura (1991), permits the individual to persevere, making him or her less likely to give up. In this respect it arises out of mastery experiences, but it also contributes to developing a further sense of mastery. *Insight* is the capacity to see the connections between affects, defenses, or cognitive strategies and behaviors; it varies greatly across individuals, depending in part on their capacity for introspection (Fonagy et al., 1995). Again, an individual's cognitive and language capacity underlies the functioning of these mechanisms.

As indicated above, these various internal structures and factors allow for interpretation of experience and, through interpretation, the assignment of meaning. Understanding of meaning is one of the main ways of accessing these structures and is the process through which therapists assist patients in seeing the connections between affects and behavior. Insight into these connections gives individuals the tools to change their behavior. I would argue then, that among the main structures for control of affect are the systems consisting of schemata, attributions, and coping responses, interacting with the individual's positive or negative self-evaluation and degree of insight. These experience-derived systems must, however, relate to the brain structures involved in the experiencing of affect.

AN INTEGRATED MODEL

I propose that the mind–brain split can be integrated as illustrated in Figure 1.1, which is a modification of a framework used by Gorman, Liebowitz, Fyer, and Stein (1989) to explain panic attacks. The first assumptions of the model are that undifferentiated states of arousal may arise in the reticular activating system and be interpreted through limbic–frontal circuits, and that through fear conditioning the amygdala, with its links to the thalamus, the prefrontal areas, the hippocampus, and the hypothalamus, generates a state of arousal in response to certain stimuli (LeDoux, 1996). Regulation of the activity in the limbic structures occurs partly genetically; partly through generalized systems such as the noradrenergic, dopaminergic, serotonergic, glutamatergic, and GABAergic systems; and partly through the influence of the prefrontal cortex and the psychological mechanisms described above. Although it is possible that some self-soothing strategies, such as thumb sucking, may have a direct impact on the limbic areas without prefrontal or frontal mediation, this model posits that perception of control through the frontal system also plays a major role in reducing the state of distress (as in panic attacks, where perceived control reduces attacks; Sanderson, Rapee, & Barlow, 1989). Conversely, a perceived lack of control increases distress. (See also Stansbury & Gunnar, 1994, and Bandura, 1991, for more complete discussions.) Following Stearns (1993) and Rapee et al. (1986), the model proposes that distress is related largely to the negative emotions of anxiety, anger, and sadness; however, it may also result from unexplained or unelaborated arousal, often connected to protracted stressful situations.

This model allows for the interaction of biological and psychological factors in the development and maintenance of psychopathology. Both genetic and experiential factors can influence the vulnerability of the individual to experiencing heightened states of distress or arousal. This model also presumes that the features distinguishing disorders

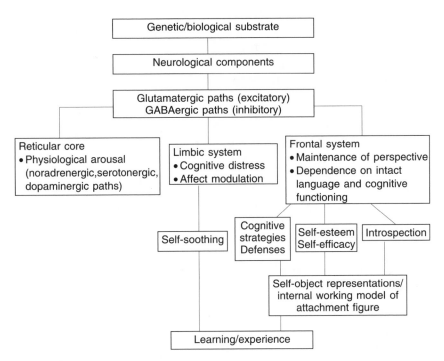

FIGURE 1.1. Conceptual diagram, integrating mind and body components. Adapted from Bradley (1990). Copyright 1990 by *Canadian Journal of Psychiatry.* Adapted by permission.

from one another arise from the interaction of the frontal and limbic systems (Fox, Schmidt, Calkins, Rubin, & Coplan, 1996; Schore, 1996). Distress produces differing types of efforts to regulate that distress (Thompson & Calkins, 1996). The regulatory strategies may be influenced by intactness of neurological pathways, functioning of neurotransmitter systems, and learning; again, this allows for the impact of both genetic and experiential factors (Rogeness & McClure, 1996; Post et al., 1996). If regulatory strategies to quell distress are successful, they may be repeated in subsequent stressful situations, reinforcing brain responses and patterns of behavior. If the strategies are unsuccessful, distress may be prolonged and result in symptoms or disorders. Symptoms reflect a combination of the experienced emotional feelings (e.g., anxiety, anger, sadness) and the efforts the individual makes to deal with those feelings (e.g., eating restriction, oppositional behavior, phobic avoidance). They may also result directly from the experience of general arousal (as in sleep disruption or psychosomatic complaints), from arousal-mediated dysfunction of the perspective-taking component of the prefrontal areas (as in psychosis), or from "wearing out" or "giving up" of the coping mechanisms (as in depression).

Arousal may be produced by stimuli from outside the individual, such as loss, trauma, abuse, or conflict, but it may also arise from the individual's evaluation of an event as threatening or uncontrollable. Some individuals (e.g., extremely inhibited children) may be sufficiently vulnerable to high levels of arousal that they experience many situations as threatening and withdraw frequently to manage that arousal. In doing so, they fail to learn other, more adaptive strategies for managing their arousal (Manassis & Bradley, 1994). If they are permitted to continue this pattern of withdrawal, they may fail to develop skills in social interaction, resulting in socially incompetent behavior (Stewart & Rubin, 1995); they also gradually find that even minor challenges feel overwhelming. Conversely, gradual exposure to challenging situations may permit the development of strategies for regulating arousal and a sense of competence or mastery in dealing with stress. Other individuals, who may be less genetically vulnerable, may experience intense arousal intermittently in situations that they regard as threatening or in situations of trauma or abuse. Development of capacities to regulate arousal in these situations depends on the response of caregivers, on temperamental variables, and on other vulnerability factors. Regulating arousal may become more difficult with prolonged states of arousal, assuming that a process analogous to kindling in cats (spontaneous seizure induction) may maintain either a high arousal state or easy arousability (Post et al., 1996). (See also Chapter 9 for studies suggesting that stress reactivity may result from prolonged exposure to stressful situations.)

The attachment system has been conceptualized as a mechanism for regulating distress. Securely attached infants are able to turn comfortably to their caregivers for alleviation of distress. Insecurely attached infants cannot do this, and so these infants need to develop their own strategies for affect regulation. Mothers of avoidantly attached infants, appear to avoid negative affect in their infants as they do in their tendency to dismissing or avoidant strategies in their evaluation of their own significant relationships (Goldberg, MacKay-Soroka, & Rochester, 1994). Avoidant infants are thus seen to use avoidance as a strategy for affect modulation. In contrast, mothers of resistantly attached infants appear to respond to negative affects but to underrespond to positive affects, thereby creating an expectancy in their infants that the mothers' attention is recruited predominantly through displays of negative affect (Goldberg et al., 1994). Infants with disorganized/disoriented patterns of attachment presumably fail to develop any reliable expectation of distress modulation by caregivers. It is reasonable to conclude that management of arousal is a developmental process that depends on genetic or biological factors, as well as on infant–caregiver attachment and other experience. Kopp (1989) has argued that the development of affect regulation strategies is a process that moves from reliance on a *caretaker*, to self-soothing behaviors, to language-based approaches. Strategies developed early in life that are used repeatedly for control of arousal can be seen as forming the components of personality structure or character defenses.

Other factors, such as self-esteem, will affect the way in which an individual interprets experience—that is, what meaning is assigned to events, and therefore how much arousal is stimulated. Furthermore, the individual's capacity for introspection can determine the ease with which connections can be made between past and present experiences, and between events and the ways they are experienced by the individual. This also will affect the assignment of meaning and have an impact on arousal. The dependence of introspection and insight on cognitive and language capacity is obvious. Just as elevated arousal can interfere with cognitive and language functions, it can also impair the capacity to maintain a perspective on one's situation (Kagan, 1989; van der Kolk, 1996). Similarly, the individual's capacity to use regulatory strategies for control of arousal may be impaired if the arousal is too intense or has too rapid an onset, as in panic attacks. Moreover, prolonged states of stress or exposure to high levels of corticosteroids may damage the hippocampus, potentially interfering with prefrontal–hippocampal connections and possible regulatory mechanisms (Kiraly, Ancill, & Dimitrova, 1997; O'Brien, 1997; see LeDoux, 1996, for a discussion of possible mechanisms).

In this model, each component part affects and is affected by the other components; this is what allows intervention in one area to have an effect on other areas. Thus interventions that alleviate general distress permit individuals to use coping strategies that they could not employ effectively when they were experiencing the arousal associated with a high level of distress. Alternatively, exposure to feared situations with opportunities for the arousal to diminish provide individuals with evidence that they can cope with their affect, or changed interpretations of experience give them a different understanding of why they are distressed. Either mechanism allows the individual to regulate affects more comfortably, which in turn reduces the intensity or duration of distress. As we attempt to design more specific interventions, and to evaluate the impact of those interventions through neuroimaging, it is important to have a conceptual framework to assess the component parts of the network that may be affected. This model provides a rough outline of such a framework.

Lastly, this model explains features common to many disorders that, when separated out, can lead to exploration of factors unique to each disorder. In the following sections I demonstrate how one can conceptualize both general distress and disorder-specific features.

SYNDROME ILLUSTRATIONS

Anxiety and Depression

The mood and anxiety disorders have been recognized as having genetic and familial links (Paul, 1988; Kendler, Heath, Martin, & Eaves, 1987; Kendler et al., 1992a). According to Kessler and Walters (1998), early-onset anxiety disorders appear to precede depression in early adulthood. Clinically, individuals with both anxiety and mood disorders give a common history of temperamental inhibition (Kagan, 1989) and are described by caregivers as not only shy but highly sensitive to affective states in others. Furthermore, they are usually seen as having difficulty expressing negative affects, except perhaps through withdrawal, moodiness, or occasional temper outbursts. Although attachment difficulties are only now being studied, they can often be elicited; some of these appear to arise in the context of mothers' anxiety or depression often related to child rearing or marital stresses (Warren, Huston, Egeland, & Sroufe, 1997; Manassis, Bradley, Goldberg, Hood, & Swinson, 1994). An insecure or anxious attachment, especially in a sensitive child, may intensify avoidant or oppositional traits as the child attempts to cope with frustration. For those children whose oppositional or avoidant behavior provokes parental anxiety or marked frustration, accompanied by lack of firm, consistent limit setting, parent–child conflict frequently ensues. Typically, such a child experiences distress related to the parent–child conflict, which may be manifested in separation anxiety, generalized worrying, or obsessive and compulsive behaviors (Hirshfeld, Biederman, Brody, Faraone, & Rosenbaum, 1997). When this pattern is prolonged or intense, and when the child feels responsible for the parent's anger or frustration (and as a result labels him- or herself as "bad" and the situation as unalterable), a depressive reaction often develops. Paul (1988) proposes a similar model with respect to the neurobiological substrate of anxiety and depression. He suggests that prolonged arousal (the anxiety state), which may be caused by antagonism of inhibitory neurotransmitters (such as GABA) or enhanced excitatory neurotransmission, eventually gives rise to depletion of norepinephrine and serotonin. Using an analogy to the "learned helplessness" model of Seligman (Maier & Seligman, 1976), which has been shown in animals to result from depletion of norepinephrine in the locus coeruleus, he posits that depression results from loss of function (due to norepinephrine depletion) in critical forebrain areas.

Depression, then, is conceptualized as sharing common roots with the anxiety disorders (Clark & Watson, 1991a, refer to this as a "shared vulnerability" to negative affectivity), but as occurring when an individual feels overwhelmed by his or her situation and perceives that "nothing works" (Maier & Seligman, 1976). This accounts for the frequent comorbidity of anxiety and depression. If the prolonged stress also produces hippocampal dysfunction or damage with concomitant memory impairment, coping may be further affected because the individual has reduced access to memories of past coping strategies (LeDoux, 1996).

Depression in children appears far less fixed than it does in adults, and it can often be alleviated through family interventions that reduce the stress related to family conflict. However, changing these conflicted patterns of parent–child interaction may not always be possible. In a British study, comorbid oppositional defiant disorder at presentation was a significant predictor of persistent psychiatric disorder in a follow-up study of depressed children and adolescents (Goodyer, Herbert, Secher, & Pearson, 1997). As an individual matures and as other significant relationships influence him or her, the individual's internal working model of self in relation to significant others may become more fixed. At the same time, the coping strategies or defenses that arise from the individual's perspective on self and others also become less flexible and may make him or her more vulnerable to an adult and more resistant pattern of depression. The dramatic increase in affective disorder in adolescent females would also suggest that hormonal changes (Seeman, 1997) and/or social factors (Zahn-Waxler, Cole, & Barrett, 1991) affect the vulnerability to distress or affect dysregulation. Finally, the fact that remission from depressive reactions becomes more difficult with successive bouts indicates that brain patterns become more fixed or more vulnerable to kindling with prolonged or repetitive distress (Post et al., 1996).

Abuse can be seen as intensifying an individual's arousal level, but also as contributing to the individual's self-perception as bad or worthy of being treated abusively—a perception that is more likely if the individual already suffers from self-esteem deficits (Cole & Putnam, 1992). A history of loss or a current loss may also contribute to the individual's distress, depending on the interpretation of the meaning of that loss and the availability of others to buffer the loss. Losses that are interpreted as a threat to one's security may produce anxiety, whereas losses that intensify a self-perception of badness may promote depression (Clark & Steer, 1996).

The longer-term importance of the trait of *emotionality* (often seen as the precursor to anxiety states) is illustrated in the findings from the Normative Aging Study, where emotionality accounted for most of the variance in later symptom reporting (Levenson, Aldwin, Bosse, & Spiro, 1988). Furthermore, the notion that difficulty managing anxiety in stressful situations (especially when it relates to conflict about hostile feelings) predisposes individuals to later vulnerability may be extrapolated from the findings of the Harvard Mastery of Stress Study follow-up. Russek, King, Russek, and Russek (1990) found that individuals who became more anxious and who developed sustained emotional reactions under stress had an increased susceptibility not only to cardiac disease but to overall future illness.

Although many interventions may alleviate the distress and permit the use of more adaptive coping strategies, they may do little to change entrenched self-perceptions, leaving these individuals vulnerable to recurrent bouts of depression or anxiety with new or recurring stresses. Conversely, however, psychotropic or psychotherapeutic reduction of the reactivity that makes these individuals more distress-prone may improve significant relationships, if significant others can respond positively to the reduced reactivity (Brown & Harris, 1978); this allows for improvement in the individual's internal working models.

Psychotic Disorders

Psychotic disorders, like anxiety and mood disorders, arise from a vulnerability to arousal that may result from a confluence of genetic and neurodevelopmental factors (Fish, Marcus, Hans, Auerbach, & Perdue, 1992; Mirsky, Kugelmass, Ingraham, Frenkel, & Nathan, 1995). However, there appears to be either a greater vulnerability to arousal or a greater impairment in the prefrontal mechanisms regulating arousal in schizophrenia than in anxiety or depression. Preschizophrenic subjects in the Israeli High-Risk Study displayed high levels of anxiety, attentional difficulties, and failure to habituate to a loud noise (Kugelmass et al., 1995). Although subjects at risk for later mood disorders also displayed high levels of anxiety, they did not display the same attentional difficulties and showed a hyporesponsive reaction to the loud noise. This difference suggests that children who later develop schizophrenia are less capable of moderating stimuli than are children who later develop mood disorders. Early negative affectivity, also seen in pre-schizophrenic children (Neumann & Walker, 1996), probably arises from a combination of (1) extreme deficits with respect to the biological bases of arousal regulation and (2) failures of the caregiving system to respond optimally to the needs of these highly sensitive and poorly regulated infants.

The types of conflict described above for anxiety and mood disorders also seem to be common in the childhood histories of preschizophrenic subjects, examined both prospectively and retrospectively. In the Israeli-High Risk Study, preschizophrenic children were described as having social difficulties; as not getting along well with parents, teachers, or peers; as having poor communication skills, as being suspicious and withdrawn; and as having low self-esteem (Mirsky, Kugelmass, et al., 1995). Although many of these individuals are exquisitely sensitive in social situations, they are often seen as awkward or insensitive. These sensitivities make it difficult for them to engage in social activities, intensifying their social withdrawal and interfering with their development of social and affect regulation skills. Family expectations for "normal" behavior (including school or work), all of which require social competence, generally produce avoidance or oppositional behavior, which results in conflict and a perceived sense of criticism. In the face of conflict and criticism, these individuals often feel overwhelmed; lacking strategies for working out interpersonal issues, they spend increasing time in fantasy. Their lack of a sense of efficacy is demonstrated by a perception that others control them (Frenkel, Kugelmass, Nathan, & Ingraham, 1995).

When these individuals move into adolescence, their distress escalates with the increasing expectations from their families and from within themselves to "behave normally." As their levels of arousal rise, their capacity to maintain a perspective on their inner world as distinct from the outer world begins to deteriorate. This may reflect a failure of prefrontal mechanisms to allow the individuals to maintain such a perspective, under the influence of chronic states of arousal emanating from subcortical pathways. Neural mechanisms may include neurotransmitter changes (Haber & Fudge, 1997) or connectivity disruptions that interfere with prefrontal–thalamic–cortical (Jones, 1997) or prefrontal–basal ganglia–amygdala (Graybiel, 1997) circuits.

Efforts to preserve self-value or to create meaning may lead these distressed adolescents to delusions of specialness. At the same time, persecutory delusions may reflect an intensification of the real-world reactions to their withdrawal and socially incompetent behavior. Moreover, their inability to deal with their own anger and frustration may produce fears of retaliation and rejection encapsulated in delusions and hallucinations. Thought disorder may be conceptualized as disorganized thinking resulting from interference with prefrontal mechanisms by high levels of arousal or distress, or as interference with a poorly developed prefrontal system by low to moderate levels of arousal.

With prolonged periods of distress and withdrawal, self-esteem and self-efficacy are impaired, and these individuals have difficulty even conceiving of having the capacity to relate to others or to meet expectations for any activity requiring social interaction. This amotivational state may gradually become the individuals' main way of coping. Effective medications can reduce the inner distress, diminishing the need for withdrawal and permitting the individuals to distinguish their inner and outer worlds more clearly. Thought disorder diminishes as the arousal is controlled. Alternate ways of achieving reduction of arousal, such as family interventions that reduce hostility and criticism, also reduce symptomatic behavior (Bebbington & Kuipers, 1994).

Disruptive Behavior Disorders

Disruptive behavior disorders may arise from a genetic vulnerability to aggressive behavior (Schmitz et al., 1995). Individuals with these disorders have often experienced insecure attachment relationships; these may interact with innate temperamental factors, such as inattentiveness and hyperactivity, to make them temperamentally difficult (Goldberg, 1997). Parental difficulty in managing the early oppositional behavior begins a pattern of parent–child conflict, with inconsistent limit setting and marked parental frustration often resulting in emotional if not physical abuse (Kendziora & O'Leary, 1993). These individuals learn that acting out their angry feelings may coerce their parents to give in, but it also results in such parental anger that most of these children feel rejected. This pattern of managing affect through oppositional, demanding behavior interferes with later relationships, including relationships with siblings, peers, and teachers. If the state of affairs is prolonged, neural circuit changes—for example, intensification of connectivity between amygdala–hippocampus "attack" circuits—may become easily activated with any kind of arousal (Adamec & Stark-Adamec, 1989). Most individuals with disruptive behavior disorders suffer from self-esteem deficits and become progressively alienated from adaptive experiences, including opportunities to engage in noncoercive relationships that would promote more adequate affect regulation and coping strategies. Substance abuse is often used as an affect-relieving strategy and can lead to dependence. Interventions that promote appropriate parental control, teach children strategies for problem solving and affect management, and remove children from delinquent associates appear effective (Kazdin, 1997).

CONCLUSIONS

The model described in this chapter, which places affect regulation in a central position in the development of psychopathology, integrates psychological and biological approaches to understanding and treating patients. This conceptualization also provides a framework for beginning to distinguish general from specific factors in the development and maintenance of psychopathology. As we advance our understanding of brain functions, revisions to this model will be necessary, especially in defining how experience and learning can affect brain physiology, neurochemistry, and structure. Newer classes of psychotropic medications will undoubtedly strive for greater specificity with respect both to arousal-reducing effects and to strengthening the prefrontal system's functioning. Psychotherapies will need to examine what aspects of interventions are most cost-effective in alleviating distress as well as in strengthening coping strategies. Furthermore, understanding how psychological structures, such as internal working models, are stored in memory and can be altered through various interventions will be the next step in this integration (for a more thorough discussion, see Crittenden, 1995; Main, 1995). Let us now proceed to a more detailed examination of the evidence in support of the model.

PART II

The Evidence

Chapter 2

An Introduction to Affect Regulation and Its Development

This chapter provides a brief overview of the literature on what constitutes affect; the aspects and functions of affect regulation; current thinking on how individuals develop the capacity to regulate affects and what factors may affect this development; the influence of affect regulation on later social competence; and the way in which internal working models may become the structures that maintain the stability of affective processing over time. I conclude with a description of the process that I see as common to the development of psychopathology—the developmental failure to learn adaptive affect regulation.

AFFECTS VERSUS EMOTIONAL FEELING: A BRIEF REVIEW

In Chapter 1, I have pointed out that emotion researchers have differed in what they regard as most basic—individual feelings or pleasant and unpleasant affects. I have opted for Frijda's (1993) position that there are two affective states, pleasant and unpleasant, and that these are elaborated into diverse feeling states that contain both cognitive and physiological components. Affect or mood has been distinguished from emotion as being less clearly related to a stimulus, longer-lasting, and more cognitively complex (Goldsmith, 1994).

The function of emotions has often been debated. There appears to be some consensus that emotions provide stimuli or events with salience (Ekman & Davidson, 1994). Over time, and presumably with increasing experience, this "attribution of relevance" function of emotions allows individuals to fine-tune their behavior through the development of cognitive–affective networks. Although there has also been debate about whether emotions can exist independently of cognition, there is some consensus that at least at the level of perceptual processing, there is always an element of cognitive activity with each emotion. Clearly there can be wide variation with respect to how much cognition takes place in the cognitive processing of a stimulus, as well as in the degree of cognitive control over responses.

LeDoux (1996) makes a distinction between the *subjective feeling of emotional behavior*, which he argues relies on the development of consciousness, and *classes of emotional behavior*, which "represent different kinds of functions that take care of different kinds of problems for the animal and have different brain systems devoted to them" (p. 127). Specifically, he describes neural networks that appraise inputs and react somewhat reflexively to certain stimuli—for example, to stimuli that threaten danger. Through conditioning and development of learned connections these neural networks respond to a variety of stimuli. He also argues that different emotions serving different functions (e.g., fear and aggression) should be studied as separate systems.

In the literature on psychopathology, affect has been most systematically studied in the two broad categories of positive and negative affect (Watson & Clark, 1994). As I have noted in Chapter 1, I view negative affect as more important than positive affect in understanding the development of psychopathology. Under the heading of *negative affect*, I include the emotions of anger and frustration, sadness and grief, anxiety and worry, and other variations on these basic feeling states. Despite my focus on the broad area of negative affect, it is my clinical experience that anger, and the anxiety and arousal related to its expression and suppression, cause the greatest distress and impairment in functioning for individuals. However, as many individuals are unaware of the specific emotions that cause their distress or negative mood, it seems more relevant to use the broader term of *negative affect* to encompass both anger and negative moods.

ASPECTS AND FUNCTIONS OF AFFECT REGULATION

Regulation of affect can be conceptualized as having adaptive and maladaptive aspects. Most modern researchers agree that affect regulation should equip individuals to respond flexibly to the demands of their environment (Campos, Campos, & Barrett, 1989; Cole, Michel, & Teti, 1994; Thompson, 1994). Thompson (1994) defines seven dimensions as important in the process of emotion regulation (as he calls affect regulation): (1) neurophysiological constituents; (2) attention processes; (3) the construal or interpretation of the event; (4) encoding of internal emotion cues; (5) access to coping resources; (6) regulating emotional demands of settings; and (7) selection of response alternatives (choosing how a specific emotion is expressed). This list is not examined in a systematic fashion here, but discussions of its elements are woven into the following chapters. The neurophysiological constituents are addressed in Chapters 3 and 7. The construal or interpretation of the event is handled in Chapters 4 and 8. The other dimensions are explored most fully in Chapter 6.

I regard the most important aspect of affect regulation related to the development of psychopathology as being how the individual deals with states of *prolonged* negative affect/arousal. For brief states of negative affect/arousal, the individual may cope by avoidance or by using strategies that reduce the arousal reasonably quickly. However, in those situations where the individual cannot use an effective coping/problem-solving strategy and the situation continues to generate negative affect, the individual will experience a chronic/prolonged state of arousal, which will be relevant in the development of psychopathology.

THE GENERAL DEVELOPMENTAL
PROCESS IN AFFECT REGULATION

The development of affect regulation is conceptualized by Kopp (1989) as a process occurring between infant and caregiver, in which regulation is initially undertaken by the caregiver but is gradually shifted to the infant, who relies increasingly on cognitive strategies as language develops. She conceptualizes a process in which the infant moves from what she calls "preadapted action systems" (i.e., behavioral schemes such as eye closing and head aversion) to more adaptive and learned strategies, eventually culminating in planful behaviors to regulate affect. She emphasizes that learned strategies can only be effectively employed when the infant is in a state of relatively low arousal, and that when highly aroused the infant will tend to revert to earlier strategies. Clearly, temperamental and developmental factors within the child, interaction with the caregiver (including the development of internal working models or schemata—see below), learning, and experience will all have an impact on this process.

Recent thinking about developmental psychopathology describes the interaction between an infant and caretaker as a series of transactions in which the caretaker influences the development of the child, and the child's behaviors affect the caretaker's responses (Sameroff, 1989). This infant–caretaker interaction is now believed to influence brain structures that contribute to temperament (Derryberry & Rothbart, 1997), affect regulation (Schore, 1996) and self-organization (Aitken & Trevarthen, 1997). If psychopathology begins to develop, not only does the experience of having an emotional illness affect the individual's sense of self-esteem and coping responses; it may also affect brain and cognitive functioning in a way that makes recovery more difficult (Post, 1992; Segal, Williams, Teasdale, & Gemar, 1996). To understand how the developing process of affect regulation can influence the development of psychopathology, we must examine this interaction and these transactions, exploring the individual within the system and also the many different levels at which the transactions occur.

LEARNING TO REGULATE AFFECTS: SPECIFIC TRANSACTIONS

The development of affect regulation occurs largely in the context of learning within the family and other important relationships. Sensitive caregiving (associated with security of attachment) helps an infant avoid the extremes of emotional states (Emde, 1989). When the caregiver reads and responds sensitively to the infant's needs, the infant develops an expectation that distress or other states of high arousal can be moderated to allow the infant a sense of control and a sense of the environment as reasonably predictable (Gable & Isabella, 1992; Sroufe, 1989a, 1989b). From this interaction, the infant perceives him- or herself as worthy of attention—the basis of self-esteem. Sensitive caregiver behavior also correlates with later higher levels of positive affect, lower levels of negative affect, greater self-esteem, and greater social competence in the child (Suess, Grossmann, & Sroufe, 1992). In contrast, insensitive caregiving is associated with more negative affect (both anger and anxiety), lower social competence, and lower self-esteem. The two types of insecure attachment labeled *avoidant* and either *resistant* or *ambivalent* are associated with hostility and with fearfulness, respectively. Avoidant individuals are seen as suppressing affect, in contrast to resistant individuals, who exaggerate affect. Sensitive caregiving has also been associated with emotional openness and with a child's capacity to label and share feelings (Greenberg, Kusche, & Speltz, 1992). The same relationships between attachment security and affect have been found in college students (Kobak & Sceery, 1988).

Empirical work supporting the relationship between attachment security and styles of affect regulation comes from examination of mother–child interactions. Goldberg et al. (1994), in a pilot study, showed that mothers of securely attached infants responded to both positive and negative affect in their infants, in contrast to mothers of avoidant infants (who tended not to respond to negative affect) and mothers of resistant infants (who responded more to negative than to positive affect). These authors concluded that infants learn that certain affects are more acceptable to their mothers, and consequently develop a style of responding that allows them to be acceptable to their mothers. The fact that insecurely attached infants display evidence of arousal despite their use of affect-suppressing strategies indicates that these strategies, although effective in the short term, may have a longer-term negative impact on levels of arousal and styles of interpersonal relating (Spangler & Grossmann, 1993).

Caregivers may also support affect regulation through *mirroring* (Field, 1989, 1994; Stern, 1985). According to this theory, supported now by sophisticated parent–child observations, mothers follow their children's behaviors and affects in a way that gives the impression that these behaviors and affects are shared. These rhythmical interactions are more obvious and coherent in healthy dyads than they are in dyads where the mothers are depressed. From these observations, Field (1994) has argued that a mother is both a behavioral and a physiological regulator, providing optimal stimulation from a sensitive reading of her infant's signals. The infant who is behaviorally and physiologically organized can then be alert, attentive, and receptive to interactions with the mother, can seek out optimal stimulation, and can avoid or avert his or her attention from nonoptimal stimulation.

In a similar vein, Sroufe (1991) describes a process of *desensitization*, in which an infant uses gaze aversion when stimulation becomes too intense or uncomfortable but returns as soon as he or she feels reorganized. He argues that if the infant uses gaze aversion constantly and fails to return to the stimulating situation, desensitization does not occur. This pattern of continued gaze aversion is commonly seen in avoidant infants. When the dyadic regulation of arousal is sensitively attuned, the caregiver responds to the infant's gaze aversion by reducing the stimulation until the infant is ready, as indicated by a return of the infant's attention. Through this process, children learn to self-regulate and can develop strategies for managing high arousal and staying organized and engaged or regaining a state of organization if they become disorganized (Sroufe, 1991). This reciprocal interaction between an infant and caregiver allows the infant to develop arousal/affect modulation and to feel that he or she is an effective partner in his or her own development. In contrast, the lack of attunement in insensitive caregiving leaves the infant in frequent negative affect states, with little sense of his or her own capacity to influence the situation.

A dysregulated infant creates added stress on the infant–caregiver dyad, promoting further insecurity and frustration in that relationship (Bates, Maslin, & Frankel, 1985). Oppositional behaviors, problems with feeding and sleeping, and irritability may become an infant's main strategies for expressing frustration—strategies that further aggravate the relationship with the caregiver. A mother's perception of her child as difficult or unsociable, or as having more control than she does, contributes to difficulties in their relationship and increases the likelihood that the child will manifest emotional or behavioral problems later (Bates et al., 1985; Bugental, 1992).

Development of affect regulation beyond the preschool period has not been as systematically studied as it has in infancy and early childhood. However, Greenberg et al. (1992) have articulated a theory focusing on the integration of behavior, emotion, and cognition over a child's first 5 years as critical to the child's later socioemotional development. Their "ABCD" (affective–behavioral–cognitive–dynamic) model proposes that the child's capacity to self-regulate depends on emotional awareness, affective–cognitive control, and social-cognitive understanding. They see the child as gradually developing self-control as he or she labels feelings, uses language to communicate needs, and develops problem-solving strategies to meet needs. The parent's role is first, through sensitive caregiving, to support the child's development of secure internal working models. Next, the parent provides language to label internal states and affects. Finally, through joint planning, negotiation, and anticipatory guidance, the parent teaches the child problem-solving strategies. Although Greenberg et al.'s model requires testing, it is entirely consistent with the other approaches described above.

AFFECT REGULATION AND SOCIAL COMPETENCE

Children who act their intense feelings out in physical ways, as well as those who escape from affectively difficult situations, are vulnerable to later socioemotional difficulties. Nancy Eisenberg, Richard Fabes, and their colleagues have been systematically examining how aspects of arousal and affect regulation (specifically, issues such as intensity of anger and mode of expression) relate to young children's perceived social competence, peer acceptance, and problem behavior (Fabes & Eisenberg, 1992; Eisenberg, Fabes, Nyman, Bernzweig, & Pinuelas, 1994; Eisenberg et al., 1996). Generally, they have found that physical expression and intensity of expression of anger are related to lower perceived competence. Children who express their anger verbally are better liked. Boys are more likely than girls to vent or seek revenge. Children who have a more accurate perception or understanding of others' behavior display more constructive coping behavior.

At a more detailed level of analysis, attentional processes (e.g., shifting and refocusing) have been found to facilitate affect regulation. Eisenberg et al. (1996) found that children who were able to make small, quick gaze aversions during a distressing film segment had lower levels of problem behavior. Generally, children high in attentional and behavioral regulation were lower in externalizing problems. Negative emotionality and emotional intensity were positively related to behavior problems.

However, Eisenberg et al. (1994) found that children who tended to escape from anger situations were perceived by teachers as lower in constructive coping (especially boys), as avoiding rather than aggressing or venting, and as low in anger intensity (especially girls). Girls who escaped from anger situations were regarded by teachers as socially skilled. The mothers of these children, however, described them as being higher in emotional negativity and intensity and as using aggressive forms of coping.

In summary, the work of Fabes, Eisenberg, and their colleagues would suggest that children with high emotional intensity and low regulation are vulnerable to developing behavior problems, but also that some children who escape regularly from situations of conflict may not be coping in the sense that they are not learning the skills to manage stressful interpersonal situations. Presumably, children who act out more overtly will be vulnerable to the development of externalizing psychopathology, while those who escape from conflictual situations may be vulnerable to the development of internalizing psychopathology. Although some of this work seems to validate common sense, it also highlights the complex interactions that need to be considered among arousal, intensity and mode of expression, and coping strategies or lacks thereof, and ultimately how all of these factors, may relate to a child's vulnerability to psychopathology.

INTERNAL WORKING MODELS (SCHEMATA) AND AFFECT REGULATION

As I have noted in Chapter 1, there is general consensus across different theoretical perspectives about the presence of internal structures that condition an individual's usual pattern of responding to interpersonal situations. These structures, which are presumed to develop in the context of relationships with caregivers, are assumed to consist of neural networks that become strengthened as patterns of interaction are repeated. These inner structures are referred to as *internal working models* in the attachment literature, and as *schemata* in the cognitive-behavioral literature.

In the early cognitive conceptualizations, schemata were presumed to be trait-like components responsible for distorted beliefs and cognitions manifested during an episode of a mental disorder, such as depression. Because of difficulties in establishing evidence for the effects of such schemata between episodes, a more dynamic way of thinking about these structures and processes—one that draws on newer theories of memory and information processing—has been developed (Segal et al., 1996). Segal et al. (1996) have proposed that schemata, which they conceptualize as associated neural networks, are latent structures that can be activated when the affect associated with a structure is elicited. These authors argue that in the case of individuals vulnerable to the development of psychopathology, these associated neural networks may be composed of interlocking negative associations that, once activated, may be difficult to contain; their continuing activation may spiral into psychopathology such as depression. Furthermore, drawing an analogy with Post's (1992) concept of kindling and sensitization at a neurobiological level, these authors propose that recurrent affective episodes sensitize the individual in such a way that these schemata are more readily accessed. The other factor that may be important is that with the activation of large neural networks of negative associations, activation of competing networks that may counteract the thoughts and feelings induced by the negative networks may be difficult. This newer conceptual framework thus suggests why disorders may become more frequent and difficult to treat with successive episodes. Presumably (although Segal et al. do not discuss this), schemata can contain not only the thoughts and memories associated with affective states, but also the associated coping responses in instances where coping has been a part of the individual's experience. Access to the neural networks linked to coping with affectively difficult situations may also be thought of as dependent on the individual's experience. Again, coping may beget better coping and lack of coping, may beget continuing adversity.

Although the Segal et al. (1996) theory arises out of a cognitive and social learning tradition, and presumes that these neural networks that can be thought to provide the structure for affective responses and coping are learned, Kendler, Kessler, Heath, Neale, and Eaves (1991) suggest that genetic factors may also be important. In a study of coping responses related to depression in the Virginia Twin Registry Study, they reported that turning to others and problem solving were largely heritable, whereas denial was best explained by factors in the family environment. Although I am, to a degree, combining affective reactions and coping in this discussion, this is a position taken by others (e.g., Kagan, 1994). It is supported by the fact that within the organism, these two components are not neatly separated; affect activation typically leads to an effort to do something (i.e., coping). In both conceptual frameworks and in efforts at measuring these constructs, confusion as to what is being measured is often a problem. This will emerge again when we look at the neurobiology underlying affects and their regulation.

THE DEVELOPMENT OF PSYCHOPATHOLOGY: A FAILURE OF AFFECT REGULATION

On the basis of the discussion to this point, I assume that for an individual who starts out with a secure infant–caregiver relationship and an easy temperament, and who lives in a stable, caring family that is responsive to the child's needs, the process of learning to regulate affects is reasonably smooth. Such a child presumably learns that the environment is responsive to his or her distress, and also over time learns ways of managing feelings in a reasonably adaptive fashion. Expression of both positive and negative affects is a comfortable part of the child's repertoire, as are a variety of adaptive coping strategies. Such a child is likely to have positive self-esteem and to experience positive affects frequently. All these characteristics will contribute to an increased likelihood of positive interactions with family members and others, including a more positive school experience. Puberty will raise issues that may at times be stressful, but this resourceful child will have learned positive coping strategies, will feel supported by family and peers, and will have a sufficiently positive view of both self and the world that he or she will seldom feel overwhelmed by affects. Furthermore, this child is not likely to experience chronic states of negative affect or to perceive situations as impossible to resolve. As this child becomes an adult, unless confronted by extreme traumas, he or she will have developed an internal working model of the self as competent and of the environment as supportive. Presumably this adult will also possess a coping repertoire, brain structures that have developed through experiences of mastery, and a sense that life may be stressful but is seldom overwhelming. Negative affects are experienced as unpleasant but tolerable.

In contrast, negative affects and prolonged periods of distress or arousal, which I argue are common to the development of most forms of psychopathology, arise from different constellations of constitutional and environmental adversity. One can presume that a child who has been exposed to caregiver hostility or who perceives the caregiver not to be accepting of his or her distress will feel rejected and angry. These angry feelings will be expressed in the interaction with the caregiver, resulting in ongoing strain in this relationship and a sense of prolonged distress in the child. This view is consistent with the literature showing the importance of early adverse experience to the development of later psychopathology.

Given the literature suggesting that prolonged states of distress produce changes at the neuronal or biochemical level, such a distressed child is likely to develop physiological patterns that reflect these early stresses and that may sensitize the child to react in maladaptive ways (Rothbart, Derryberry, & Posner, 1994). Furthermore, patterns of coping (reliance on affect-suppressing or affect-exaggerating strategies) may predispose the individual to react to future stresses in maladaptive ways. Extremes of temperamental traits will affect the early interaction between child and caregiver, making the child appear to be difficult, and in so doing enhancing the likelihood that this relationship will be further strained. Temperament (again, especially at the extremes) may influence the coping strategies used, as well as the intensity and manner in which the child expresses feelings (see Chapters 3 and 6). Other innate capacities, such as intactness of central nervous system structures, intelligence, and language abilities, may have a positive or negative impact on this process.

Beyond those beginnings in infancy, trauma and abuse may make contributions to this developing process. Beeghly and Cicchetti (1994) report that maltreated toddlers are deficient in *internal-state language*— that is, the ability to talk about feelings in self and others. Because abused children are more likely to have an insecure attachment relationship with their caretaking figures, these children may experience combined adversities that interfere with their learning to regulate affects.

The child's developing schemata about him- or herself in relationship to important others will continue to exert an influence on how the child expects the world to react to feelings, and consequently on how he or she expresses feelings. Although schemata or internal working models are presumed to be relatively stable, their reworking is undoubtedly a part of normal development. With exposure to others outside the family, peers, teachers, coaches, and ultimately partners in intimate relationships become important in this reworking (Brown & Harris, 1978).

The process of affect regulation appears to go further and further off track for those children who perceive the caregiving environment as uninterested in their distress or unavailable to alleviate their distress; whose dilemma is compounded by a difficult temperament, adverse living situations, or other stresses; and who lack supports to buffer or ameliorate their distress. Although as infants they may adopt strategies that allow them to maintain a relationship with their caregivers (e.g., avoidance), in so doing they fail to experience themselves as learning to regulate negative affect states comfortably. Moreover, they begin to develop an inner model of the world as failing to respond to their needs and of themselves as unworthy of caregiver attention. They may attend to stimuli in a way that aggravates their situation— avoidance in fearful children and aggressive retaliation in abused children. Their angry feelings are easily aroused, and the fact that they have few adaptive strategies for coping contributes further to their own sense of being ineffective. For some this leads to a reluctance to express negative feelings directly and a tendency for feelings to be manifested in nonverbal ways as tensions increase.

In the toddler period, when most children are learning to negotiate with parents and when negative affects are easily aroused, these children may be oppositional as a way of dealing with their negative feelings. Parents who respond with intense frustration and inconsistent limit setting to these oppositional behaviors may inadvertently reinforce the children's oppositional way of dealing with negative affects. (For a fuller discussion of these transactions, see Bugental's [1992] description of the "threat-oriented family system," and the discussion of Bugental's model in Chapter 4.)

As these frustrated children move into the arena of peer interaction, they will be more likely to encounter further rejection. A fearful child may attempt to cope through a lack of assertion or withdrawal, while a more aggressively acting-out child may attempt to coerce peers into meeting his or her needs. In either case, the experience does little to enhance the development of adequate social skills. School may become an added stress, as the fearful child puts pressures on him- or herself to do well and the aggressive child resists the intrusions of yet another authority perceived as unfair and uninterested.

Although various factors may serve to ameliorate the severity of these patterns, they may be difficult to reverse once they are put in motion, unless a child's caregivers can act to assist the child in developing new patterns of interaction.

LONGER-TERM OUTCOMES
OF AFFECT DYSREGULATION

The importance of the failure to develop adaptive self-regulatory strategies is evident in a follow-up of children of depressed mothers (Zahn-
Waxler, Iannotti, Cummings, & Denham, 1990). Dysregulated aggression (out-of-control behavior) at age 2 predicted externalizing behavior
problems at age 5 and child reports of internalizing difficulties at age 6.
Follow-up of the New York Longitudinal Study sample shows that
these negative interactions in early and middle childhood continue to
exert a negative impact on the parent–child relationship into adolescence, although this impact diminishes in early adulthood (Tubman &
Lerner, 1994). If new interactions can alter children's internal working
models and assist in the development of coping strategies that permit
the resumption of successful social interaction with parents and peers,
presumably these children can get back on track. However, for many
the process is slow and trying, and requires an immense amount of parental work and patience. (See Webster-Stratton & Spitzer, 1996, for a
description of parenting a child with conduct disorder.)

Furthermore, adolescence intervenes before some distressed children have achieved adequate coping or social skills, and at this point it
may be harder for parents to assist their children in making up for the
deficits incurred in childhood. Efforts by the parents to address the adolescents' behavioral difficulties may provoke withdrawal. Moreover,
as the adolescents perceive their own incompetence in social interactions, they gravitate toward others who are also lacking in adaptive
coping or social skills and may become involved in antisocial or self-
destructive behaviors (Dishion, French, & Patterson, 1995).

Adult mental illness may develop out of these early failures at affect regulation and social interaction, although Brown and Harris
(1978) have shown that a supportive marital relationship can ameliorate the impact of early adversity. Dishion, French, and Patterson
(1995) cite studies showing that for an individual with conduct disorder, marrying a nonantisocial individual and getting a stable job can
help reverse the antisocial pattern. In cases, where there is little intervention, one can presume that as adolescents and young adults these
individuals suffer prolonged states of negative affects, experience
themselves as inadequate in social interaction, often behave in ways
that provoke negative affects from others (especially their families),
and see few ways of alleviating their distress. The specifics of their disorders are elaborated in the chapters on each major group of disorders.
My thesis is that such states of negative arousal or general distress are

common to all disorders and arise, with a multitude of variations, from the general process described above.

Personality can be conceptualized as the consolidation of patterns of emotional experiencing and responding, described as affective–cognitive schemata, that determine interpersonal behaviors (Izard, Libero, Putnam, & Haynes, 1993). These patterns may be intensified at times of stress, resulting in the magnification of personality traits that may be less obvious or troublesome when the stress remits. Presumably, when individuals meet criteria for a personality disorder, these patterns of expectation and response are maladaptive and have become crystallized in a way that prevents both insight and change from occurring through natural mechanisms (although time and experience may promote some change).

Having provided this outline of the development of affect regulation and how it can be disrupted, in the following chapters I expand upon this framework by reviewing the literature on temperament; attachment and other caregiver variables; stress, trauma, and abuse; and coping mechanisms as they relate to affect regulation and psychopathology. I then review the neurobiology of affect regulation and the findings related to psychopathology. I conclude this section of the book with a consideration of what we can surmise about affect regulation from the psychotherapeutic literature.

Chapter 3

Constitutional and Genetic Factors

The relationship between life stresses and psychological illness has been well documented. It is equally clear that individuals vary considerably in their responses to life stresses. Research attention has shifted to understanding the variables that mediate the relationship between stress and illness (Gannon, Banks, Shelton, & Luchetta, 1989). These authors have reported that individuals with greater physiological arousal to or slower recovery from a laboratory stressor exhibited a stronger relationship between environmental stress and symptoms than those who were less reactive or faster to recover. As there was no direct relationship between psychophysiological reactivity and symptoms, they have concluded that their results support a buffering or vulnerability model in which psychophysiological reactivity mediates the relationship between stress and illness.

In this chapter, I examine some of the constitutional and genetic factors that may predispose individuals to respond differently to affective stresses. Following from the findings of Gannon et al. (1989), the discussion here centers on factors affecting psychophysiological reactivity to psychological stressors. Because of the more extensive literature on factors that predispose individuals to the development of internalizing disorders, the primary focus in this chapter is on the internalizing disorders. I also examine, albeit more briefly, those factors that may make a child more vulnerable to the development of externalizing disorders.

BACKGROUND

Since early history, people have been observed to differ with respect to constitution or temperament; for example, ancient Greek authors described the sanguine, choleric, phlegmatic, and melancholic dispositions. Although many of these notions of personality types were dismissed because of the conceptual framework on which they were based (body humors), scientific interest in temperament has gradually expanded over the last 40 years. Diamond (1957) described four constitutionally based temperaments shared by all primates: fearfulness, aggressiveness, affiliativeness, and impulsiveness. Following the pioneering work of Chess and Thomas (1984) and Buss and Plomin (1984), and more recently that of Kagan and associates (Kagan, Reznick, Clarke, Snidman, & Garcia-Coll, 1984; Kagan et al., 1987; Kagan, Reznick, Snidman, Gibbons, & Johnson, 1988; Kagan, Reznick, & Gibbons, 1989), evidence has accumulated for inherited factors appearing early in a child's life that condition responses to social and emotional stimuli. (For a recent review, see Rothbart & Bates, 1998.) This work has been supported by similar findings in nonhuman primates (Higley & Suomi, 1989; Bolig, Price, O'Neill, & Suomi, 1992), in dogs (Scott & Fuller, 1965), and in rats and mice (Fuller & Thompson, 1960).

Much of the work on temperament has focused on emotional responses. For example, Allport (1961) defined temperament as "the characteristic phenomena of an individual's emotional nature, including his susceptibility to emotional stimulation, his customary strength and speed of response, [and] the quality of his prevailing mood" (p. 34). Some investigators, such as Eysenck (1967), Strelau (1994), Gray (1991), and Cloninger (1987), have focused on the concept of nervous excitatory and inhibitory processes. This work, which originated in Pavlov's theories of brain strength (the capacity to regulate excitability) and from studies of autonomic nervous system functioning, has been applied more often to theories of personality than to psychopathology. (See Buss & Plomin, 1984, for an overview of the historical origins of this work, and McBurnett, 1992, for a more recent review and for applications to child psychopathology.) Despite the variety of approaches some common themes have emerged. I concentrate here on those traits that differentiate individuals best with respect to stress reactivity, and that, by implication, make them more or less vulnerable to psychophysiological arousal.

Although the original nine dimensions of temperament identified in the New York Longitudinal Study have not held up to empirical validation (Buss & Plomin, 1984), factor analysis of some of the scales derived from Chess and Thomas's framework have yielded factors that appear to be consistent with factors derived from other temperament research. These include sociability/shyness (slowness-to-warm up) and emotionality (difficultness). Buss and Plomin (1984) have demonstrated modest heritability for sociability and for emotionality. Fearfulness, a component of Buss and Plomin's emotionality, has been shown to be heritable in a number of studies (see Buss & Plomin, 1984, and Plomin & Stocker, 1989, for reviews) and was one of the most enduring personality traits in the Fels Research Institute longitudinal study (Kagan & Moss, 1962). Bates, Bayles, Bennett, Ridge, and Brown (1991) defined two components of difficult temperament, one of which (reactivity to novelty) was related to later internalizing symptoms and the other (resistance to control) to externalizing symptoms. Reactivity to novelty identifies the withdrawing and fearfulness that are discussed largely under the heading of *inhibition* below. Children exhibiting resistance to control are less well studied from a temperamental perspective, but they are discussed in the final section of the chapter.

STUDIES OF INHIBITION AND ITS RELATIONSHIP TO THE INTERNALIZING DISORDERS

Kagan has labeled temperamentally fearful children *inhibited* (Kagan et al., 1984). Although there are semantic problems with the term *inhibition* (see Plomin & Stocker, 1989, for a discussion of the issues), Kagan's work has formed the basis for the association of a temperamental trait with both anxiety and mood disorders, and it constitutes the most coherent and systematic body of developmental work relating a trait to vulnerability to psychopathology. I review the studies of inhibition as a trait, studies of its association with psychopathology, theories about its neurobiological basis, and the animal studies that provide confirmatory evidence for a heritable trait influencing an individual's threshold of emotional arousal. I conclude my review with a brief look at the interactions of inhibition with the effects of socialization. Much of the discussion of inhibition is based on various chapters of the edited volume *Perspectives on Behavioral Inhibition* (Reznick, 1989) and on the series of papers on the longitudinal study of inhibited and uninhibited children by Kagan and his collaborators (Kagan et al., 1984, 1987, 1988, 1989).

Research on Inhibition as a Trait

Kagan and his collaborators define *inhibition* in both theoretical and operational terms. Reznick et al. (1989) provide the following theoretical definition: "vulnerability to the uncertainty caused by unfamiliar events that cannot be assimilated easily" (p. 30). Their operational definition focuses on specific age-related behaviors in specific contexts. Generically, Reznick et al. (1989) define the inhibited child as "one who tends to be slower to explore an unfamiliar situation or object, spends more time proximal to the parent and is more likely to retreat from unfamiliarity" (p. 47). In Kagan and colleagues' research, the term is operationalized for children at different ages in different situations. For example, the inhibited child at each age, in contrast to the uninhibited child, emits fewer spontaneous vocalizations when initially introduced to a strange person, takes more time to emit the first vocalization, and remains longer within arm's length of the parent during the observation period in the strange playroom. These authors have focused on children at the extremes of the inhibited–uninhibited distribution, and have argued that they are categorically different from children within the middle range of the distribution of this trait (Kagan et al., 1989). Although the evidence supporting inhibition as a categorical variable is open to criticism (most temperamental traits are regarded as continuous variables), most would agree that it is the individuals at the extremes of a distribution who are most vulnerable (Rothbart & Bates, 1998). Kagan's group's approach to defining groups of inhibited and uninhibited children has been to select populations scoring in the upper and lower 15–20% of a sample on an aggregate index of inhibition.

Kagan (1989) credits Jung with prescience regarding the biological basis for the trait of inhibition, in that Jung regarded introverts as having a poorer "restitutive" capacity than extroverts. The Pavlovian tradition, articulated recently by Strelau (1994), defined individual differences according to strength of the nervous system. Although Kagan (1989) uses different language, his framework is similar, in that he views the central feature of inhibition as a "greater arousal of the sympathetic and hypothalamic–pituitary–adrenal axis following challenge and unfamiliarity" with a greater requirement for "time to adapt to unfamiliar situations" (p. 4). Kagan's argument for a biological basis for this trait is based on similar findings in animals (including behavioral and physiological variables), familial studies that support a connection with anxiety and mood disorders, and brain research that has begun to elucidate physiological differences in transmission patterns in limbic circuits in so-called "defensive" and "nondefensive" cats (Adamec & Stark-Adamec, 1989). Specifically, Kagan (1994) proposes that this enhanced reactivity to novel or challenging situations is mediated by a lower threshold for arousal in the amygdala and/or its connections with the hypothalamus and sympathetic nervous system. (See also Kagan, Snidman, & Arcus, 1992.)

Kagan attributes some of his early interest in inhibition to findings from the Fels Research Institute longitudinal study, in which shyness/ timidity in unfamiliar situations was the only trait preserved from age 3 through adolescence (Kagan & Moss, 1962). Similarly, behavioral timidity in unfamiliar situations and a high and stable heart rate were the best-preserved characteristics in a follow-up study of infants and children from 3 through 29 months of age (Kagan, Kearsley, & Zelazo, 1978).

Beginning in the late 1970s, Kagan, along with Reznick, Snidman, Garcia-Coll, and others, began following two cohorts of children selected as extremely inhibited and extremely uninhibited (Garcia-Coll et al., 1984). Mothers of 305 European American children aged 21 months were interviewed by telephone about their children's temperaments, especially their inhibition or lack of inhibition; from this sample, 117 children were selected for laboratory testing. On the basis of each child's response to a variety of unfamiliar situations, such as exposure to a female stranger, exposure to a robot, and separation from the mother, two subgroups (consisting of 28 extremely inhibited and 30 extremely uninhibited children) were recruited. Selection into these two groups was based on consistent responses across situations on measures such as latency to interact with the unfamiliar adult, retreat from the unfamiliar adult or object, clinging to the mother, or crying. These children were retested with the same battery 1 month later. A second cohort of 62 children was first seen at 31 months and assessed in a similar fashion. At 4 years of age, 43 of the original 58 children were reassessed with a battery including heart rate measures, cognitive tasks, and observation of play with an unfamiliar peer. The second cohort was reassessed at 3½ years. At 5½ years both cohorts of children were observed again with an unfamiliar peer, in their classrooms, and in a room with toys thought to convey a sense of risk. When these children were 7½ years old, 22 of the originally inhibited youngsters and 19 of the originally uninhibited ones were observed in a play group of 8–10 unfamiliar children. They were also assessed on several cognitive measures, some of which were designed to be emotionally arousing. Salivary cortisol was measured, and the heart rate measures were repeated.

The main findings were that the behavioral measures of inhibition showed reasonable consistency over time. The behaviorally inhibited children tended to remain inhibited; the uninhibited youngsters tended to remain uninhibited; and there was a modest correlation between the behavioral measures of inhibition and some of the physiological measures indexing sympathetic activity. Specifically, a high and stable heart rate (little variability between beats), particularly under demand situations, correlated significantly with behavioral inhibition. Behaviorally inhibited children showed greater increases in salivary cortisol with stress than did the uninhibited children. Furthermore, the inhibited children with high cortisol levels at home and in the laboratory were reported by their mothers to have unusual fears (e.g., fear of being alone, nightmares, fear of the bath) not reported by mothers of children in the other groups (Kagan et al., 1987). At 7½ years of age, however, heart rate variables and cortisol levels did not discriminate between the inhibited and uninhibited groups as well as they did at 5½ years.

More boys than girls changed from inhibited to uninhibited (Kagan et al., 1987). Those children who became less inhibited over testing intervals were more likely to have been in the less extreme parts of the continuum with respect to physiological variables and to have been encouraged by their parents to be more outgoing (Kagan et al., 1987). Inhibited compared with uninhibited children showed more disruption of cognitive functioning both after exposure to affectively threatening stimuli and following a cognitively demanding task that involved some failure (Kagan, 1989). All of the formerly inhibited children made more errors after exposure to threatening as opposed to neutral stimuli, whereas two formerly uninhibited girls who at 7½ years were displaying inhibited behavior did not perform more poorly either after exposure to threatening stimuli or following the stress situation (Kagan, 1989). The inhibited children observed in their classrooms were more isolated, withdrawn, and quiet than the uninhibited children (Gersten, 1989).

Based on the number of children screened in the original recruitment process (305, from whom 28 extremely inhibited children were selected), Kagan et al. (1984) have estimated that roughly 10–15% of European American children can be described as inhibited. When Kagan's group examined a normative sample of 100 infants seen at 14 months, 20 months, and 32 months, they found a similar proportion of children defined by their earlier measures as inhibited. When the extremes of that population were followed up, there was reasonable continuity of the trait of inhibition. There was less continuity in the less extreme range of the population. As in the earlier work, girls were more inhibited than boys; there was also a higher proportion of blue-eyed children among the inhibited group (Kagan et al., 1989; Reznick et al., 1989). Moreover, the inhibited children were overrepresented in the group of children who refused to come in for subsequent interviews. Measures of inhibition were correlated with parent-reported approach–withdrawal on the Toddler Temperament Scale (Carey & McDevitt, 1978; Fullard, McDevitt, & Carey, 1978), with the fear scale of the Infant Behavior Questionnaire (Rothbart, 1981), with the unadaptable scale of the Infant Characteristics Questionnaire (Bates, Freeland, & Lounsbury, 1979) and with the shyness scale on the Emotionality, Activity, Sociability Temperament Survey for Children (Buss & Plomin, 1984). The authors have concluded that these four questionnaires provide "realistic contemporaneous descriptions" (p. 47) of a child's inhibited behavior (Reznick et al., 1989).

Broberg et al. (1990) reported on a sample of 144 Swedish children assessed at 16 months and followed for 2 years. The measure used in this study was a composite index of inhibition derived from behavioral observation and maternal report of temperament on Rothbart's (1981) Infant Behavior Questionnaire. The authors reported stability for the trait of inhibition over the 2-year period, and also noted that inhibited children engaged in less high-quality peer play. Inhibited children had more difficulty in the initial adjustment to day care, but this difference disappeared over the time of the study.

In Kagan and colleagues' normative sample reported above, there was a low positive relation between mother-reported variables such as irritability, sleeplessness, chronic constipation, and marked fear of strangers and of separation in the first year of life, and behavioral inhibition at 14 months. The relationship between these signs and behavioral inhibition at 32 or 48 months was not significant. In a longitudinal study of infants from 4 months through 14 months of age, Kagan et al. (1992) found that the 23% of the sample who displayed high motor activity and frequent crying displayed more fearful responses to a variety of unfamiliar events at 9 and 14 months than did infants with low motor activity and minimal irritability.

Behavioral Inhibition and Psychopathology

The finding that 10–15% of children in a normative sample appear to be inhibited contrasts remarkably with the finding in one study that approximately 80% of children born to parents who had panic disorder and agoraphobia were described as inhibited. The findings for children of parents with mood disorders were intermediate between those for the children of parents with this anxiety disorder and the children of normal controls (Rosenbaum et al., 1988). This connection of inhibition with anxiety and mood disorders has been pursued further in longitudinal research by Rosenbaum, Biederman, and their colleagues (see Chapter 9 for details). Moreover, Rosenbaum, Biederman, Hirshfield, Bolduc, and Chaloff (1991), further examining the relationship of behavioral inhibition to panic disorder, found that parents from the original longitudinal cohort of Kagan and collaborators reported higher rates of social phobia, history of a childhood anxiety disorder (including avoidant and overanxious disorders), and a persistence of childhood anxiety disorder into adulthood, compared with parents of uninhibited and normal comparison children.

In a more recent follow-up of children with *high reactivity* (largely consistent with the notion of *inhibition*) versus children with *low reactivity*, Kagan, Snidman, Zentner, and Peterson (1999) reported an association between high reactivity in infancy and anxious symptoms at 7 years of age. Highly reactive children who developed symptoms of anxiety at age 7 were differentiated from highly reactive but nonanxious children by the presence of fearful behaviors at 2 years as well as other physiological indicators at age 7, such as higher diastolic blood pressure and greater magnitude of cooling of the temperature of the fingertips to cognitive challenge (a measure of sympathetic reactivity). These studies provide good support for the belief that behavioral inhibition can be seen as a predisposing factor to anxiety disorders and probably to mood disorders as well.

Negative emotionality is a term often used to refer to inhibited children. This is taken to mean greater proneness to distress and slower recovery from arousing situations. Such children are often described as "difficult" by parents. Negative emotionality has been shown to relate to the development of both internalizing and externalizing problems in preschoolers, and in the case of internalizing problems it appears to interact with exposure to parental conflict (Shaw, Keenan, Vondra, Delliguardi, & Giovanelli, 1997). Stevenson-Hinde and Glover (1996) found negative mood, worries and fears, and problem behavior in preschool boys and girls were associated with high levels of shyness as assessed in both home and laboratory settings. High-shyness boys differed from medium- and low-shyness boys and all groups of girls in higher levels of acting-out behavior as rated by teachers.

Beyond the descriptions of the inhibited children in the longitudinal studies, other work has highlighted the impact that a trait such as inhibition may have on other aspects of development. Asendorpf (1991), in a longitudinal study of 87 children observed in peer play at 4, 6, and 8 years of age, reported that children described as inhibited by their parents spent progressively more time in solitary passive play; in contrast, their not-inhibited peers spent longer time in social behavior. Rubin, Stewart, and Coplan (1995), in a follow-up study of socially withdrawn children, have shown a correlation of social withdrawal with felt insecurity, negative self-perceptions, dependency, and social deference. Furthermore, social withdrawal, when combined with negative self-appraisal, predicted internalizing difficulties in late childhood and adolescence. In a longitudinal study of children

from age 3 to 15, examining the relationship between early temperament and behavior problems, Caspi, Henry, McGee, Moffitt, and
Silva (1995) found that the factor "sluggishness" was associated with
anxiety and inattention in girls and with fewer competencies in adolescents of both sexes. "Sluggishness" was descriptive of children
who reacted passively to changing situations, withdrew from novelty, and failed to initiate action. Although we have no way of comparing this concept directly to behavioral inhibition, the behavioral
description is clearly similar.

Kagan (1989) has speculated that inhibition may become fairly
fixed by about age 7; he cites the findings from his group's longitudinal study that those children who were consistently inhibited at earlier
assessments were most likely to be inhibited at age 7. He has raised the
question that a mechanism such as *kindling* (spontaneous seizure induction; see Adamec & Stark-Adamec, 1989; Post et al., 1996) might account for the apparent fixity of this trait. However, given the impact
that isolation from peers has on a child's self-esteem, and the fact that
low self-esteem may in itself interfere with a child's capacity to approach challenging situations, it is reasonable to assume that an inhibited child may find coping with the tendency to withdraw from stressful situations increasingly difficult.

Neurobiological Basis for Behavioral Inhibition

The theoretical basis for the trait of inhibition is thought to be a lowered threshold for activation of the limbic system to situations of unfamiliarity or challenge (Kagan, 1989). Based on the increased excitability
of the amygdala–hypothalamus connection in defensive cats (Adamec
& Stark-Adamec, 1989), Kagan has speculated that inhibited children
have a similar physiological vulnerability. This is felt to account for the
peripheral signs of sympathetic arousal (e.g., a high and stable heart
rate and elevations of cortisol) observed in challenging or stressful situations. Heart rate and its variation appear to track or reflect the
behavioral state of inhibition, as the consistently inhibited children in
Kagan and colleagues' research maintained a high or increasing heart
rate over the test periods, in contrast to those children who became less
inhibited and showed a drop in heart rate or those who became more
inhibited and showed a rise in heart rate (Kagan, 1989). Although these
physiological differences were hypothesized to be due to higher levels
of central norepinephrine or greater turnover of this neurotransmitter
in the locus coeruleus, in light of the more recent studies on stress reactivity and change in cortisol receptors in the hypothalamus and amygdala, it seems likely that changes such as these could precede the

norepinephrine turnover differences. If so, inhibition might be better understood as enhanced stress reactivity related to inadequate modulation of the stress response at the level of the hypothalamic–pituitary–adrenal axis. (See Chapter 5 for further details.)

Activity in the locus coeruleus produces enhancement of the signal-to-noise ratio (Segal, 1985; Panksepp, 1993). Children seen clinically with internalizing disorders are typically described by their parents as "sensitive" (Bradley, 1985; Zucker & Bradley, 1995). Suomi (1991a) has commented on a similar sensitivity in "reactive" monkeys (equivalent to inhibited). LaGasse, Gruber, and Lipsitt (1989) tested infants on their sucking responses to sweet solutions. Highly avid neonates (displaying enhanced responsiveness to increasing sweetness) were more likely to be inhibited when tested in their second year. Rothbart and Bates (1998) review other studies that support the link between sensitivity and susceptibility to distress. Kagan (1989) cites work on sensory detection differences between introverts and extroverts, showing better performance for introverts on certain tasks. Assuming that inhibited children are similar to introverted adults, he speculates that behaviorally inhibited children may have a similar sensitivity reflecting enhanced signal-to-noise detection because of greater norepinephrine activity.

Such a mechanism, though speculative, would provide a possible explanation for the heightened sensitivity reported by parents of children with anxiety disorders—a factor that sometimes makes them more challenging for their parents. Although this sensitivity has been poorly studied, it has been a remarkable feature of the early histories of children I have seen in an anxiety disorders clinic. Their intense and extreme reactions to normal sensory stimuli (e.g., singing, clapping, other sounds, lights, and the feel of clothes) and to others' moods confuse their parents, especially those who themselves have never experienced such reactions. These children react to such stimuli with intense crying and efforts to remove themselves from the situation. Conflict, especially if it involves high levels of expressed emotion, causes upset and produces either withdrawal or efforts to stop the conflict. Loud voices, especially when perceived by the children as anger directed at them (a frequent perception in young children), often produce a belief that they are bad. Given their relative helplessness and limited capacity to clarify the meaning of their parents' anger, this perception of threatening and negative responses may intensify their arousal. This situation becomes compounded by the fact that many parents of these children are themselves anxious and in situations of uncertainty may react intensely out of their own sense of confusion and powerlessness (Bugental, 1992).

Animal Studies

As noted earlier, heritable differences have been demonstrated in animals for defensive or fearful behaviors. Animals demonstrating these differential patterns of reactivity include rats and mice, dogs and cats, and different species of nonhuman primates (Kagan, 1989). Higley and Suomi (1989) provide an overview of their work, as well as that of other researchers, on temperamental reactivity in nonhuman primates. The main findings are that reactivity is a relatively stable trait over time, is manifested in behaviors similar to those observed by Kagan and collaborators in children (e.g., proximity to an attachment source, latency to approach stimuli in an unfamiliar setting), and correlates with a high and stable heart rate and cortisol elevations under stressful situations. Furthermore, reactive monkeys are more prone to display behaviors that parallel anxiety and depression when exposed to the stressors of maternal separation (related to mating) or social separation during adolescence (Suomi, 1991a, 1991b; see Chapter 9). Although reactivity has a strongly heritable component, it can also be induced by environmental manipulations. Peer-reared monkeys show higher levels of reactivity than mother-reared monkeys, as measured by more clinging to attachment objects (e.g., a favorite peer) and less social play. M. T. McGuire, Raleigh, and Pollack (1994) have shown a similar behavioral consistency with respect to social competence (a concept similar to the "confident-to-fearful" factor of Stevenson-Hinde, Stillwell-Barnes, & Zunz, 1980, in vervet monkeys). This tendency to be cautious in approach to novel stimuli can also be induced by maternal overprotectiveness in vervets (Fairbanks & McGuire, 1993).

Prenatal stress has been hypothesized to induce more fearful behaviors in offspring. The primate work on prenatal stress is reviewed briefly by Clarke, Soto, Bergholz, and Schneider (1996). In monkeys this induction of emotionality is often accompanied by other abnormalities, such as reduction in attention and motor coordination, and has been mimicked by injections of adrenocorticotropic hormone (Schneider, Coe, & Lubach, 1992). Because this hormone cannot cross the placental behavior, this effect has been presumed to result from elevations of cortisol, which can cross the placental barrier. Behavioral inhibition (increased stress reactivity) has also been demonstrated in rats prenatally exposed to alcohol *in utero* (Kaneko, Riley, & Ehlers, 1993), and exposed to artificial rearing (Kaneko, Riley, & Ehlers, 1996–1997). Because of the presence of event-related potential abnormalities in the amygdalae and hippocampi of these exposed rats, the authors suggest that damage or dysfunction in these structures from elevated cortisol may account for the long-lasting effects on affective behavior.

Normatively, the development of "freezing" behavior (also referred to as "behavioral inhibition") in adrenalectomized rat pups has been shown to be dependent on the presence of corticosterone at a critical period in early development. Behavioral inhibition, in this context, is an important part of the animal's defense repertoire. In animal studies, the fact that corticosteroids are necessary for the developmental organization of this behavior but at elevated levels can induce an atypical responsiveness suggests the need to examine the timing and levels of corticosteroids as possible biological variables affecting its expression in humans.

Socialization Effects

As noted above in regard to the animal studies, fearfulness or inhibited behavior can be produced through variations in the caretaking environment. Although the impact of attachment is discussed more fully in Chapter 4, Kagan (1989, 1994) has often pointed out that those children who change from inhibited to uninhibited appear to have parents who promote more outgoing behavior. Furthermore, Kagan (1994) argues that the actualization of the inhibited temperamental disposition requires environmental stressors. In a different vein, Stevenson-Hinde (1989) argues that the greater persistence of inhibited behavior in girls is partially a result of parents' greater tolerance for this behavior in girls as opposed to boys. It is also important to note that inhibited children do not typically display socially avoidant behavior within familiar contexts—that is, at home or with friends. However, their pattern of avoidance of challenging situations may display itself at home in a reluctance to engage in difficult tasks or tasks in which they feel less competent or unsure of themselves. This pattern has been noted as a precursor to the various oppositional behaviors that often accompany anxiety disorders (see Chapter 9).

The degree of arousal experienced by inhibited children appears dependent on the situation and the degree of perceived control in that situation. In a study using salivary cortisol as a measure of arousal, inhibited children in contrast to uninhibited children showed little evidence of arousal on beginning school, but more arousal later in the school year (Stansbury & Gunnar, 1994). The authors note that in contrast to the uninhibited children who were very involved in active, stimulating activities, the inhibited children, initially avoided such activities and presumably were able to regulate their stress response through this mechanism. In another study, Gunnar's group found that fearful children displayed arousal on exposure to novel stimuli only if they were insecurely attached to their accompanying caretakers (Nachmias, Gunnar, Mangelsdorf, Parritz, & Buss, 1996). These studies point to the importance of the context and the resources available to children in regulating distress—an issue that may be more relevant for children with a temperamental disposition to easy arousal.

STUDIES OF TEMPERAMENTAL FACTORS RELATED TO THE EXTERNALIZING DISORDERS

Research on Lack of Inhibition and Other Factors as Traits

In their original theorizing about the trait of inhibition, Kagan et al. (1984) proposed that those children at the opposite end of the spectrum—that is, highly uninhibited children—were at risk for the development of behavior disorders. In a follow-up of his two cohorts, his group did demonstrate a difference between inhibited and uninhibited adolescents with respect to externalizing behaviors (Schwartz, Snidman, & Kagan, 1996). In contrast, Cole and Zahn-Waxler (1992) have recently proposed that behavior disorders should be conceptualized as disorders stemming from anger dysregulation. The temperamental predisposition, distress to restraint or goal frustration, appears moderately stable and is related to externalizing problems in preschoolers (Bates & Bayles, 1984; Bates et al., 1985; Bates, 1994). Furthermore, Caspi et al. (1995) demonstrated that their factor "lack of control," which included ratings of extreme instability of emotional responses, restlessness, and impulsive and uncontrolled behavior at age 3, predicted externalizing problems and lack of competence in adolescence. Diamond's (1957) original heritable traits included aggressiveness and impulsiveness.

Recent studies have supported Diamond's belief that aggressiveness has a significant heritable component. In a twin study of problem behavior in early and middle childhood, Schmitz et al. (1995) demonstrated significant heritability for aggression. In follow-up studies of preschoolers, aggressiveness is one of the more stable traits and is predictive of later externalizing problems (Campbell, Pierce, Moore, Marakovitz, & Newby, 1996; Olweus, 1979). Impulsiveness has been studied largely in the context of attention-deficit/hyperactivity disorder (Thapar, Hervas, & McGuffin, 1995) and is also emerging as having a heritable component (Cadoret, Yates, Troughton, Woodworth, & Stewart, 1995b; Zahn-Waxler, Schmitz, Fulker, Robinson, & Emde, 1996). Both aggressiveness and impulsiveness tend to be part of the factor "difficultness" that has been connected with the development of be-havior disorders (Thomas, Chess, and Birch, 1968).

Hare (1975), expanding Eysenck's and Gray's work, has stated that psychopaths, who are at the extreme end of the behavior disorder spectrum, have temperamental characteristics (identifiable by the Hare Psychopathy Checklist) that make them categorically different from others who engage in antisocial behaviors. These characteristics in-clude a low arousal level and a failure to learn from experience. Pur-suing this train of thought, Wootton, Frick, Shelton, and Silverthorn (1997) examined the interaction between quality of parenting and the presence of "callous/unemotional" traits in predicting conduct prob-lems. They found that ineffective parenting was associated with con-duct problems only in children not displaying these traits, whereas children with these traits had a high level of conduct problems regard-less of the quality of parenting received. Although these dimensions were measured in children 6 to 13 years old (i.e., too late for these to be true measures of purely constitutional traits), this work, together with other findings on the role of temperament in the development of psy-chopathology, is highly suggestive that those children who are at an extreme with respect to certain traits are less amenable to parents' de-mands.

Developing the ideas of Eysenck and Gray with respect to herita-ble dimensions of personality, Cloninger (1987) has proposed a tridi-mensional model of brain–behavior relationships. Simplistically, he proposes that three interactive systems determine a person's response tendencies. These systems are harm avoidance (serotonergic), novelty seeking (dopaminergic), and reward dependence (noradrenergic). On the basis of high versus low activity in each of these systems, Clonin-ger can categorize most personality types and much of psychopatho-logical behavior. He describes antisocial personality disorder as the re-sult of high novelty seeking, low reward dependence, and low harm avoidance. Similarly, he would explain traits such as impulsivity as due to high novelty seeking and low harm avoidance, and opposition-al behavior as due to low reward dependence and low harm avoid-ance. Although Cloninger's conceptual framework has not yet been well tested, teacher ratings of a large sample of Swedish children on these three dimensions predicted adult outcome, including criminality (Sigvardsson, Bohman, & Cloninger, 1987). (Cloninger's theory is de-scribed more fully in Chapter 7.) Although Cloninger proposes that these systems predispose an individual to react in a specific manner, he states clearly that what determines psychopathology is the interac-tion of these personality substrates with the individual's experience.

Neurobiological Factors Related to Temperamental Vulnerability to Externalizing Behaviors

In contrast to Kagan's work with respect to the trait of inhibition, the biological underpinnings for externalizing behaviors have been somewhat less well studied. However, Raine (1997) has recently reviewed the psychophysiological evidence for underarousal in antisocial boys and concludes that findings on skin conductance and heart rate justify characterizing antisocial boys as underaroused. Furthermore, in a follow-up of a cohort of antisocial boys from ages 15 to 29, those boys who desisted from criminal activity had higher electrodermal and cardiovascular arousal and higher electrodermal orienting than the persistently criminal group (Raine, Venables, & Williams, 1995). Similarly, Mezzacappa et al. (1997), in following a cohort of "at-risk" boys, found that anxiety and antisocial behavior were predictably related to enhanced and diminished levels of mean heart rate, respectively. Although the anatomical underpinnings have not been examined systematically, Bechara, Tranel, Damasio, and Damasio (1996) report deficits in patients with frontal lobe damage in the production of anticipatory skin conductance responses; they suggest that these deficits are correlates of their insensitivity to future outcomes.

However these traits arise, there is evidence that children vulnerable to developing externalizing symptoms are temperamentally more difficult. This "difficultness" may take the form of extreme reaction to restraint, high novelty seeking, low harm avoidance, low reward dependence, or a combination of these traits. What is clear is that children with these temperamental traits are challenging to parents, and that especially in the context of adverse rearing conditions, these children are more vulnerable to the development of psychopathology (Thomas et al., 1968; Patterson, 1982; Kendziora & O'Leary, 1993; Cole & Zahn-Waxler, 1992).

SUMMARY

The evidence from both human and animal studies indicates strongly that stress reactivity has a heritable component and that this trait predisposes individuals to the development of internalizing disorders. Such individuals display an enhanced and more persistent response to stressors. These physiological reactions appear to make them more likely to withdraw from stressful situations. Their affect regulation will be influenced both by their more intense and prolonged arousal and by their tendency to withdraw. The biological basis for this trait is being investigated; it seems likely to involve limbic structures such as the amygdala and hippocampus and their connections, including the noradrenergic system. The possible association of enhanced perceptual sensitivity with norepinephrine turnover may permit better understanding of the trait of sensitivity, which can act as both a strength and a weakness in individuals with behavioral inhibition. It is equally clear that the trait of behavioral inhibition on its own does not predict psychopathology, but does increase the likelihood of psychopathology, given other (environmental) circumstances.

The temperamental basis of externalizing traits is less well studied but also suggests a strong heritable component, possibly involving several factors such as impulsivity, aggressivity, and attentional difficulties. The basis has been defined as distress to restraint in infant studies and suggests a greater experience of anger in situations of frustration. A caregiving situation that exacerbates these traits is likely to produce difficulties with affect and self-regulation and to set the stage for externalizing disorders.

Chapter 4

The Caregiving Environment

Despite constitutional or genetic vulnerabilities to difficulties with affect regulation, the caregiving environment plays a major role in determining how an individual responds to affect-provoking situations. I show in this chapter that failures of caregiving—specifically, insecure attachment and exposure to parental anger and hostility— produce difficulties with affect regulation and leave the developing individual exposed to elevated levels of arousal. Given our relatively newly emerging understanding that the environment can affect the development of neurotransmitter systems (Kraemer et al., 1989) as well as the formation of mental representations that guide behavior (Main, 1995), I presume that such early influences can have an enduring effect on the individual.

THE ATTACHMENT SYSTEM

This part of the chapter focuses primarily on the attachment literature. In describing this literature, I have drawn heavily upon Magai and McFadden's book *The Role of Emotions in Social and Personality Development* (1995), as well as the edited volumes *Attachment Theory: Social, Developmental, and Clinical Perspectives* (Goldberg, Muir, & Kerr, 1995) and *Attachment and Psychopathology* (Atkinson & Zucker, 1997). Issues of separation and loss are discussed within the review of the attachment literature, as these issues first arise in the context of the infant–caregiver attachment relationship. Attachment insecurity is presumed to involve a degree of feared loss of this important connection.

Since John Bowlby's seminal theorizing about the importance of the parent–child relationship in establishing a sense of security in the child, empirical studies have demonstrated that security of attachment is related to the development of psychopathology (Sroufe, 1989a, 1989b; Goldberg, 1997; Crittenden, 1995; Main, 1995). The mechanism by which the attachment relationship exerts its influence is much less clear. However, emerging evidence suggests that affect regulation constitutes an important part of the relationship between attachment and psychopathology (Sroufe, 1989a, 1989b; Kobak & Sceery, 1988; Cassidy, 1994; Goldberg et al., 1994; Goldberg, 1996; Shaw et al., 1997).

Brief Overview of Attachment Theory and Research

Bowlby, a psychoanalyst, formulated attachment theory from his observations of the reactions of young children separated from their parents. Influenced by the emerging discipline of ethology, he theorized that the infant's need for the caregiver, as expressed in protest at separation, is a survival mechanism that maintains the infant in proximity to the caregiver. The attachment relationship provides the infant with a sense of what Bowlby called "felt security." During the phase in which the infant moves away from the caretaker to explore the environment, he or she is seen to use the caregiver as a "secure base." The expectations that the developing child internalizes about the reliability and predictability of the caregiver are conceptualized as internal working models or schemata. Bowlby's three-volume work *Attachment and Loss* (1969, 1973, and 1980) provides a full discussion of his theory.

Mary Ainsworth, who worked with Bowlby, developed a systematized approach to the measurement of the attachment relationship (Ainsworth, Bell, & Stayton, 1971). The Strange Situation procedure which assesses the child's behaviors in a series of mildly stressful separations and reunions from the mother, has permitted the development of a classification system for parent–child attachment. A *securely* attached child is generally positive in the presence of the main attachment figure, shows distress at separation, and shows relief when reunited with the caregiver. In contrast, the two main patterns of *insecure* attachment, *avoidant* and *resistant* (or *ambivalent*), are marked by emotional negativity and a failure to use the caregiver as a source of emotional support or soothing. In the avoidant pattern, the child shows little distress at separation and at reunion fails to approach the caregiver for comfort. The resistantly attached child displays markedly ambiva-

lent reactions to the caregiver and fails to be comforted by the caregiver's return. With further examination of this process, subcategories
of each of the attachment groups have been defined. In addition, a
separate category, *disorganized/disoriented*, has been created from the
difficult-to-classify subjects in the original three-category system (Main
& Solomon, 1990).

In her original Baltimore study, Ainsworth and her colleagues
(Ainsworth et al., 1971) set out to examine one of the original principles from Bowlby's theory of attachment—namely, that caregiver sensitivity predicts security of attachment. Bowlby defined this sensitivity
as the caregiver's ability to read and respond appropriately to the infant's attachment messages. Ainsworth et al. confirmed that sensitive
responding on the part of caregivers (in this case, mothers) was related
to secure attachment, and further described the insensitive behaviors
of the mothers of the insecurely attached children. Generally, these included less affection and tenderness, and in the case of the mothers of
avoidantly attached children, rejection and aversion to bodily contact.
In contrast, the mothers of securely attached children were deemed to
be accepting of their children's positive and negative feelings and of
those feelings within themselves. Furthermore, they were seen as co-
operating with or facilitating their children's efforts at self-regulation
and as being emotionally available to the children.

Although the caregiver characteristics of sensitivity and contin-
gent responsivity are thought to be the main factors promoting the development of a secure attachment relationship, it is presumed that
caregivers who behave in a sensitive, responsive way toward their infants are themselves securely attached. Thus secure caregivers would
be expected to rear securely attached children. This stability of attachment across generations has been demonstrated (Main, 1995). Main
and Goldwyn (1984) developed the Adult Attachment Interview (AAI),
using the same theoretical base as Ainsworth used for the infant classification system. The category *autonomous* is equated to secure, *dismissing* to avoidant, *preoccupied* to ambivalent/resistant, and *unresolved
about loss or trauma* to disorganized. Studies using the AAI with parents
and the Strange Situation with their infants have shown that autonomous mothers are more likely to have securely attached children than
are dismissing or preoccupied mothers (Zeanah et al., 1993). These
continuities have been demonstrated when an adult's state of mind is
assessed prior to a child's birth, as well as in assessments during the
offspring's infancy and childhood. (See Main, 1995, for an overview.)
Benoit and Parker (1994) have demonstrated stability of attachment
categories across three generations.

Further, van IJzendoorn and Bakermans-Kranenburg (1996) conducted a meta-analysis of studies using the AAI with mothers, fathers, and adolescents in clinical and nonclinical groups. This analysis showed that mothers, fathers, and adolescents in nonclinical groups did not differ from one another or from AAI norms in the distribution of attachment patterns; however, those in clinical groups showed higher levels of insecure attachment. Moreover, in studies using the AAI and the four-category Strange Situation procedure, the proportion of mothers in nonclinical groups classified by the AAI as autonomous (55%), dismissing (16%), preoccupied (9%), and unresolved (19%) did not differ from the proportions of infant–mother dyads in nonclinical groups classified by the Strange Situation: secure (55%), avoidant (23%), ambivalent (8%), and disorganized (15%).

There has been ongoing debate about the extent to which child characteristics, such as temperament, influence attachment categories. (Kagan, for example, would argue that attachment categories reflect the infant's style of emotional expression; see Karen, 1990.) Using Ainsworth's system of lettering for her three attachment categories, Belsky and Rovine (1987) did demonstrate that more expressive infants were more likely to be categorized as B3 and B4, the subcategories of B (secure attachment) more closely related to C (resistant), whereas less expressive infants tended to be categorized as B1 or B2, the subcategories of B more closely related to A (avoidant). Izard, Haynes, Chisholm, and Baak (1991) also reported that an infant's emotionally expressive behavior in mildly stressful situations was a predictor of the attachment relationship. A recent study found that attachment and behavioral inhibition (a child factor thought to influence attachment) are independent constructs, but that their interaction can influence arousal (Nachmias et al., 1996). However, in a meta-analysis of attachment studies examining parent versus child factors, van IJzendoorn, Goldberg, Kroonenberg, and Frenkel (1992) concluded that parent factors have a much larger influence on the distribution of child attachment patterns than do child factors.

Despite the apparently large effect of the relationship with the parent and other parent factors, there is evidence that child constitutional factors do play a role in determining an infant's security or insecurity of attachment. Grossmann (1995), reviewing subgroups in his and his coworkers' longitudinal study of attachment, described a subgroup of avoidant children with reasonably sensitive mothers. His colleague Fremmer-Bombik and he (Fremmer-Bombik & Grossman, 1993) found that as newborns these infants were highly irritable and rated lowest in the sample on orientation ability. Grossman also reported that the presence of disorganized/disoriented attachment correlated with the newborns' orientation and state regulation and not with maternal sensitivity. Goldberg (1996) has attempted a rapprochement between the opposing positions of van IJzendoorn and his colleagues and of Grossmann and his coworkers by suggesting that what is actually being measured in the Strange Situation is affect regulation, and that attachment to the parent and temperament should interact in the area of affect regulation.

A recent intervention study does suggest that maternal sensitivity can buffer the impact of infant characteristics on security of attachment. van den Boom (1994) trained a high-risk sample of mothers of irritable infants to respond sensitively to their infants' behavior. The intervention group had higher levels of securely attached infants than did the nonintervention group. Although irritability is not temperament, it is linked to the concept of infant difficultness, and this study does suggest that maternal skill can override some temperamental traits to produce a securely attached (and thus, perhaps, well-regulated) infant. What has not been adequately explored in this debate (but is suggested in Grossmann and colleagues' findings) is whether extremes of temperament or constitutional factors might have a more influential effect. Lastly, Sroufe (1991) has demonstrated that adults behave differently toward secure and insecure children, in a fashion that would tend to confirm their expectations and strengthen their internal working models of self and others. Thus Eagle (1995) and Belsky, Rosenberger, and Crnic (1995) have proposed that temperament may affect attachment through its impact on mother–infant interaction. (See also Rothbart & Bates, 1998, for a more complete discussion of temperament and attachment.) To return, however, to Goldberg's notion that both temperament and attachment should have an impact on the development of affect regulation, a more important point may be suggested by the Nachmias et al. (1996) study—namely, that the interaction of an insecure attachment relationship with inhibition may be what produces difficulties in regulating distress.

As would be expected, maternal characteristics beyond the issue of sensitivity and responsivity have been shown to affect attachment. Belsky et al. (1995), in reviewing these studies, conclude that most of these distal factors (maternal personality variables such as anxiety and depression, the marital/couple relationship, and support outside this relationship) exert their impact through their effect on mother–child interaction.

A maternal characteristic that correlates both with insecure mother–child attachment and with difficult child temperament is physiological reactivity to an infant's cry (Frodi, Bridges, & Shonk, 1989). Mothers who showed increased reactivity (as measured by heart rate, skin conductance, and blood pressure) to an infant's cry in prenatal testing were more likely to rate their babies as difficult than easy and tended to be more punitive and rigid in child-rearing attitudes. When their babies were tested in the Strange Situation procedure at 12 months all the babies rated as easy by their mothers were in the secure category. Similarly, Donovan and Leavitt (1989) found that mothers who overestimated their control of termination of an infant's cry were more likely to be depressed and to show elevation of their heart rate with impending infant cries at 5 months, and to have an insecure attachment with their babies at 16 months. Both of these studies suggest that maternal reactivity may be a direct contributor (among other factors) to maternal stress, which may in turn interfere with sensitivity to an infant's cries. Furthermore, given the likelihood that some degree of physiological reactivity is heritable, these reactive mothers may be more likely to have more reactive babies—a combination that may increase the chance of an insecure attachment. This issue has been raised as well in a study of the offspring of women with nonorganic psychosis by Persson-Blennow, Binett, and McNeil (1988).

Despite these maternal variables, Crockenberg (1981) has shown that social support is the best predictor of secure attachment and is most important for mothers of irritable babies. She argues that social support may mitigate the impact of maternal unresponsiveness through the provision of substitute caregivers. This is consistent with a finding by Adler, Hayes, Nolan, Lewin, and Raphael (1991) that low-risk mothers who perceived their social networks as less supportive during pregnancy were likely to see their 1-year-old infants as more difficult. However, in this low-risk sample none of the antenatal variables, including social support, predicted insecure attachment or other outcome measures. This is consistent with the finding by Belsky et al. (1995) that security of attachment correlates negatively with number of risk factors, including parental personality, the marital/couple relationship, and support outside this relationship.

In Ainsworth's original study (Ainsworth et al., 1971) securely attached infant–mother dyads accounted for about 65% of the total sample, with avoidantly attached representing the next largest category at about 20%. Resistantly attached infant–mother dyads composed about 10% of the sample. These rough proportions have been replicated in samples across the world, with the main difference being a higher rate of avoidantly attached dyads in Western Europe and of resistantly attached dyads in Israel and Japan. (See Magai & McFadden, 1995, for actual percentages.) In a more recent meta-analysis of precursors, concomitants, and sequelae of disorganized attachment, van IJzendoorn, Schuengel, and Bakermans-Kranenburg (1999) reported that about 15% of infants of middle-class families displayed a disorganized attachment pattern. In low-socioeconomic-status (low-SES) and clinical groups the percentage rose significantly, and it approached 50% in cases of maltreatment. Although there is some variability in the stability of attachment classifications over time, there is also relative continuity, especially in families not undergoing significant stress (Campos, Barrett, Lamb, Goldsmith, & Stenberg, 1983). It is presumed that consistency of attachment patterns over time is the product of the relative stability of the internal representations that maintain behavioral responses. It is also clear that changes in attachment categories may take place over time, probably in relation to experience and to how the individual deals with that experience (Fagot & Pears, 1996).

Attachment and Psychopathology

Although Bowlby did not explicitly conceptualize insecure attachment as psychopathology, his original formulation indicated clearly that an insecure attachment can be seen as creating a vulnerability to later psychopathology. Cross-sectional studies have shown higher levels of insecurity in clinical and "at-risk" groups, but now longitudinal studies are confirming these findings. Examination of attachment relationships in individuals with emotional disorders has been facilitated by an adaptation of the Strange Situation procedure for preschool children (Cassidy & Marvin with the Attachment Working Group of the MacArthur Network, 1992), as well as by measures such as the AAI and other questionnaire and Q-sort measures for adults.

Cross-Sectional Studies

Goldberg (1997) reviewed the data from published and unpublished studies available at that time that assessed attachment in normal, at-risk, and clinical samples of children. In a medically diagnosed sample of children followed up from infancy, avoidant attachment was connected with both internalizing and externalizing psychopathology. In a cross-sectional study of Romanian adoptees, most of whom had suffered fairly marked deprivation prior to their adoptions, securely attached children had lower Child Behavior Checklist (CBCL) scores than insecurely attached children. This effect was accounted for largely by children with disorganized/controlling attachment patterns. (In the preschool assessment of attachment, disorganized is replaced by *controlling*, which is thought to be the developmental outcome of disorganization in infancy; see Main, Kaplan, & Cassidy, 1985.) In a third at-risk sample, consisting of preschool children of mothers with an anxiety disorder (Manassis et al., 1994), 80% of the children were insecurely attached (predominantly disorganized/controlling). Three of the 20 children, all of whom were from the insecure group, met criteria for an anxiety disorder. In two clinical samples (infants referred to an early intervention program, and children with gender identity disorder) the proportion of subjects with insecure attachment was high but confounded by the fact that the rate of insecure attachment in the "normal" controls was also much higher than in standardization samples. The children with gender identity disorder were also compared with a psychiatrically referred clinical group, 83% of whom were insecurely attached (predominantly avoidant and disorganized/controlling); in contrast, the children with gender identity disorder were roughly evenly distributed across avoidant, secure, and resistant/ambivalent groups. Goldberg concluded that there appeared to be increased rates of insecure attachment in defined clinical populations, with children in the at-risk populations (except for children of mothers with an anxiety disorder, who were comparable to the clinical samples) falling in between the clinical groups and "normal" samples. Goldberg also commented on the predominance of disorganized/controlling attachment relationships in the clinical samples as probably more relevant to the development of psychopathology, but cautioned against extrapolating too much from these largely cross-sectional studies.

van IJzendoorn and Bakermans-Kranenburg (1996), in their meta-analysis of AAI studies, found high levels of insecure representations in the mothers of clinically referred children and in clinical groups of adolescents and adults. Work is also emerging demonstrating high levels of insecure attachment in subjects with various mental disorders and their offspring. Torgersen and Alnaes (1992) studied subjects with borderline personality disorder; Pettem, West, Mahoney, and Keller (1993) studied depressed subjects; Manassis et al. (1994) studied mothers with anxiety disorders and their children; Field (1989) studied children of depressed mothers; and Cassidy (1992) studied subjects with generalized anxiety disorder.

Study of "at-risk" children has been a major interest in the attachment literature because of the obvious connection between factors known to influence child outcomes, such as poverty and abuse, and the theoretical assumptions that there are interferences in the parent–child relationship in these situations. Studies of abused and neglected children have demonstrated high levels of insecure attachment, especially disorganized attachment since the newer four-category system has been used (Cicchetti & Toth, 1995). Children from low-SES backgrounds display higher rates of insecure attachment in the second year of life, but not necessarily in the first year. This is similar to findings on children of depressed mothers, where the prevalence of insecure at-

tachment in the first year is not remarkably different from that of normal controls but does diverge significantly by the second year. (See
Field, 1989 and 1994, for reviews.). van IJzendoorn and Bakermans-
Kranenburg (1996) meta-analysis found higher than expected levels of
insecure relationship patterns on the AAI among mothers in low-SES
samples, as well as in the clinical groups.

Follow-Up Studies

Insecurely attached children (defined as such in infancy) show greater
deficits in a variety of socioemotional domains (generally as measured
in early childhood). These include more negativity and fearfulness;
lower self-esteem; poorer social competence; less empathy and compliance; and, in cases of disorganized attachment, more disorganized and
bizarre behavior (Main et al., 1985; Suess et al., 1992; Sroufe, 1991; see
Magai & McFadden, 1995, for an overview). More recently, Fagot and
Pears (1996) reported on a longitudinal study with the Strange Situation at 18 months, the Crittenden (1992) attachment measure at 30
months, and the CBCL (Achenbach, Edelbrock, & Howell, 1987) and
other behavior ratings at age 7. Consistent with the description above,
they found higher ratings on the CBCL at age 7 for insecurely attached
children (particularly the coercive/resistant children, Crittenden's
term for resistant/ambivalent attachment in preschoolers) as defined
in the assessment of attachment at 30 months. (See also Moss, Rousseau, Parent, St.-Laurent, & Saintonge, 1998.) Shaw, Owens, Vondra,
Keenan, and Winslow (1996) reported that disorganized attachment in
infancy, along with maternal personality risk and exposure to child-
rearing disagreements, predicted child aggression at age 5. In the same
longitudinal study of high-risk mothers, Shaw et al. (1997) demonstrated that disorganized attachment classification along with child
negative emotionality, negative life events, exposure to child-rearing
disagreements, and parenting hassles predicted the development of
preschool-age internalizing problems. van IJzendoorn et al. (1999), in
their meta-analysis, reported a moderate relationship between disorganized attachment and later conduct problems.

Main (1995) has also suggested that the disorganized/disoriented
group may be the most vulnerable to the development of psychopathology. She bases this on the association of this pattern with child maltreatment and a theoretical argument that children with disorganized/
disoriented attachment are exposed to parents who are frightening or
frightened. A child who is threatened/frightened by a caregiver is left
in an untenable situation (presumably in a state of extended arousal); a
child whose caregiver expresses a state of being frightened in the con-

text of the child's behavior may experience a sense of being powerful but bad. This latter state may also be presumed to induce a sense of arousal in the child. Liotti (1995) argues that the disorganized/ disoriented pattern is relevant to the development of psychopathology through the induction of dissociated states.

The notion that the relationship between attachment and child psychopathology is not entirely direct is well illustrated by Radke-Yarrow et al. (1995), who compared outcomes (at 6 and 9 years) for two groups of children: offspring of mothers with major depression or bipolar disorder, and children from a control population. They concluded that maternal psychopathology interacts with the attachment relationship to affect later developmental outcomes. Counterintuitively, they found that securely attached children of mothers with major depression were uniquely vulnerable to later problematic behavior. Furthermore, they found an absence of anxiety symptoms in insecurely attached children of mothers with bipolar disorder. They provided some explanation for these findings, in that most of the latter children were relatively assertive and not locked in a helpless dependency on their unavailable mothers. For the children of severely depressed mothers, they found that the majority of the depressed mothers were affectively engulfing and that the children, many of whom were inhibited, responded with dependent neediness.

Although the evidence for the connection between insecure attachment and psychopathology is largely correlational at present, it is consistent with attachment theory. That is, it appears that an insecure attachment relationship with one's primary caregiver acts as a vulnerability factor for the development of psychopathology. The next section describes one of the theoretical bases on which this vulnerability may rest.

Attachment and Affect Regulation

Ainsworth took Bowlby's notion of the attachment relationship and conceptualized attachment security as the base from which the child learns to explore the world (Bretherton, 1995). Subsequent attachment researchers have expanded and clarified this notion of a secure base largely within the framework of affect regulation. Bowlby's concept of an internal working model presumed that the infant learns to respond to the parent's signals, including those about affects, in a way that will promote maintenance of the attachment relationship. Main (1995) and others have developed the notion that the infant learns to regulate affect through the use of strategies that promote proximity to the caregiver. Thus, in the most optimal situation—a secure attachment relationship—the infant can express both positive and negative affect and has the presumption that the caregiver will respond to distress signals. In the situation of an avoidant attachment, the infant experiences the caregiver as rejecting and insensitive to the infant's needs and affects. This is presumed to account for the infant's lack of display of negative affect and avoidance of the caregiver on reunion in the Strange Situation. It is presumed that the avoidant infant does not experience the caregiver as interested in or able to alleviate his or her distress. In the situation of resistant attachment, the infant perceives the caregiver as preoccupied and emotionally unavailable. The infant's strong displays of negative affect are seen as a way of obtaining the caregivers' attention. Cassidy (1994) has recently reviewed the empirical basis for seeing affect regulation as a strategy for maintaining the attachment relationship. From this perspective, she concludes that the evidence is good that individuals with avoidant or dismissing attachment relationships tend to suppress affect, particularly negative affect. Although it has been presumed that individuals with resistant or preoccupied attachments exaggerate or magnify affect, the evidence for this is less clear.

Although the original theorizing about attachment and affect regulation emphasized the notion of a goal-corrected system in which the infant's behaviors served to maintain proximity to the caregiver, it is also possible to view the infant's responses within a social learning framework. This presumes that the infant learns behaviors that are reinforced by the caregiver. Although these approaches are not incompatible, the social learning approach requires an examination of maternal response to infant affect. As indicated in Chapter 2, Goldberg et al. (1994) have demonstrated in a pilot study that mothers of securely attached infants do respond equally to positive and negative affect, whereas mothers of avoidantly attached infants fail to respond to what little negative affect is expressed by their infants, and mothers of resistantly attached infants respond more to negative affect than to positive or neutral affect.

These findings are consistent with Izard et al.'s (1991) study, in which they showed that a mother's emotional expressiveness predicts mother–child attachment. In this longitudinal study of 114 white mother–infant dyads followed from birth through 13 months, they showed that mothers of more securely attached infants reported experiencing fewer negative emotions and more positive emotions. They were also more open in expression of negative emotions around their children and were rated as more sociable, nurturant, and empathic. In contrast, mothers of insecurely attached infants reported experiencing more negative emotions but were less open in the expression of these around their infants. Somewhat surprisingly, but of theoretical interest, these mothers reported expressing more positive emotions around their infants. As reported above, the insecurely attached infants generally displayed more sadness and anger, cried, demanded attention, and showed distress in a mildly stressful or frustrating condition of physical limitation. However, in the condition in which mothers displayed negative emotions (sadness or anger), the securely attached infants displayed more anger than the insecurely attached infants. These findings do suggest that a mother's greater comfort with expression of negative affect may encourage a child's comfort with negative affect. Furthermore, the insecurely attached child receives conflicting messages about affect and, particularly in the avoidant attachment situation, learns to suppress negative affect. Lastly, the mother's reduced experience of positive affect diminishes the opportunity to share positive affect.

Sroufe (1989a, 1989b, 1991) has theorized that the process of developing affect regulation is a developmental progression in which the caregiver initially does all the regulating, through sensitive responsiveness to infant signals of distress and interest, with a gradual transition to the infant's having the capacity to regulate his or her own affects. If this theory is correct, the development of strategies of affect regulation may be influenced by caregiver response as well as by the infant's capacity to respond. In studying depressed mothers and their infants (children vulnerable to the development of psychopathology), Field (1989, 1994) has articulated a theory that combines maternal responsiveness and infant behaviors to produce a more comprehensive view of the ways in which variables studied as part of the attachment system may interact with child factors to produce affect dysregulation.

On the basis of work by Hofer (1995), who has demonstrated that a mother rat acts as a physiological regulator for her pups, Field has proposed that a primary caregiver acts as an emotional regulator for an infant. Extending the animal work to humans, Field (1994) has reported a series of studies examining the behavior of infants subjected to either physical separations from their mothers (maternal hospitalization for the birth of a sibling, a mother's conference trip) or emotional unavailability (the still-face paradigm in the laboratory, maternal depression). She has shown that maternal hospitalization, with reduced availability (due to the mother's caretaking duties with the newborn sibling) on the mother's return, is more stressful for an infant than a mother's conference trip (which presumably does not interfere with mother's availability on return). Physiological and behavioral indices suggest a continuing state of dysregulation for a period of time after the mother's return in the case of hospitalization.

In the still-face paradigm, mothers are asked to assume a still face or depressed look and not to respond to their infants. Infants become quite agitated (both behaviorally and physiologically) in this situation, and this agitation may continue for some time following the mothers' resumption of normal behavior. When depressed mothers are asked to maintain a still face, their infants appear less disturbed. This difference has been interpreted as due to these infants' greater familiarity with still-face behavior. Moreover, in the still-face paradigm these infants do not show the heart rate elevations of the infants of nondepressed mothers, despite showing cortisol elevations. Field (1994) interprets this as a state of learned helplessness. Notably, observations of the mothers' behaviors when asked to maintain a still face suggest little difference from their normal facial expression. The interactions between depressed mothers and their infants are generally less positive than those between nondepressed mothers and their infants. When infants of depressed mothers are exposed to more animated strangers, they do not increase their level of positive interaction—an effect interpreted as a generalization of their depressed style of interacting to other adults. What has been surprising to Field and her colleagues is the apparently negative effect these "depressed infants" have on the behavior of the nondepressed stranger, who performs less optimally in interaction with these infants than with infants of nondepressed mothers.

Reviewing the attachment literature on children of depressed and nondepressed mothers, Field (1989) notes that although the attachment relationship of infants and depressed mothers does not differ from normal in the first year, it does deviate in the direction of more insecure attachment by the second year. Cicchetti and Aber (1986) see this increase in insecure attachment in the second year as due to maternal stress consequent on a developing toddler's behavior, which then interferes with the security of attachment. In explaining these findings, Field refers to the normal sensitive attunement between mother and infant, which is lacking in the depressed mother–infant dyad. Depressed mothers appear unresponsive because of either their withdrawn behavior or their intrusiveness and hostility; in either case, they fail to provide the modulation of feeling states needed for the development of effective affect regulation. Field acknowledges that genetic factors within a child may make the child more vulnerable to affect dysregulation, but she also emphasizes that the child of the depressed mother begins to behave in a fashion that may induce less positive interactions with others. In a similar model, Tronick and Gianino (1986) see a mother's lack of regulation as causing an infant to be in a chronically negative state of affect arousal. They also propose that the child of a depressed mother gradually internalizes an expectation of the mother's not being able to meet his or her needs and of the self as not being worthy of attention. As noted earlier, this chronically negative affect state may be presumed to have an enduring effect on brain structure and function (Post, 1992; Segal et al., 1996).

Because not all infants of depressed mothers are insecurely attached and not all mothers of insecurely attached infants are depressed, the impact of maternal depression on infant affect regulation cannot be simply extrapolated to other situations of insecure attachment. However, this paradigm does provide evidence for the deleterious effect that insensitive caregiving can have. Furthermore, maternal depression is quite common and can be presumed, at least in its more severe forms, to interfere with the infant's capacity to regulate arousal and to expose the child to prolonged states of negative affect that appear to leave him or her vulnerable to developing psychopathology.

Arousal has been assessed empirically through measurement of heart rate, changes in cortisol secretion, and skin conductance. Because there is not a clear association between these measures and behavior, it has been difficult to assess how stressed individuals may be in any one situation. Infants showing significant behavioral distress (e.g., crying) may show little cortisol elevation. Conversely, infants with little behavioral evidence may show physiological evidence of distress. Despite reduced behavioral signs of distress, avoidantly attached infants in one study did display heart rate elevations in the Strange Situation procedure (Spangler & Grossmann, 1993). Moreover, their heart rate did not decrease with object manipulation and increase on looking to their mothers, as it did in securely attached infants. The authors interpreted their findings as evidence that an avoidantly attached infant does not use the mother as a secure base, but evasively avoids her when the attachment system is activated. Cortisol responses in these infants confirm that they were more stressed by the separation experience than were the securely attached infants.

Gunnar et al. (1989) have argued that the cortisol elevation seen in avoidantly attached infants is a reflection of inadequate coping strategies. Because of conflicting evidence in the literature about the impact of the quality of the attachment relationship on physiological indicators of distress, Gunnar et al. (1989) have reformulated the issue. In some studies, securely attached children show a more reactive cortisol response than do insecurely attached children; furthermore, there is a relationship between cortisol reactivity and social competence, such that more competent children show greater cortisol reactivity. Gunnar et al., borrowing from the coping literature, suggest that securely attached children are more likely to use approach strategies in stressful situations. Although approach strategies may initially be more stressful, children using approach strategies become more competent over the longer term. These authors argue that the degree of control a child experiences in a challenging or stressful situation is what determines how much stress and how much cortisol elevation will be produced. Furthermore, what is emerging as an important indicator of stress reactivity is the ability to bring cortisol levels back to baseline, which may reflect control over the situation or coping strategies that reduce the perceived stress (Gunnar & Barr, 1998). Stress-reactive individuals demonstrate a more prolonged elevation of cortisol after the stress than do nonreactive individuals.

From this perspective, it is logical to presume that insecurely attached infants who can use an avoidant strategy may be able to control their arousal, but that they may be more vulnerable to increases in their arousal whenever they are in a situation where it may be difficult to use avoidance. As a consequence of their prolonged use of avoidance, they will be less likely than securely attached infants to develop more effective coping strategies (which are largely developed through approach and exposure) and consequently will be less competent in social domains. Moreover, this failure to develop effective coping strategies, which would allow them to modulate both their stress and cortisol elevations, leaves them more vulnerable to future stresses. The fact that the disorganized infants in the Spangler and Grossmann (1993) study, who would be presumed not to have an organized strategy for dealing with the distress of separation, showed the largest changes in cortisol secretion would support the notion that the cortisol response reflects the adequacy of the coping response. Similar skin conductance changes have been reported for college students who use deactivating strategies (equivalent to avoidant dismissing attachment) when asked about attachment and separation issues (Dozier & Kobak, 1992).

Despite the present focus on the caregiving environment, evidence would suggest that the interaction of factors within the child and the environment is most likely to be relevant in understanding the development of psychopathology, especially as it depends on the adequacy of affect regulation (Sameroff, 1989; Nachmias et al., 1996). In fact, Erickson, Sroufe, and Egeland (1985) have shown that securely attached children with behavior problems, in comparison to those without, have mothers who have less support in their relationships and more difficulty setting limits on their children's behavior. Conversely, mothers of insecurely attached children without behavior problems, compared to those with behavior problems, have more supportive relationships, appear more sensitive to their children, and are better able to set limits on their children's behavior. The Shaw et al. (1996) study, reported above, confirms the importance of an interaction of child–environment factors: Infants with disorganized attachment who were perceived by their mothers as difficult showed higher levels of aggression at age 5 than those who were not perceived as difficult. Clearly, these studies suggest that the attachment relationship is only a part of the picture and has to be seen in that light.

Rutter (1989) has demonstrated that psychopathology arises most commonly when an individual is exposed to a number of risk factors, including a number of parental variables. An insecure attachment relationship, particularly a disorganized/disoriented pattern, could be conceptualized as a mediating factor for several of those variables and also as a risk factor in its own right. Belsky et al. (1995) have also shown that the risk of developing an insecure attachment is affected by the number of risk factors to which a mother–child dyad is exposed. The study by Nachmias et al. (1996), which shows that the combination of an inhibited child and insecure attachment is what produces cortisol elevations upon exposure to stress, does suggest either that more than one factor may be needed or (as has been suggested earlier) that one factor may have to be at an extreme level to produce the sort of impairments in arousal modulation that contribute to the development of psychopathology. Calkins and Fox (1992) have argued that a complex interaction between distress reactivity and maternal caregiving is what produces failures in the development of affect regulation. The interaction of biological and rearing effects has also been shown to be important in developmental outcomes in methadone-exposed infants (Bernstein & Hans, 1994) and in the development of criminal behavior (Raine et al., 1996). The presence of situational stress is another important factor, which will be dealt with in Chapter 5.

Animal Studies

Since the early studies by Harlow and associates with various forms of surrogate rearing in rhesus monkeys, it has been clear that monkeys deprived of their mothers over critical early periods are less able to manage stressful situations than are mother-reared monkeys (Suomi, 1991a, 1991b). Isolated monkeys display a variety of maladaptive responses to stresses, including heightened levels of fear and aggression, and are more likely to be abusing as mothers. Even peer-reared monkeys who may appear normal in nonstressful situations display more extreme reactions to social separations than do mother-reared monkeys. These reactions have been shown to persist into adulthood. Suomi (1991a, 1991b) has suggested that the peer rearing is akin to insecure attachment, in that it leaves a young monkey with less effective strategies for managing stressful situations. As adolescents, these peer-reared monkeys show more aggression toward strangers, have lower levels of 5-hydroxyindoleacetic acid (a serotonin metabolite) in their cerebrospinal fluid, and are more likely to be expelled from their social group than are mother-reared monkeys (Suomi, 1995). Moreover, infants raised by mothers in a variable foraging situation (which is stressful for the mothers) display more extreme reactions when exposed to stressful situations than do infants raised by mothers in situations where there is no uncertainty about the food supply.

Studies in which infant monkeys are raised by foster mothers who differ in their nurturance reinforce the importance of maternal sensitivity, but emphasize the interactional nature of the resulting adaptation. Inhibited or highly reactive infant monkeys are more susceptible to the effect of punitive maternal behavior. Conversely, these same monkeys, when raised by highly nurturant mothers, become leaders within their groups (Suomi, 1995).

From these studies, Kraemer (1992) has articulated a theory that builds on Hofer's (1995) work. Kraemer believes that the attachment system provides a psychobiological regulation that is reflected in the development of neurotransmitters. Because the surrogate-reared monkeys display an initial deficit in norepinephrine, followed by a supersensitivity to norepinephrine, he postulates that the effect of the attachment system is to regulate the development of patterns of neurotransmitters (Kraemer et al., 1989). When this regulation is less than adequate, the developing organism does not have an adequately functioning system for managing arousal and dealing with stress. (See Chapter 5 for a more complete discussion of this issue.)

Summary of the Work on Attachment

Although none of the above-described studies provide definitive proof that the attachment system acts as a mechanism for the developing organism to regulate affect, the general thrust of the studies is in the same direction. We can presume that attachment may act at a psychobiological level, as suggested by Kraemer (1992); at the level of social learning; and also at the level of the development of internal working models or schemata. It appears that insecurely attached individuals are more vulnerable to difficulty in managing stress. Whether this vulnerability is best explained as a neurotransmitter supersensitivity, a failure to learn adequate coping strategies, a deficit in internal working models, or a combination of all three will have to await more empirical tests of the various theories. What is important for the present thesis is that an emerging body of evidence suggests that the attachment system plays a role in the development of affect regulation, and that individuals with insecure attachment have a greater likelihood of experiencing prolonged arousal when under stress. In the chapters on specific syndromes in Part III, I show how the various facets of the caregiving system may interact with other factors to produce different forms of psychopathology. Because attachment theory does not encompass all aspects of the caregiving environment, it is important to discuss other aspects of parenting that have been shown to relate to the development of psychopathology.

DYSFUNCTIONAL PARENTING

I have arbitrarily separated attachment difficulties from dysfunctional parenting, in order to emphasize the other large literature on caregiving problems that have been shown to have an impact on child psychopathology. Dysfunctional parenting can encompass the affectionless control shown by Baumrind (1989) to contribute to later psychopathology, as well as the varieties of inconsistent, neglectful, and rejecting parenting styles that have also been found to contribute to it (Kendziora & O'Leary, 1993). I focus first on two models that have been empirically validated: those of Gerald Patterson and Daphne Bugental.

Patterson's and Bugental's Models of Dysfunctional Parenting

Patterson's work has shown that inconsistent discipline and coercive interactions between parent and child are related to conduct disorder (Dishion, French, & Patterson, 1995). Patterson describes a sequence of behaviors between parent and child that, with multiple repetitions, reinforces the child's demanding and oppositional behavior and allows the child to escape from the parent's demands. The parent deals with the child's coerciveness through talking (critical and harsh comments), but is inconsistent (often gives in), thus reinforcing the child's coercive behavior. Although the child gets what he or she wants, it is at a cost to the relationship, which becomes highly negative. The more demanding the child, the more the parent's frustration becomes apparent and interferes with more constructive parenting. Patterson and coworkers have subjected various aspects of their model to empirical testing and have generally good support for most aspects of it. (Dishion, French, & Patterson, 1995, review this evidence.)

Bugental (1992) has articulated a model that differs from but is not inconsistent with Patterson's framework. Her model provides a way of understanding how dysfunctional parenting may develop and be maintained when a parent perceives a child as difficult, which, as I have noted above, is often the situation with an insecure attachment relationship. Bugental cites the cognitive-behavioral literature showing that the affect experienced in a situation is partially dependent on the cognitive interpretation of the situation. A parent's frustration with a child may be related to the extent to which the parent believes that the child has control over his or her behavior. Furthermore, Bugental has shown in her own work that a parent's level of perceived control in a situation with a child affects the parent's arousal level. Parents who are anticipating interaction with unresponsive children and who see themselves as having low control over the children's behavior show higher levels of arousal (increased skin conductance and heart rate) than do parents who see themselves as having more control over their children's behavior. As this increased arousal may lead to a narrower focus of attention, such parents may be more likely to react emotionally rather than thoughtfully in situations with children whom they perceive as not under their control. This conceptualization suggests that such situations may access automatic as opposed to controlled cognitions. (See Chapter 7, especially the theories of LeDoux [1992, 1996] about the role of brain structures in automatic vs. controlled processing.) Automatic cognitions are thought to operate through processes that provide rapid access to an affective/cognitive schema, which in turn conditions later perceptions and reactions. Thus, for example, a parent who perceives a situation with a child as fitting a pattern that has in the past been difficult and arousing may react preemptively with frustration and a sense of helplessness. This reaction may then interfere with more constructive problem-solving approaches to the situation.

Against this background, Bugental (1992) proposes the following model for what she terms "threat-oriented family systems." Certain child features or behaviors are seen by the parent as challenging; these include ambiguous, unusual, or aversive behaviors. These child behaviors elicit an automatic parental schema, which produces defensive arousal, negative affect, and problem-focused (as opposed to solution-focused) ideation. A parent with a schema low in threat-orientation will not react automatically with the same affective arousal and will have more access to solution-focused cognitions. A parent with a highly threat-oriented schema is more likely to "lose the battle" with the child, because such a parent perceives herself as the victim and the child as in control. Bugental also describes efforts by highly threat-oriented parents to deal with the situation in advance. These include false smiles and ingratiating behaviors which Bugental believes the children interpret negatively. This produces negative affect in the children and more avoidance and unresponsiveness, thus confirming the parents' beliefs about these children and their behavior. With increases in the intensity of arousal and negative affect, the likelihood of emotionally and physically abusive behavior directed at these children increases. Drawing on both her own and others' work, Bugental provides substantial support for her model.

Stocker (1995) provides support for the negative impact of a conflicted parent–child relationship on later behavior disorder. She examined differential relationships between parents and siblings, and compared these with measures of mother-rated temperament and child adjustment. Children whose relationships with both parents were described as more conflictual and less close than those of their siblings had more emotional temperaments and more problem behaviors than did other children in the sample. Children who were closer than their siblings to either parent had ratings falling between those of children who were less close to both parents and those of children who were closer to both parents.

I believe that the conceptual frameworks of Patterson and Bugental are nonspecific with respect to later childhood disorders (i.e., relevant to both internalizing and externalizing disorders). The critical elements are that the relationship between parent and child becomes skewed, with internal working models evolving that lead to further negative and nonsupportive interactions. The ongoing interaction between parent and child is one in which the child is perceived by the parent as difficult and the child perceives the parent as hostile and critical. This conflicted parent–child relationship may contribute to depression in the parent (Brown, Bifulco, & Andrews, 1990), as well as to either internalizing or externalizing disorders in the child (Messer & Gross, 1995; Ge, Best, Conger, & Simons, 1996). Because this type of interaction is seen commonly in child and adolescent psychiatric disorders, I believe that this pattern is the most likely descriptor of the dysfunctional parenting and early adverse experiences that have been related to the development of psychopathology. It provides a way of understanding the high levels of expressed emotion that are now being reported for both internalizing and externalizing disorders, as well as an explanation for the frequent comorbidity of disorders (particularly the co-occurrence of conduct disorder or oppositional defiant disorder with anxiety and depression). With respect to affect regulation, this framework provides an explanation for why a developing individual may be exposed to high levels of negative parental affect. I review the literature on expressed emotion before speculating how this exposure to parental negative affect influences the child's development of both self-esteem and affect regulation.

Exposure to Criticism and Conflict

Exposure to high levels of expressed emotion (abbreviated in this discussion as EE) has been seen as an important factor in relapse in schizophrenia and in other major psychiatric disorders. (See Kavanagh, 1992, for a review.) The mechanism through which exposure to EE exerts its effect is not clear. In the original studies (Brown, Birley, & Wing, 1972; Vaughan & Leff, 1976), three components in the attitude or behavior of the significant adult toward the patient were identified: critical comments, hostility, and emotional overinvolvement. There is a tendency for these attitudes and behaviors to correlate with one another and to correlate with rejection and lack of warmth as perceived by the patient (McCreadie, Williamson, Athawes, Connolly, & Tilak-Singh, 1994). Hooley and Teasdale (1989), in a longitudinal study of subjects with unipolar depression, found that although high EE, marital distress, and perceived criticism from the spouse were all related to relapse, the best predictor of relapse was perceived criticism. These studies are consistent with the older literature on risk factors for childhood disorders, in which lack of parental warmth and hostility were related to childhood disturbance (Rutter, Graham, & Yule, 1970).

Since the beginning of study in this area, there has been a presumption that exposure to high levels of EE—especially negative or critical comments directed at the patient—produces arousal beyond an optimal level (Brown et al., 1972). Although there are problems with the measurement of arousal (as discussed in connection with the attachment research), studies generally confirm that subjects exposed to or in the presence of high-EE relatives are more aroused than subjects in the presence of low-EE relatives (Sturgeon, Turpin, Kuipers, Berkowitz, & Leff, 1984; Tarrier, Barrowclough, Porceddu, & Watts, 1988; Tarrier, 1989; Altorfer, Goldstein, Miklowitz, & Nuechterlein, 1992). The difficulties in this literature have to do not only with the measurement of arousal (behavioral or physiological indices and even which physiological measure to use), but with the status of the patients at the time of assessment (psychotic vs. remitted) and changes over time in EE status of relatives—changes that do not seem closely matched by physiological indices of arousal in the patients. There has also been some controversy as to whether the relatives' EE is reactive to the patients' behavior. Nuechterlein, Snyder, and Mintz (1992), in analyzing variables predictive of relapse in schizophrenic patients, have established that EE may be both a mediating variable contributing to relapse and a response to living with such patients. Kavanagh (1992), reviewing the literature on EE and schizophrenia, concludes: "Psychophysiological evidence demonstrates that people with schizophrenia do experience powerful emotional reactions in response to negative interactions" (p. 609). He also provides a model that attempts to explain some of the inconsistencies in the literature. This interactive model proposes that aversive behaviors exhibited by a patient and related to anger, anxiety, or depression produce critical responses in relatives, especially when they may not understand the patient's illness. This may lead to withdrawal and increases in psychotic symptoms. If Kavanagh's model is correct, it would be reasonable to assume that this pattern of interactions could become increasingly stressful and frustrating for both the patient and relatives, and may account for the greater correlation between EE and symptomatology at the time of admission.

The study of EE's effects on children has roughly paralleled the research on adults. In an early study, Doane, West, Goldstein, Rodnick, and Jones (1981) followed disturbed adolescents into early adulthood and found that parental affective style (as measured by support, criticism, guilt induction, and intrusiveness) was related to psychiatric status at follow-up. It has been shown that parents of children with disruptive behavior disorders or obsessive–compulsive disorder have high levels of EE and psychiatric disorder, compared to parents of controls (Hibbs et al., 1991). The percentages of high EE were 88% for parents of children with disruptive behavior disorders, 82% for parents of children with obsessive–compulsive disorder, and 41% for parents of the control children. Presence of a psychiatric disorder was the only predictor of high EE in fathers, while for mothers a child's diagnosis was a stronger predictor than a mother's psychiatric diagnosis. In a community survey of 108 preadolescent children, Stubbe, Zahner, Goldstein, and Leckman (1993) found higher levels of disruptive behavior disorders in families where parents expressed high levels of criticism. Anxiety disorders were elevated in those families where parents expressed high levels of emotional overinvolvement. Asarnow, Goldstein, Tompson, and Guthrie (1993) found that high EE in families was related to persistence of mood disorders in depressed children. Vostanis, Nicholls, and Harrington (1994) measured maternal EE in parents of children with conduct disorder, emotional disorders (anxiety and depression), and controls. They found that maternal warmth distinguished the three groups (conduct disorder < emotional disorders < controls). Maternal criticism distinguished the group of children with conduct disorder, but also was associated with child behavior ratings across the sample. In addition, at a 9-month follow-up, mothers of children with conduct disorder expressed significantly less criticism and more warmth (Vostanis & Nicholls, 1995). Lastly, Hibbs, Zahn, Hamburger, Kruesi, and Rapoport (1992) examined parental EE and autonomic activity in a sample of children with disruptive behavior disorders or obsessive–compulsive disorder, compared to normal controls. They found higher skin conductance (a measure of autonomic reactivity) in children with two high-EE parents. Particularly in the obsessive–compulsive disorder group, fathers' EE and mothers' psychiatric diagnoses were related to higher autonomic reactivity in the children.

A related but different approach has been to examine the impact of adult conflict on children's behavior. Cummings, Iannotti, and Zahn-Waxler (1985) exposed 2-year-old children to background scenarios between two unfamiliar adults, the themes being friendly and angry interactions. Most children responded to the angry interaction with some form of distress, and in some children there was a subsequent increase in aggression with the peer playmate. Children who were exposed to a repeat of the angry scenario displayed even more distress and aggression. The investigators interpreted this increased responsiveness as the induction of emotional reactivity in the exposed children. Extending this work to 4- and 5-year-olds, El-Sheikh, Cummings, and Goetsch (1989) found that systolic blood pressure increased in response to anger and that the heart rate response patterns differed across three groups described as "angry/ambivalent," "concerned/ distressed," and "unresponsive." Shaw et al. (1997) also demonstrated that exposure to child-rearing disagreements was a predictor of internalizing problems in a preschool sample of children of high-risk mothers.

Pursuing differences in individual responses to interadult anger, Ballard, Cummings, and Larkin (1993) found that sons of hypertensive parents showed greater systolic blood pressure reactivity than sons of normotensive parents. Moreover, marital distress and overt maternal anger predicted behavioral responses to interadult anger better than did family history of hypertension. They concluded that vulnerability to stress (such as parental anger) may be related to specific familial histories and backgrounds. Interestingly, when children also witness the resolution of conflict, their arousal is modulated (Cummings, Simpson, & Wilson, 1993).

That the negative effects of parental conflict are not short-lived is apparent from a study by Henning et al. (1997), who surveyed undergraduate students about their experience of witnessing their parents' physical aggression as children. Those who reported witnessing such aggression acknowledged higher levels of current distress than those without such experience did. This effect was still present even when the impact of other variables (e.g., divorce, SES, physical abuse of the child, parental alcoholism, and nonphysical discord between the parents) was controlled for. The authors point out that although their findings provide support for the notion that witnessing interparental physical aggression plays a traumatic role, a substantial portion of the variance of such aggression on adult adjustment was mediated through decreased parental caring and warmth during childhood. One can presume that children living in homes where there is a high level of conflict with little resolution may experience prolonged states of hyperarousal. How this arousal is expressed is undoubtedly influenced by both familial and child factors. However, it does appear that children can be sensitized to anger, resulting in greater arousal when exposed to subsequent stimuli.

The mechanism(s) for the impact of EE and exposure to interadult anger on the individual must be speculative, as research cannot provide definitive answers at this time. However, from the studies discussed above, one can presume that EE and exposure to interadult anger cause distress and increase arousal. It appears that some children act aggressively in these situations, while others withdraw. These reactions may be temperamentally influenced and learned. As suggested in the discussion of attachment, prolonged states of arousal may have an influence on the development of neurotransmitter systems, but they may also influence a child's opportunities to learn about affects and coping strategies. Withdrawal deprives the child of opportunities to learn adaptive strategies for working out conflict and can interfere with the development of social skills; these strategies and skills are both learned in an interpersonal context. Learning about affects may also be impaired if the individual experiences high levels of arousal when attempting to explore or discuss feelings. This may occur if an individual is highly sensitized to specific affects and fears the arousal accompanying these feeling states. Withdrawal may be perceived as the only solution. Furthermore, difficulties in affect *recognition* in schizophrenia and other psychiatric disorders may develop as an easily aroused individual is exposed to high EE or high levels of parental conflict, which make affects very uncomfortable. The natural avoidance response may thus interfere with the individual's opportunity to learn about the subtleties of facial affect expression. This in turn may be an impediment to more adaptive forms of affect regulation. Lastly, prolonged stress (such as that which may occur in sensitive individuals exposed to high levels of conflict) may actually impair hippocampal development and functioning, as high levels of corticosteroids are known to produce hippocampal cell loss. This may render such exposed individuals more vulnerable, as cognitive strategies for dealing with their distress may be impaired through hippocampal damage (O'Brien, 1997).

CONCLUSIONS

The evidence from the attachment literature suggests that insecure attachment is a vulnerability factor that may interfere with the development of optimal affect regulation and predispose children to the development of psychopathology. Other factors in the caregiving environment—such as dysfunctional parenting in general, and exposure to high levels of EE and to interadult conflict in particular—may make independent contributions to affect regulation difficulties. These factors may act at several different levels, producing increased levels of arousal within the individual and interfering with the development of adaptive affective coping strategies. Because of the transactional nature of development, many of these factors may be presumed to interact with individual factors. Over time and with the development of the individual, these processes can be presumed to affect neural development, potentially leading to a decrease in behavioral and affective flexibility with prolonged adversity.

Chapter 5

Stress, Trauma, and Abuse

This chapter discusses the effects that stress in general and two severe forms of stress in particular—trauma and abuse—can have on arousal and its regulation, and thus on the development of psychopathology. I begin by defining how I use the terms *stress*, *trauma*, and *abuse*. I then provide a brief summary of the research linking stress in general to vulnerability to mental disorders, followed by a description of the neurobiology of the stress response. (This description is somewhat more detailed than the mentions of neurobiology in chapters to this point; nonspecialist readers may wish to peruse Chapter 7 before proceeding with this section.) The roles of trauma and of abuse in generating affect dysregulation are then discussed, with particular emphasis on the potential these severe types of stress create for posttraumatic stress disorder (PTSD) and for intergenerational abuse, respectively; brief descriptions of possible neurobiological factors are also provided.

DEFINING STRESS, TRAUMA, AND ABUSE

As Lazarus and Folkman (1984) point out, defining stress is complicated by whether the focus is on the individual experiencing the stress or on the agents causing the stress. For our purposes, I have chosen their definition of stress that encompasses both domains. They define psychological stress as "a relationship between the person and the environment that is appraised by the person as taxing or exceeding his or her resources and endangering his or her well-being" (p. 21). In particular they emphasize the importance of the individual's cognitive appraisal of a situation as contributing to his or her judgment of its stressfulness. Trauma can be conceptualized as an extension of this definition in which the individual experiences an event as overwhelming and the self as threatened and helpless. Clearly I imply a continuum of events and reactions from mild stress to severe and overwhelming trauma. Abuse refers to physical, sexual, or emotional maltreatment (including severe neglect) of an individual. Here, as well, the individual's appraisal of the situation may be the critical factor in determining the amount of stress generated.

STRESS AND ITS RELATIONSHIP
TO PSYCHOPATHOLOGY

The study of stress and its relationship to psychopathology has a long history, the most salient findings of which are highlighted here. Various stressful life events have been associated with the onset of mental disorders (Kendler, Kessler, et al., 1995; Brown & Harris, 1993; Brown, Harris, & Eales, 1993). Rutter (1989) has shown that there is an additive effect: The likelihood of developing a disorder is relatively small with one stressor, but quite high with four or more stressors. It is also clear that not all individuals develop mental disorders in the context of stressors. As indicated in Chapters 3 and 4, it is now believed that genetic factors and early childhood experience affect an individual's reactivity to stress. Brown, Harris, and their coworkers have shown in an elegant series of studies that early adverse experiences (loss, separation from parents, and neglectful or abusing environments) make women more vulnerable to developing a mood disorder in the context of a significant life stress (Brown & Harris, 1993; Brown et al., 1993). This group has also demonstrated the existence of a life history trajectory that increases this vulnerability; it consists of early adverse experiences, premarital pregnancy, and a nonsupportive marital relationship (Harris, Brown, & Bifulco, 1987). Kendler, Kessler, et al. (1995), examining factors related to onset and recurrence of depression in the Virginia Twin Registry study, concluded that genetic factors appear to increase vulnerability to stress. (For a more complete discussion, see Chapter 9.) What seems clear is that stress can beget stress. Some of this may arise from the development of maladaptive internal working models, which predispose an individual who has experienced dysfunctional relationships in the past to develop further maladaptive relationships. It is also possible to conceptualize the linkage of stress to later stress as mediated through maladaptive neurobiological stress responses and inadequate coping responses. It is likely that all of these formulations have merit.

It was initially believed that specific relationships might exist between certain types of stressors and certain disorders (e.g., loss and depression). However, it now appears that although adverse life events are definitely increased prior to onset of a disorder, event–disorder relationship are relatively nonspecific. There may nevertheless be a degree of specificity related to how the individual perceives the stress (Hammen & Goodman-Brown, 1990). It is clear that adverse life events increase physiological stress responses, and that if stresses are prolonged, affected individuals experience increased vulnerability to the development not only of psychopathology but also of cardiovascular and other physical problems (Sapolsky, 1994). Some of the physical effects appear to be mediated through elevations of catecholamines, as well as through activation of the hypothalamic–pituitary–adrenal (HPA) axis and corticosteroid elevations. One of the major factors provoking a physiological stress response or sustaining such a response is perceived unpredictability or lack of control (Gunnar & Barr, 1998). Therefore, to the extent that the individual continues to perceive the situation as uncontrollable, it will continue to generate a stress response.

Gunnar and coworkers, in a series of studies on infants, have shown that the behavioral manifestations of stress are not always correlated with the physiological responses (Gunnar, 1992; Gunnar & Barr, 1998). Gunnar has argued that although some of these differences may reflect cultural differences in child rearing, the coherence of behavior and physiology may also reflect the infant's capacity to organize an effective response to his or her situation. In their series of studies, Gunnar and collaborators have shown that most infants display a gradual reduction in their cortisol response to the stress of medical exams and inoculations over their first 2 years of life. However, some infants continue to display significant elevations of cortisol with stressful situations at 18 months (Gunnar, Brodersen, Krueger & Rigatuso, 1996). When a large sample of infants were assessed for temperament, attachment classification, and reactivity, these investigators found that a secure attachment buffered the cortisol elevation only in those infants who were described as fearful. Furthermore, those infants who displayed the highest cortisol elevations were predominantly insecurely attached. Lastly, those infants who at an early age displayed large differences between their behavioral response (crying) and physiological response to inoculations were more likely to be classified later as insecurely attached, to have less responsive mothers, and to have higher pretest cortisol levels (Gunnar, Brodersen, Nachmias, Buss, &

Rigatuso, 1996). These studies are consistent with the animal work in which the maternal caregiver appears to be a physiological regulator of the infant (Hofer, 1987, 1995). Although some infants may be genetically more vulnerable to difficulty with moderating their stress response, this work does suggest that the quality of maternal caregiving may play a significant role in a young child's capacity to develop that regulation.

Although adverse events appear to be associated with the *onset* of disorders, there is now research evidence that their role in provoking *recurrences* may be less salient; this work suggests that the individual's system is sensitized by the initial stress, so that minor difficulties may provoke symptoms and recurrence of illness (Post, 1992). Post, Weiss, and Smith (1995) discuss the sensitization of neural processes (such as may occur in learning), as well as *kindled* processes (in which subthreshold stimuli delivered over a period of time lead to a triggered seizure and eventually to autonomous seizure activity). They have developed their model from the effects of cocaine in inducing behavioral sensitization (increased reactivity to subsequent doses) and seizures. Although speculative, this model provides one way of understanding the possible neurobiological bases of psychopathological symptoms as they emerge following a series of stressful events and how they may evolve over time. If the model is correct, interventions would be expected to have differing levels of efficacy, depending on when they were delivered in this evolving series of neural events.

In their review article, Gunnar and Barr (1998) also note that elevated levels of glucocorticoids appear to interfere with attention and focusing, as well as with remembering new information. Because children who exhibit higher cortisol levels under normal situations have more trouble with sustained attention than do children with lower cortisol levels, and these same children are also less well regulated behaviorally than the low-cortisol children, Gunnar and Barr suggest that early experience leading to glucocorticoid dysregulation may have an impact on memory, attention, and self-control. (See also Jacobvitz & Sroufe, 1987.)

NEUROBIOLOGY OF THE STRESS RESPONSE

The psychobiological bases of the stress responses are gradually being elucidated, largely through studies of animals. It is well established that stress induces secretion of epinephrine (E) and norepinephrine (NE) from the adrenal medulla and NE from terminals in the sympathetic nervous system (SNS). (See Johnson, Kamilaris, Chrousos, &

Gold, 1992, for a review.) In addition, corticotropin-releasing hormone (CRH), released by the paraventricular cells of the hypothalamus, stimulates secretion of adrenocorticotropic hormone (ACTH) by the pituitary, which in turn induces release of glucocorticoids from the adrenal cortex. Typically, with reduction of the stress, the HPA stress response is turned off through a negative feedback process in which increased circulating glucocorticoids reduce the release of CRH. This negative feedback effect appears to occur largely through glucocorticoid effects on receptors in the hippocampus and hypothalamus. The release of adrenergic substances tends to be more immediate and short-lived, in contrast to the glucocorticoids, which appear within minutes to hours and tend to have a longer-lasting impact on the system.

Although the short-term effects of increased glucocorticoids prepare the organism for action through changing the normal homeostatic balance in a number of physiological systems, these changes have a negative impact on the organism when the stress becomes chronic. The negative physiological effects of chronic or sustained stress appear to result more from the glucocorticoids than from E or NE, although depletion of NE has been linked to the development of learned helplessness, which is considered an integral part of the depressive reaction (Johnson et al., 1992). Sapolsky (1994) postulates that many of the harmful effects, such as elevations in blood pressure, cardiac effects, and gastrointestinal effects, arise from imbalances in the body's response to the need to conserve resources versus the need to maintain other functions. What may be most important from the perspective of the development of psychopathology is the capacity to turn off the stress response, since chronically high levels of glucocorticoids have a deleterious effect on many systems as well as on the brain, particularly the hippocampus (O'Brien, 1997; Sapolsky, 1994). If we assume that such effects could occur early in life, this may provide a way of understanding how early adverse experience can increase vulnerability to later stresses.

Gunnar and Barr (1998) review the effect of stress on the developing organism. Experience affects the development of CRH-producing cells and receptors for the corticosteroids. Different authors have used different labels for these receptors. Simplistically, the mineralocorticoid receptors (Type I) bind aldosterone (which regulates salt balance) and also play a role in the tonic regulation of the HPA axis through binding glucocorticoids (De Kloet, 1991). The glucocorticoid receptors (Type II) bind glucocorticoids, which regulate a variety of metabolic processes; most importantly for present purposes, they regulate the phasic aspects of the HPA axis and are intimately involved in the regulation of the stress response. De Kloet (1991) provides an extensive discussion of the studies (primarily on animals) with respect to these two types of receptors. Type II receptors appear to be more affected by early experience than are Type I receptors. When Type II receptors are activated in the hippocampus and hypothalamus, they reduce CRH production, thus turning off the stress response. Although with brief CRH stimulation adults experience increased energy and concentration, if Type II receptors are stimulated for a prolonged period, the opposite occurs. In animal research (see Meaney et al., 1996), early experience can affect the ability of the brain to regulate CRH, and with it the magnitude and duration of glucocorticoid elevations and the animal's capacity to manage stress. Repeated exposure to stress-inducing situations modifies the activity of the HPA axis, in some cases sensitizing the system and in other cases desensitizing it.

Meaney et al. (1996) review work from their own laboratories as well as that from others on various stressful manipulations in young rats. A brief handling experience (mild stimulation) that takes place during the first 2 weeks of life reduces adrenal steroid responses to stress and increases glucocorticoid receptor density in the hippocampus and frontal cortex. This response wanes over the first 3 weeks, becoming ineffective by days 15 to 21. These authors conclude that there is a sensitive period for this effect of mild stimulation to reduce the HPA response to stress. The handled rats are less fearful, anxious, and reactive in novel environments than are the nonhandled rats. In other studies, Meaney et al. have shown that repeated lengthy separations from the mother during the first 2 weeks of life produce increases in plasma ACTH and corticosterone responses to either restraint or novelty, in comparison to nonseparated controls. Animals exposed to brief separations, similar to those used in the handling experiments, show reduced plasma ACTH and corticosterone responses. The effects of longer maternal separations appear to be mediated by decreased glucocorticoid receptor binding in the hippocampus and hypothalamus, both sites for regulation of CRH synthesis.

In both these paradigms (handling and maternal separation), the effects endure throughout the lives of the rats, such that the experimental rats display decreased or increased responses to stress. These investigators have shown that these effects involve an altered rate of glucocorticoid gene receptor expression, which results in changes in the sensitivity of the system to the inhibitory effects of glucocorticoids on the synthesis of CRH in hypothalamic neurons. These changes then determine how responsive the HPA system is to stress. In the hippocampus, prolonged elevation of glucocorticoids results in shrinking of dendrites and loss of neurons which affects regulation of the HPA axis.

(See O'Brien, 1997, and Sapolsky, 1994, for reviews.) This reduction in the brain's capacity to turn off the stress response appears to be mediated by loss of glucocorticoid receptors; over time, with increasing stress and glucocorticoid elevations, it may have a cumulative and damaging effect on the brain. In this way, at least in rats, we can see how early experience can program neural systems to overrespond to stress and perhaps to become increasingly vulnerable to minor stresses. (See also Post, 1992.)

There is evidence from animal studies that prenatal stress operates in a similar way to increase catecholamine activity, although not all studies support HPA axis dysregulation (Meaney et al., 1996; Schneider et al., 1998). Elevation of maternal glucocorticoids produces reduction of glucocorticoid receptors in offspring, which in turn is related to less effective HPA responses to stress, including more fearful behavior and lessened ability to sustain attention. In rats and monkeys, these effects can be modified by the quality of maternal caretaking and by handling (Meaney et al., 1996). High-quality maternal behavior can increase glucocorticoid receptors and improve the HPA response to stress, resulting in less fearful offspring behaviors. Conversely, if maternal behavior is suboptimal, the HPA response to stress is increased, resulting in more fearful behavior and an enhanced catecholamine reaction to stress.

According to De Kloet (1991), there is a complicated interaction between corticosteroid receptor balance and homeostatic control, including control over the monoaminergic systems. He describes a balance between mineralocorticoid (Type I) and glucocorticoid (Type II) receptors in both hypothalamic and limbic neurons, which he feels is instrumental in control of the stress response. He cites work in different strains of rats showing reduced emotional and adrenocortical reactivity related to the balance between these receptors in the hippocampus. Although a complete review of De Kloet's ideas is beyond the scope of this discussion, he makes several interesting observations. He notes that these receptors are distributed in many brain regions (the hypothalamic and limbic areas being important for regulation of the HPA axis, as noted above). Importantly, however, glucocorticoid receptors play a role in mediating the action of glucocorticoids on the three main monoaminergic neurotransmitter systems—the serotonergic, noradrenergic, and dopaminergic systems. Furthermore, work in animals shows that although the interactions between glucocorticoids and the monoamine systems are complex, glucocorticoids (through Type II receptors) activate and sensitize these systems during development and stress. Corticosteroids also control responsiveness to these neurotransmitters at the postsynaptic level. Finally, De Kloet describes a reduction in glucocorticoid receptors in the hippocampus with age. Although other parameters of this system also change with age, De Kloet suggests that the degree of aging is related to the failure of the balance of these two receptor types in the hippocampus to adjust to changing environmental conditions. These interesting ideas all require testing in humans, but they speak to the highly complex interactions that are undoubtedly part of the stress response within the brain.

Although the focus up to this point has been on the HPA system, the SNS clearly plays a role in the stress response, and I turn to a more detailed examination of this now. Increased sympathetic discharge resulting from activation of the locus coeruleus (LC) (the main NE tract) and SNS produces arousal, vigilance and anxiety (Johnson et al., 1992). Although acute stress results in secretion of NE from SNS neurons and of both NE and E from the adrenal medulla, chronic, intermittent stress produces increased rates of catecholamine synthesis in the adrenal medulla, sensitization of the catecholamine system to *novel* stressors, and reduction of the SNS response to *familiar* stressors. Inescapable or uncontrollable stress, as in the paradigm that produces learned helplessness, appears to involve a depletion of NE and/or of the enzyme responsible for its synthesis, tyrosine hydroxylase. There are interactions among the catecholamine systems, with the LC/NE system activating the dopamine system (mesocortical and mesolimbic branches) with stress. At the same time, the LC/NE system is activated by serotonin and acetylcholine, and inhibited by gamma-aminobutyric acid (GABA) and the opioid peptides. As indicated above, because the catecholamines are partially under the control of the HPA axis, dysregulation of the HPA axis or inability to shut off the stress response will have an impact on activity in these systems.

Changes in dopamine and its receptors, particularly in the frontal and prefrontal cortices, may also be important in stress. Although we can only speculate on the underlying mechanism, exposure of monkeys to noise stress in one study produced impairment in prefrontal cortical function, which was related to hyperdopaminergic indices (Arnsten & Goldman-Rakic, 1998). Once more this may represent a dysregulated response that becomes long-lasting with changes in receptors. Such a change may be relevant in schizophrenia, where increased activation of dopaminergic systems is seen to be relevant to understanding symptomatology. This also demonstrates some of the different paths that can become sensitized through early experience.

Another mechanism for sensitization of responses appears to reside in the amygdala. In rats, when glucocorticoids are placed into brain ventricles over several days, increased CRH activity is evident in the amygdala. This activity, which may correlate with activation of both the central and peripheral catecholamine systems, can produce fearful and hypervigilant behaviors. Schulkin, McEwen, and Gold (1994) hypothesize that chronic activation of the central nucleus of the amygdala through CRH, whether related to stress or the effects of elevated glucocorticoids, produces a state of what they call "allostatic load" or "arousal pathology." They define allostatic load or arousal pathology as a state of chronic anticipation of negative events, and suggest that this sustained physiological response may underlie many psychopathological states such as melancholia. In contrast to the negative feedback on CRH production that occurs with elevation of glucocorticoids in the hypothalamus and hippocampus, glucocorticoids exert a positive feedback effect on CRH in the amygdala. Thus increased circulating glucocorticoids may have a chronic activating effect on the amygdala, producing a sustained negative affective state, as is seen in some forms of depression.

Figure 5.1 illustrates what is currently known about the neurobiological components of the stress response in animals. Clearly if these findings apply to the development of humans, we may begin to understand how stress reactivity can emerge in both positive and negative directions, and how subsequent experience may either facilitate or remediate an individual's reactivity. It is also likely that for some individuals, especially those who may be genetically vulnerable to difficulties with stress regulation and who are in suboptimal caretaking situations, the neurobiological underpinnings of this system may become severely dysregulated at an early age. This reactivity may further interfere with the relationship with a caretaker, thus intensifying the stress and reducing the chances for a reversal of the reactivity and for optimal growth.

TRAUMA

Like the study of stress and psychopathology, research on the effects of trauma in the development of psychopathology has a long history. Only now, however, are these effects beginning to be understood in all their complexity, from the biological to the intrapsychic. The recent volume *Traumatic Stress: The Effects of Overwhelming Experience on Mind, Body, and Society*, edited by van der Kolk, McFarlane, and Weisaeth (1996), provides a current overview of this area.

Traumatic experiences have been associated with a variety of psychopathological reactions, including eating disorders, self-mutilation, substance abuse, and aggressive behavior, as well as personality disorders (e.g., borderline personality disorder) (van der Kolk, 1996). These

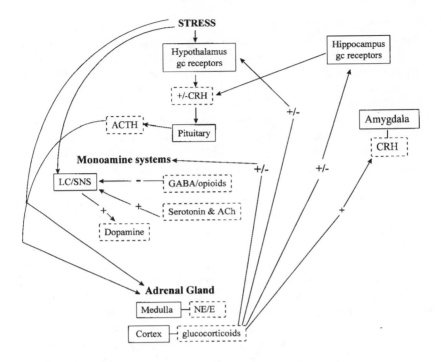

FIGURE 5.1. Neurobiological components of the stress response in animals. gc, glucocorticoid receptor; CRH, corticotropin-releasing hormone; ACTH, adrenocorticotropic hormone; LC/SNS, locus coeruleus/sympathetic nervous system; GABA, gamma-aminobutyric acid; NE/E, norepinephrine/epinephrine; ACh, acetylcholine; +, increased; –, decreased.

associations have been derived largely from retrospective accounts of patients, in which the impact of the trauma has sometimes been difficult to distinguish from the effects of other deleterious life or rearing experiences. The diagnosis of PTSD has, in contrast, been relatively well studied in a prospective fashion, as large cohorts of individuals exposed to a variety of traumatic stressors are being followed systematically. The study of this disorder and of the other reactions associated with extreme stress provides a model from which we can draw inferences about the development of psychopathology in general, as well as about the biological and psychological concomitants of an individual's responses to stressful life events.

The emergence of symptoms following a traumatic event is seen as resulting from "people's inability to come to terms with real experiences that have overwhelmed their capacity to cope" (van der Kolk &

McFarlane, 1996, p. 4). This reaction is moderated by a variety of factors including the nature of the trauma, preparation for the event, support after the event, and individual vulnerability factors. Presumably, also, the timing of stressful life events—that is, whether such events occur during development or maturity—will differentially influence the individual's response (Pynoos, 1993). An infant witness to the traumatic death of a parent will experience this trauma differently and have access to different coping strategies than will a mature, well-integrated individual who experiences a tornado destroying his or her house. The long-term impact of such events can also be presumed to differ. However, there are similarities in the immediate posttraumatic responses of most people. These acute stress reactions include anxiety, panic, freezing, agitation, confusion, intrusive memories of the event, a sense of numbing, and dissociation (Shalev, 1996; Solomon, Laor, & McFarlane, 1996). Many of these symptoms decrease with time, leaving only a proportion of those exposed to trauma with more chronic symptoms (such as PTSD) and other reactions (such as depression) (McFarlane & Yehuda, 1996).

Vulnerability to the development of a more long-standing reaction (PTSD) is related to a family history of psychiatric disorder; previous history of PTSD, anxiety, and/or depression; prolonged childhood separation from parents; the degree of distress at the time of the trauma, including dissociative reactions; and prolonged arousal following the event (McFarlane & Yehuda, 1996; Breslau & Davis, 1992). In particular, history of exposure to an earlier trauma, particularly multiple traumas or an assaultive experience, increases the likelihood of developing PTSD with a new trauma (Breslau, Chilcoat, Kessler, & Davis, 1999). This list of individual vulnerability factors suggests that those individuals with a preexisting likelihood of more intense arousal to stress or of difficulty in modulating arousal will have more difficulty in resolving the experience of a traumatic event. van der Kolk and McFarlane (1996) do suggest that "it is likely that effective treatment of one problem, such as physiological reactivity, will have widespread beneficial effects on the overall system, and can secondarily decrease intrusions, concentration problems, numbing, and the way victims experience themselves and their surroundings" (p. 17).

The heightened arousal that accompanies the traumatic experience typically diminishes over time. In some individuals, however, this arousal is prolonged and is accompanied (or, indeed, provoked) by persistent intrusive memories, which appear to produce a state of being retraumatized. These "relivings" of the trauma may be associated with specific reminders of the original event, but may also become so autonomous that the individual experiences a sense of being unable

to control the arousal and intrusive memories. Many individuals attempt to cope by avoiding situations that threaten to induce intrusive
memories and their accompanying arousal. Numbing of experience
appears to result when avoidance fails to control the arousal (Foa,
Riggs, & Gershuny, 1995). Those individuals whose symptoms persist
remain physiologically and psychologically overreactive (Breslau &
Davis, 1992; Morgan, Grillon, Southwick, Davis, & Charney, 1996), although some persons with PTSD appear to alternate between hypo-
and hyperresponsiveness. Although PTSD was originally conceptualized as a "normal" reaction to extreme stress, more recent findings
suggest that PTSD represents an interaction between vulnerability factors (both genetic and experiential) and a stress that is perceived as
overwhelming (Yehuda & McFarlane, 1995).

van der Kolk and McFarlane (1996) describe six key features affecting individuals with PTSD, which they believe are important in understanding the complexity and persistence of this disorder:

> (1) They experience persistent intrusions of memories related to the
> trauma, which interfere with attending to other incoming informa-
> tion; (2) they sometimes compulsively expose themselves to situations
> reminiscent of the trauma; (3) they actively attempt to avoid specific
> triggers of trauma-related emotions, and experience a generalized
> numbing of responsiveness; (4) they lose the ability to modulate their
> physiological responses to stress in general, which leads to a de-
> creased capacity to utilize bodily signals as guides for action; (5) they
> suffer from generalized problems with attention, distractibility, and
> stimulus discrimination; and (6) they have alterations in their psycho-
> logical defense mechanisms and in personal identity. This changes
> what new information is selected as relevant. (p. 9)

The intrusive memories and the avoidance of trauma-related triggers
have been discussed above. McFarlane, Yehuda, and Clark (cited in
van der Kolk & McFarlane, 1996) speculate that the avoidance of and
withdrawal from other (non-trauma-related) stimuli, which are understood as attempts to avoid feelings generally, eventually produce central nervous system changes similar to those resulting from prolonged
sensory deprivation. The compulsive reenactment of the trauma may
lead to harm to others, self-destructiveness, and revictimization. The
inability to modulate physiological arousal produces extreme responses to a variety of stimuli, including intense negative reactions to
even minor stimuli, as well as a generalization of threat (the world is
seen as generally unsafe). Their lessened ability to use body signals reliably leads to difficulty in interpreting feelings and a concomitant
over- or underreaction to many events. The general interference with

attention produces difficulty in sorting out relevant from irrelevant cues and ultimately a general loss of flexibility in cognitive processing. Finally, the change in how they view themselves and the world leads to a bias in perception and processing that can profoundly affect their interpretation of all subsequent experience (van der Kolk & McFarlane, 1996). As is evident from this discussion, the interaction of prolonged arousal with disturbance in information processing and a changed view of the self in the world interferes dramatically with efforts at recovery and makes sense as to why PTSD, once established, is very difficult to treat.

The biological substrates of PTSD that have been studied suggest that this reaction can be conceptualized as a conditioned response involving the amygdala, LC, thalamus, and hippocampus. The failure of this response to extinguish in the absence of further trauma has been seen as due to the persistence of the intrusive memories with their accompanying arousal, and may represent the failure of the sensory cortex to inhibit a kindling-type reaction in the amygdala. Further sensitization of the fear response maintains the elevated arousal and general vulnerability to a variety of stressors. This sensitization probably involves many neurotransmitter systems (Charney, Deutch, Krystal, Southwick, & Davis, 1993). In addition to the prolonged arousal, difficulties in concentration and attention are common. Interference with hippocampal function has been demonstrated with high levels of glucocorticoids (part of the physiological response to stress; see above) and with high-intensity stimulation from the amygdala (van der Kolk, 1994), and is thought to represent one pathway producing deficits in concentration, attention and memory. Recent neuroimaging studies (cited in van der Kolk, 1996) of subjects with PTSD have shown increased activation of right-hemisphere structures and decreased activation of Broca's area (language center) in the left hemisphere; these studies have led to the speculation that the memories of the traumatic event are stored in such a way that there is no integration of the feeling of the event with the interpretation of the event. This would account for the sense of uninterpretable terror when memories are activated.

Although the emphasis in this book is on demonstrating the presence of heightened arousal and difficulties with affect modulation across various conditions or situations relevant to the development of psychopathology, it is also clear that in many disorders, the way in which experience is interpreted is central both to modulation of arousal and to the later continuation of difficulties or development of symptoms. This is clearly the situation in PTSD (van der Kolk & McFarlane, 1996). Both the working models of self and others with which an individual confronts a traumatic experience, and the reworking of those models, will affect the individual's ability to achieve a perspective on his or her experience. As conceptualized by van der Kolk (1996), resolution of the acute stress reaction appears to be dependent on an individual's ability to develop a narrative of the traumatic experience that no longer has the capacity to threaten. This appears to allow the individual to gain control over the sense of powerlessness accompanying intrusive memories, and simultaneously to decrease his or her arousal. Similarly, the development of coping strategies will have an impact on how the individual deals with both the acute stress and the longer-term sequelae. Thus both the internal schemata of the individual and his or her coping strategies will affect how the person attempts to regulate arousal and manage the negative feelings (e.g., anxiety, anger, and depression) that are common accompaniments to PTSD.

ABUSE

The experience of abuse can be seen as a variant of the experience of trauma. What may be particularly important, however, is that when a developing child experiences abuse at the hands of the caretaker, its impact may be more extreme. Clearly, it must influence the development of the child's sense of self and the child's attachment security (Crittenden & Ainsworth, 1989). Maltreated children are more likely to have insecure (particularly disorganized) attachments than are nonmaltreated children (Cicchetti & Toth, 1995). Furthermore, abuse may interfere with the development of adaptive coping strategies and of other aspects of cognitive functioning, such as attention and impulse control; the earlier the abuse, the more extreme its effects (Erickson, Egeland, & Pianta, 1989). Maltreated toddlers display deficits in their use of feeling-state words (Beeghly & Cicchetti, 1994) and in communicative behavior (Cicchetti, 1989). Abused children also appear deficient in the development of social skills and empathy, and are more likely than nonabused children to overrespond to situations that elicit negative affect (Feshbach, 1989). They display more aggressiveness in interactions with peers (Mueller & Silverman, 1989), but in spite of this, they are also more likely to be victimized by their peers (Schwartz, Dodge, Pettit, & Bates, 1997). If the abuse of a child is prolonged, it can be presumed that the fear response will not extinguish and that the child will be highly sensitized to threat. The development of behavioral and emotional symptoms may further interfere with socialization, learning opportunities, and peer interaction (Cicchetti, 1989). Within this framework, the development of personality disorders—especially the more severe varieties, such as antisocial and borderline personality

disorder—can be related to experiences of abuse, especially in temperamentally vulnerable individuals (Shaw & Bell, 1993).

Recent imaging studies have shown deficits in hippocampal volume both in subjects with PTSD and in women exposed to abuse in
childhood. There is a tendency for these deficits to be more right-sided
than left-sided, but this literature is not definitive. Stein, Koverola,
Hanna, Torchia, and McClarty (1997) who found a left hippocampal
deficit to be correlated with severity of dissociative symptoms in
women abused in childhood, provide a brief review of these studies.
These authors raise the issue that these findings may be a result of the
trauma/abuse or may be a risk factor for the development of symptoms. Teicher et al. (1997) have found preliminary evidence for abnormal cortical development in abused children. Using retrospective EEG
reports on a sample of children seen at a psychiatric hospital, they
found an increased prevalence of left-sided (predominantly fronto-
temporal) EEG abnormalities. Using EEG coherence measures, they
then examined 15 child and adolescent psychiatric inpatients with a
history of intense physical or sexual abuse, as well as a sample of
healthy volunteers. They found greater left-hemisphere coherence,
which they interpret as reflecting diminished left-hemisphere differentiation, in the abused group than in the controls. Although these findings need replication, they do suggest that early abuse may create significant neurodevelopmental changes. To what extent these apparent
deficits can be reversed with treatment remains an important question.

The fact that experiences of abuse in childhood make one more
likely to be an abusive parent (Kaufman & Zigler, 1989) has led to theories of intergenerational transmission. Although these cannot be explored here in depth, there is evidence that mothers who have been
abused and have been unable to develop a self-reflective capacity are
more likely to be abusing parents themselves (Pianta, Egeland, &
Erickson, 1989). It is possible to speculate that, as with the experience
of the development of PTSD, the capacity to create a narrative of an
abusive experience that permits a non-self-blaming perspective may
allow the individual to moderate affect more successfully, and thus
may reduce the likelihood of his or her becoming a perpetrator of
abuse. As an illustration of this, Bugental, Mantyla, and Lewis (1989)
have shown that mothers who attribute more power to their children
than to themselves (which can be conceptualized as impaired self-
reflection) in a situation of conflict experience more intense negative
affect and arousal. If such an individual is less empathic and more
likely to overreact to negative affect, the possibility of an abusive response to a child's noncompliant behavior is increased. Other factors,
such as low self-esteem and lack of parenting skills, may add to a par-

ent's likelihood to act abusively with a noncompliant child. Although simplistic, this formulation does permit some understanding of how abuse may be transmitted across generations as part of a failure to develop adequate affect regulation skills.

CONCLUSIONS

Stress, trauma, and abuse can be conceptualized as being on a continuum, with some stress being normative and necessary for optimal growth and development. As the intensity of stress increases, and especially if it is perceived as overwhelming the individual's coping responses, the likelihood of symptoms' developing also increases. How these symptoms are manifested may depend on prior history of stress exposure, history of previous coping responses, temperament, and support. When stress is in the form of trauma or abuse, its impact is likely to be far more damaging, affecting the individual's self-esteem and internal working models. The neurobiology of the stress response is still being defined, but appears to involve sensitization of neural networks and probably down- or up-regulation of glucocorticoid receptors. From the perspective of psychopathology, enhanced stress reactivity (which may be heritable or related to early stresses) appears to predispose an individual to symptoms that may result from failure to turn off the stress response and concomitant dysregulation of catecholamines and other neurotransmitters. Affect regulation is impaired under situations of chronic arousal; this is especially important in the developing individual, where learning effective coping strategies may require some distance from the stress. Alternatively, tolerable levels of stress—levels that are not overwhelming or do not induce major reactions like dissociation or extreme avoidance—may permit a sense of mastery and adaptive coping to develop.

Chapter 6

Coping: Learning and Experience

As indicated in Chapter 2, emotional responses must be flexible, responsive to the situation, and adaptable to changing conditions so that the individual can function optimally (Thompson, 1994). Clearly, we presume that in psychopathology emotional responses are not optimally flexible, responsive to the situation, or adaptable. How these maladaptive coping responses emerge is an important question. In this chapter I describe how coping strategies (which I equate with learned emotional responses) are thought to develop normally and how they are affected by attachment, temperament, and learning, as well as by other variables (e.g., intellect and language functioning).

The process of learning to regulate affect can be conceptualized as involving (1) recognition and labeling of specific emotions and emotional cues in self and others, and (2) the development of strategies to control uncomfortable levels of arousal in oneself and to mediate interpersonal situations. According to Lazarus and Folkman (1984), these strategies can be simplistically divided into *emotion-focused* and *solution-focused* approaches. Strategies that focus on how to manage affect as opposed to dealing with the source of the stress (problem-solving or solution-focused strategies) are generally held to be less adaptive although they may be adaptive, in situations where the individual can do nothing about the situation. Optimally, the individual can select flexibly from a variety of strategies (both emotion-focused and solution-focused) the one most appropriate to a particular situation.

GENERAL PRINCIPLES IN THE DEVELOPMENT
OF COPING RESPONSES

In Chapter 2, I have described briefly Kopp's (1989) theory of affect regulation as a process that moves from parent to child control. Here I describe in more detail her ideas about how the child develops coping responses. Her first principle is that affect regulation initially involves an "action system or behavioral scheme" (p. 344), such as playing with an object or self-distraction, to reduce heightened levels of arousal. The next principle is that affect regulation involves two levels of adaptive cognitive responding. The first of these levels is described as pre-adapted, using elemental cognitive processes; the second level utilizes more advanced cognitive processes, such as planning and organization. Examples of the preadapted programs include crying, eye closing, and head aversion. According to Kopp, the child gradually learns associations between various behaviors and responses both from the caregiver and within him- or herself that produce relief from arousal. At the level of more advanced cognitive strategies, the child learns what has caused his or her distress and how to react or behave to modify or avoid that distress.

The third principle is that the developing individual is reliant on external support to learn to regulate arousal. Kopp regards the child's gradual development of strategies for affect regulation as arising initially out of reflexive behaviors, which are replaced by more elaborate methods as the child matures with respect to attention and cognition. The caregiver's responses shape the infant's behaviors; the caregiver attempts at times to soothe and at other times to socialize. From the cognitive-developmental perspective, Kopp emphasizes that "with language, children can state their feelings to others, obtain verbal feedback about the appropriateness of their emotions, and hear and think about ways to manage them" (p. 349). Obviously this presupposes an environment that has encouraged the child to learn about, to express, and to discuss feelings. However, the control of affect through verbal means gives the child improved capacity to tolerate frustration and delays in achieving desired goals. Furthermore, learning verbal strategies for affect regulation enables the child to relate both to parents and peers in a way that promotes further social learning and acceptance. The transactional nature of this process is illustrated vividly when aspects of this process in either the child or the environment can cause the whole course to go "off track," as we will see below.

The term *social referencing* refers to the process by which the infant "checks out" with the caregiver how the caregiver is responding to a particular situation (Campos et al., 1989). This process is presumed to be an initial regulator of the child's behavior, including emotional responses. One can presume that when this process is working optimally it allows the child to get quick feedback about behavior, or at least about how the parent is regarding that behavior. However, temperamental factors (e.g., inattention and high levels of sensitivity) may interfere with the optimal functioning of this feedback system.

Exposure is another factor thought to be important in the development of coping strategies (Campos et al., 1989). Simplistically, children who are seldom exposed to certain emotions may have difficulty in developing comfort with these feelings and will have diminished opportunities to learn to regulate themselves. Conversely, children exposed to chronically high levels of anger may experience such high levels of arousal that they cannot learn effective coping strategies (Cummings & Davies, 1994).

In the development of individual regulatory structures, Cicchetti and Tucker (1994) emphasize the self-organizing tendencies of all organisms as they strive to create coherence of self and experience. These may "best be understood by considering the child's continually evolving personality structures, which lead him or her to adopt a set of social and private strategies to maintain the integrity of the self" (p. 547). From this perspective, a child may choose coping strategies that maintain the integrity of the self but that nonetheless will be perceived by others as maladaptive (e.g., gender identity disorder). But let us begin at the beginning, with temperament and other constitutional factors.

THE INFLUENCE OF TEMPERAMENT
AND OTHER CONSTITUTIONAL FACTORS

Derryberry and Rothbart (1997) provide an elegant integration of how temperamental variables influence self-organization, which they conceptualize as a broad or overarching framework that influences the individual's efforts at self-regulation or coping. They define four motivational systems for which the neural bases are beginning to be understood: (1) appetitive and approach behavior, (2) fearful or defensive behavior, (3) frustrative and aggressive behavior, and (4) affiliative and nuturant behavior. These motivational systems (all of which have a heritable component) consist of neural networks in limbic structures that have evolved for appetitive, defensive, aggressive, and nurturant purposes.

The other component critical to the development of self-regulation is attention. Derryberry and Rothbart (1997), drawing on the work of Posner and Rothbart (1992), describe three attentional networks. The

first network, involving norepinephrine projections from the locus coeruleus to the cortex, is responsible for general alertness. The second, a
posterior system involving the superior colliculus, the pulvinar nucleus
of the thalamus, and the parietal lobe, regulates engaging and dis-
engaging of attention. The third system, located in the frontal regions
and anterior cingulate, has been conceptualized as providing "effortful
control"—a way of moderating more reactive (posterior) systems. Other
authors (Schore, 1996; Ryan, Kuhl, & Deci, 1997) have also argued that
the frontal cortex plays a critical role in affect regulation. Schore (1996)
has proposed that the attachment representations are primarily located
in the right frontal cortex and, as discussed below, regulate the individual's choice (predominantly at a subconscious or unconscious level) of
coping strategies. Ryan et al. (1997) conceptualize the right frontal cortex
as facilitating positive affect through the internalization of an autonomous self. They regard this right frontal cortex representational capacity
as developing in the context of supportive empathic parenting. Clearly,
some form of guidance from the frontal cortex (probably right-sided) as-
sists in the development of mature coping.

In discussing developmental processes within and among the four
motivational systems and the three attentional systems, Derryberry
and Rothbart (1997) propose

> that as the child develops, cortical synapses are progressively stabi-
> lized to form representations that provide input to subcortical motiva-
> tional systems. These cognitive representations provide motivational
> circuits with more detailed information that enhances their ability to
> evaluate complex situations and to regulate behavior accordingly. Al-
> though cortical representations depend in large part upon environ-
> mental inputs, their stabilization also depends upon activity within
> the underlying motivational systems. In a sense, the motivational cir-
> cuits can function as specialized learning mechanisms, guiding the de-
> velopment of cortical representations in light of underlying appetitive
> and defensive needs. This leads to progressive differentiation of rep-
> resentational and response processes, but in a manner that is integrat-
> ed or organized in terms of the central motivational functions. (p. 639)

Using this framework, the authors describe how fearful or defensive
traits predispose an individual to greater attention to negative cues
and greater negative affect. In contrast, the approach-oriented individual is slow to disengage from positive cues and displays more positive
affect. Because of their differing tendencies to focus on positive or negative aspects of their environments, individuals with these biases will
store information differently.

As discussed above, these motivational and attentional biases shape cognitive representations through enhanced cortical connectivity. These cortical representations then feed back to limbic motivational systems sharpening detection and guidance capabilities. Although this fine-tuning appears geared to adaptive coping, Derryberry and Rothbart (1997) point out that the heightened sensitivity to threat cues in the anxious individual may worsen anxiety, whereas a reward-oriented child who disengages slowly from positive cues may become more impulsive or demanding. These systems can and do influence each other, with defensive behaviors muting or diverting a child from approach or aggressive behavior. Presumably, these systems are reasonably balanced in the optimal situation; the individual can attend to both positive and negative cues and can approach or avoid, depending on which is more adaptive in a particular context. Achieving this balance may depend on adequate functioning of the frontal attentional system, which facilitates effortful control. According to Derryberry and Rothbart (1997, p. 643), "These executive attentional functions allow the child to rely on an increasing range of conscious representational context, to more flexibly coordinate this context, and to generate behaviors aimed at future states of affairs (Posner and Rothbart, 1992)." As an example, the inhibited child who learns coping strategies that permit exposure to feared situations is using the anterior "effortful control" system to counteract the more reactive attentional systems, which may be slow to disengage from worries or threat cues. Implementation and repetition of these coping strategies will help the child achieve exposure to the feared situation; this may permit the development of new cortical representations that assist in the control of anxiety.

Although we assume that temperament is largely an inherited predisposition to respond, there is increasing evidence that prenatal factors (e.g., stress) may also influence such traits as attention, emotional reactivity, and exploratory behavior (Clarke & Schneider, 1993; Clarke et al., 1996; see Chapter 3). Jacobvitz and Sroufe (1987) also provide evidence that attentional difficulties can arise from overly intrusive caregiving. Stiefel, Plunkett, and Meisels (1987) examined emotional arousal and regulation in preterm infants, separated into three risk groups by severity and chronicity of respiratory illness; they found that the high-risk infants showed a greater sensitivity to distress arousal at low levels of stress, and less ability to modulate distress once aroused, compared to those at low and moderate risk. Together, these studies indicate that deficits in attention, heightened emotional reactivity, and inhibition in exploratory behavior, whether present from birth or developing early in a child's life, will influence the individual's choice of responses in a particular situation.

Derryberry and Reed (1996) point out how temperamentally based perceptual biases may affect behavior. To an extroverted individual, who is typically reward-oriented, the world may look different than it does to an introverted individual, who is punishment-avoidant and who preferentially sees threat cues. Not only do such individuals interact differently with their world, but they perceive and process the events in their lives differently. These differences presumably will affect the choice of coping strategies, as the goals for such individuals also differ. Derryberry and Reed also emphasize the importance of the capacity to shift attention in order to self-regulate. Those persons who are unable to shift attention may experience more negative affect. Conversely, they point out that the other extreme—that is, too much shifting—may mean no opportunity for learning. What they regard as optimal is flexible attending, in which the individual can perceive the threat but also the source of relief. Too much arousal, or too frequent or intense periods of arousal, may interfere with perceiving relief or with developing solution-focused coping strategies.

Temperament-Biased Coping Strategies in Externalizing Disorders

Attention deficits interfere with an individual's opportunity to learn. This may involve learning about the emotional responses and cues of others (as in the process of social referencing, described above), as well as learning coping responses. Presumably, when attentional difficulties are combined with hyperactivity and impulsivity (as in attention-deficit/hyperactivity disorder or (ADHD), there is a greater likelihood that children will fail to learn strategies for regulating themselves in a more general way (Tannock & Schachar, 1996). Meichenbaum (1977) regards these children as having deficits in the development of coping strategies, especially when they lack adequate verbal strategies for self-regulation. Because hyperactivity, impulsivity, and attention deficits are often comorbid with language disorders, such children may be quite impaired with respect to developing verbal coping strategies (Cohen, 1996).

Oppositional and acting-out behaviors may become these children's main way of dealing with their anger, also resulting in a projection of blame on others as a way of maintaining their own self-esteem (part of Cicchetti & Tucker's [1994] self-coherence). This may eventually result in the cognitive distortions of threat attributions in situations of uncertainty, described for antisocial children and adolescents by Dodge (1993). Such attributions produce negativity and aggressive responses in many interpersonal situations. These children experience rejection by peers and fail to develop adaptive social skills for managing interpersonal situations (Dishion, Loeber, Stouthamer-Loeber, & Patterson, 1984). They are thus left with a combination of deficits and distorted response tendencies.

These coping strategy problems result in further peer rejection, difficulties in relationships with parents and siblings, underachievement at school and work, and increased vulnerability to associating with deviant peers (Dishion, French, & Patterson, 1995). Self-esteem deficits inevitably accompany such interactions, although many of these children evince an inappropriately high self-regard. Individuals involved in such patterns are also more likely to become involved in substance abuse (Dishion, French, & Patterson, 1995), perhaps as a way of alleviating the discomfort attached to their various dilemmas, and also as a form of risk taking. The pattern of coping through use of mood-modifying substances may replace other strategies despite the negative consequences.

Temperament-Biased Coping Strategies in Internalizing Disorders

As indicated in Chapter 3, the natural response tendency of inhibited individuals is to avoid situations of novelty or challenge (Stevenson-Hinde & Glover, 1996). Coping through avoidance reduces the opportunities to engage in such situations, which would normally lead to skills for managing discomfort in those situations. If inhibited children are allowed to avoid and fail to develop strategies to manage their discomfort, they may learn to rely on avoidance as their main strategy for coping. Obviously, this further reinforces restricted exposure and further interferes with coping skill development. Some inhibited children may also attempt to manage through controlling situations so that they do not have to worry about the unpredictable. This may result in excessive ordering behavior, needs to know about what is going to happen in advance, and refusal to try new things (e.g., new foods or new activities). These avoidant and controlling behaviors make inhibited children challenging for their parents, and the results are often conflicted parent–child interactions. As with children who have ADHD, temper tantrums and oppositional behavior may become general strategies for managing anger (Stevenson-Hinde & Glover, 1996).

If inhibited children continue their avoidance into the school-age period, this response tendency may become fairly fixed in their neural networks (Kagan, 1989). The ongoing avoidance, as a coping strategy, continues to reduce opportunities to learn social skills and to become assertive in social interactions. It may also result in procrastination with respect to homework and other chores that the children may perceive as difficult or challenging. Such coping skill deficits may be joined by cognitive distortions, such as beliefs that the individuals cannot cope, cannot do homework, and are disliked by peers. From a social information-processing perspective, Dodge (1993) hypothesizes that in the case of childhood depression, early adverse experience creates an internalized expectancy (schema); when this schema is activated by a stressful experience, it leads a child to attend to depressogenic cognitions that may induce a depressive reaction. Depressed children tend to attribute self-blame in a situation more readily than do nondepressed children, despite being angry about another's behavior. These cognitive distortions perpetuate low mood and withdrawal.

Inhibited children, particularly those who are insecurely attached (see below), often fail to develop ways of talking about their feelings (especially negative or angry feelings) and may even have trouble labeling their various affect states. From a social referencing perspective, their sensitivity appears to make them hypervigilant about parental negative affects; in contrast to children with ADHD, they may overreact to parental cues. At the extreme end of the spectrum of inhibition, these children become highly disadvantaged in social and interpersonal situations (Rubin, Stewart, & Coplan, 1995). They are rejected by peers, partly because of their lack of social skills and partly because of their withdrawal (which usually includes lack of eye contact, often interpreted as lack of interest by peers). For some this leads to depression and further withdrawal, often to engrossment in fantasy, and to very limited opportunities to correct their situation. For others (boys more than girls), peer rejection, family conflict, and the accompanying low self-esteem may lead to aggressive and oppositional behaviors (Rubin, Coplan, Fox, & Calkins, 1995). By adolescence, these youth may have resorted to fantasied solutions so long to manage their feelings of anger and sadness that their capacity to assess reality accurately may be impaired.

In both of the temperamental pathways described above, children are more likely to attempt emotion-focused coping strategies (e.g., distraction) than solution-focused strategies. This may occur because emotions become intense and require attention quickly in their own right. In less intense situations and with parental support, children may develop the capacity to reflect on a situation and to see it as a problem that can be addressed. The development of solution-focused coping strategies may require some distance from emotional arousal, as well as adult guidance through either modeling or the provision of direct teaching.

THE ROLE OF ATTACHMENT AND CAREGIVING

As indicated in Chapter 4, the attachment system has been conceptualized as a system for affect regulation. Simplistically, the categories of attachment can be seen as overarching reaction patterns for regulating feelings in the company of a particular caregiver. The securely attached child can express both positive and negative emotions, and perceives the caregiver as responding to his or her happiness and distress. The child in an avoidant attachment relationship avoids the expression of negative feelings, sensing that the caregiver will not attend to or be interested in his or her distress. The child in a resistant/ambivalent attachment relationship appears to intensify the expression of negative affect, having learned that this will elicit caregiver attention (Goldberg et al., 1994). The child with a disorganized attachment does not have a reliable expectation of what the caregiver will do and may attempt a variety of strategies to elicit attention. Each of these attachment patterns is accompanied by an internal working model that sets up expectancies of caregiver behavior and that presumably, with time and development, creates neural networks to guide the child's behavior.

The securely attached child has an awareness that he or she can count on the caregiver to alleviate distress. Presumably, this creates a freedom to learn about feelings, to label and experience feelings, and to learn coping responses (Greenberg et al., 1992). Although a securely attached child may develop maladaptive coping strategies, such a course may require an extreme temperament, dysfunctional parenting behavior, or abuse or other traumas. Greenberg et al. (1992) report on their own work studying attachment, affect regulation, and frustration tolerance in 5-year-old children. They found that more secure children were more emotionally open, and that coping behavior during a frustrating task was related to both security of attachment and to emotional openness.

In contrast to the securely attached child, the avoidantly attached child is conditioned to avoid negative affect, and this may interfere with his or her experiencing, labeling, and learning about such feelings. Learning coping responses to manage negative affects is more problematic when one cannot express, label, and discuss such feelings. One can presume that an avoidantly attached child will, as a consequence, be less likely to develop solution-focused strategies and more likely to use emotion-focused coping. In this attachment pattern, the child's awareness that the caregiver attends preferentially to positive affect may condition the child to exhibit pseudodisplays of positive affect to cover up negative affect. This defensive utilization of positive expression, at its extremes, may lead to manic/hypomanic reactions and a defensive belief that one can cope through dramatic avoidance strategies (e.g., gender identity disorder or eating disorders). Also in extreme cases, or if defensive positive expression is combined with temperamental inhibition, this pattern increases avoidance of situations that require assertion and problem solving, ultimately leading to more frustration and hostility because of the inability to manage interpersonal situations competently. As described above in connection with inhibition, coping skill deficits arise from prolonged avoidance. In contrast, cognitive distortions may develop as an individual engages in maladaptive repetitive patterns that reinforce a distorted view of the self in interaction with others. Crittenden (1995), however, has proposed that avoidant children are more likely to use cognition as a way of coping with emotional situations, in contrast to resistant children, whom she sees as using emotion as a preferred coping strategy in situations of stress. Neither of these types of coping responses is highly adaptive because of its inflexibility.

In the case of the resistantly attached child the caregiver attends to intense expressions of negative affect, but fails to provide equal validation of the child's positive affect (Goldberg et al., 1994). This skewed responsivity may predispose the child to exaggerated displays of negative affect, which may ultimately lead the parent to both frustration and a tendency to ignore real distress. The child may have more difficulty learning to use positive affect to buffer negative affect and to self-soothe, as attachment to the caregiver is maintained through negative affect. With time, these intense reactions may become the child's main way of managing anger. It is reasonable to assume that the predominant strategy will be emotion-focused as opposed to solution-focused, since the intensity of interaction in such dyads may interfere with opportunities to learn problem-solving strategies.

Disorganized attachment predisposes children to both internalizing and externalizing problems (Ogawa, Sroufe, Weinfield, Carlson, & Egeland, 1997; Shaw et al., 1996, 1997). As indicated above, these children do not have a stable pattern of affect regulation. The fact that disorganized attachment frequently occurs in situations of abuse (Cicchetti & Toth, 1995) suggests that trauma may play an equally large role in such a child's development of coping strategies, increasing the development of dissociative defenses (Ogawa et al., 1997) and non-language-based strategies (Cicchetti & Beeghly, 1987). The absence of a stable pattern of affect regulation presumably leaves such children vulnerable to periods of arousal for which there is no clear relief. This vulnerability, together with the unpredictability of the caregiver's response, will produce confusion, difficulty deploying attention, and problems with self-soothing. It is speculated that this lack of a stable pattern is more likely to produce extremes of affect, which make development of solution-focused coping responses more difficult.

Beyond formal attachment studies, there is evidence that the affective quality of the parent–child relationship does affect cognitive development (Estrada et al., 1987). These authors suggest that the affective quality of this relationship may influence the child's cognitive development through affecting the parent's tendency to support the child's problem-solving efforts; through affecting the child's social competence, and therefore the child's communication with adults; and, lastly, by affecting the child's tendency to explore and persist at tasks. Clearly, all these mechanisms can affect the child's development and choice of coping responses.

Marital/couple conflict is another caregiver behavior likely to affect child coping responses. Cummings and Davies (1994) review children's responses to situations of interadult anger. They define three basic patterns. The first is described as concerned and empathic, but such children are able to use their parents (usually their mothers) to reassure themselves. The second is angry/ambivalent. In this second pattern, children appear very upset but may also display inappropriate positive affect, such as laughter. These children are also more likely to behave aggressively toward playmates following exposure to background anger. The last group is described as unresponsive. As they avoid their mothers after the exposure to interadult anger, they are presumed to be suppressing or internalizing feelings. Cummings and Davies also discuss work showing that older children are more likely to become involved in mediating disputes; although one might regard this as solution-focused coping, it may put a heavy burden on these already stressed children. Girls tend to become involved in supporting and comforting their mothers, in contrast to boys, who tend to increase their aggressive behavior. Although we can only speculate about the mechanisms involved, it is clear that children who witness high levels of sustained interparental conflict become sensitized and tend to react to anger in subsequent situations with patterns that develop out of these initial experiences. Along with disorganized and avoidant attachment, early neglect and abuse, and stress reactivity, Ogawa et al. (1997) found that witnessing violence in infancy predisposed subjects to later dissociative behaviors.

THE ROLE OF LANGUAGE AND COGNITION

The link between language disorders and childhood psychiatric disorders is clear. (See Stevenson, 1996, for an overview.) Children with established speech and language disorders have a higher prevalence of emotional and behavior disorders than do those without the former disorders. Conversely, children with psychiatric disorders have a higher than expected prevalence of unsuspected speech and language disorders (Cohen, 1996). The strength of the association between language disorders and psychiatric disorders is greater in individuals with low IQ, which would seem to reinforce the notion that cognitive difficulties contribute more to emotional disorders than vice versa. The specifics of the association, however, suggest that mechanisms may differ with age and other variables. Preschool children with language disorders are more likely to develop internalizing disorders in middle childhood. Reading disability, often connected with language disability, is more strongly related to later conduct disorder, however (Stevenson, 1996). The mechanism for this association is unknown, but is a subject of current debate and research. With respect to coping strategies, it seems reasonable to presume that children with language disorders will have trouble developing language-based approaches to affect regulation. Furthermore, because solution-focused strategies are generally language-based, it will be hard for them to develop and use these more adaptive strategies. As well, many children with language disorders are vulnerable to attentional difficulties, and so they may have trouble learning both emotional cues and strategies for self-regulation.

Work with deaf children may throw some light on this complicated area. Greenberg et al. (1992) report on their study of deaf school-age children (a group at increased risk for psychopathology), which found high levels of behavior problems and social-cognitive deficits. The authors assessed emotional understanding, problem solving, and behavior problems in deaf children aged 6–9 and 9–12 before and after an intervention aimed at improving their emotional understanding and problem solving. At baseline (particularly in the older children), there was a correlation between better emotional understanding and social problem-solving skill, and between social competence and reduced behavior problems. In comparison to controls, children receiving the intervention improved in role taking, social problem solving, emotion recognition and labeling, and frustration tolerance. These gains were correlated, as expected. The gains in emotional understanding, role taking, and problem solving were related to improvements in externalizing behavior problems and emotional adjustment. The results of this study lend support to the authors' "ABCD" (affective–behavioral–cognitive–dynamic) model, which posits that a child's coping (as manifested in behavioral and emotional self-regulation) is dependent on emotional awareness, affective–cognitive control, and social-cognitive understanding.

Alexithymia, a term coined by Sifneos (1973) and studied systematically by Taylor, Bagby, and Parker, (1997), refers to a deficit in emotion language. Although not systematically examined with respect to an association with formal language disorder, the concept implies that such individuals are impaired with respect to their ability to label and discuss their feelings. Taylor et al. (1997) see this deficit as a developmental failure in affect regulation, and as the primary mechanism that makes these individuals vulnerable to psychosomatic and a variety of other psychiatric disorders.

Although I have focused here on the likelihood that language problems interfere with the development of coping strategies, it is also possible that emotional and behavior disorders interfere with language acquisition. This could arise through a number of possible mechanisms, such as kindling in the limbic system, or simply arousal that is sustained long enough to interfere with attentional processes. The possibility that a disorder of attention such as ADHD interferes with learning coping responses has already been mentioned. Furthermore, parenting a temperamentally challenging child is more likely to produce conflict that may interfere with the parent–child relationship, thus further reducing opportunities for constructive dialogue and learning. Trevarthen and Aitken (1994) discuss their view that the experience of sharing emotions and ideas with the caregiver is critically important for the infant's learning. They cite the withdrawal behavior of infants of depressed mothers as removing the infants from this opportunity for joint emotional interchange and for learning. Once more, such mechanisms are likely to interfere with the development of adaptive coping responses. Recognizing the complexity of all the factors involved, Greenberg et al. (1992) conceptualize coping ability as influenced by constitutional factors, the sensitivity and responsiveness of the caregiving environment, any traumas a child has experienced, and cognitive and linguistic stimulation. This transactional conceptualization acknowledges that these systems are highly interactive in complicated ways, particularly during the early years of rapid cognitive and social development.

THE ROLE OF PEER RELATIONSHIPS

As children mature, they rely increasingly on peers as a source of information and learning. Having close friendships can also buffer adversity within the family to some extent. Children who are acting out or who have failed to learn reciprocal and mutual peer relationship skills may miss out on valuable learning opportunities, as well as opportunities to enhance their self-esteem in close friendships. Very inhibited children may miss the opportunities to learn prosocial skills in the context of the mutual give and take of friendship. Children who become marginalized may become more vulnerable to association with deviant peers, especially if those peers encourage acting out of angry feelings. Clearly, this is an opportunity for children to learn both adaptive and maladaptive coping strategies. Because exploration of early psychosexual feelings takes place largely within a peer context, those adolescents who have not been able to develop a supportive peer network may lose out further in the opportunities to establish a sense of psychosocial and psychosexual competence. If these deficiencies are compounded by early difficulties with affect regulation and maladaptive coping skills, such individuals may become vulnerable to serious decompensation in adolescence, when expectations for "normative" behavior become more intense. The most vulnerable adolescents— those who develop severe mood disorders and psychoses—typically have a history of poor premorbid functioning, including withdrawal from peers.

SUMMARY

Adaptive coping responses are learned through a process that begins in infancy with empathic attunement of caregiver responsiveness, a reasonably intact neurobiology, and nonextreme temperament. The process continues with the development of adequate language skills; a parenting system that encourages understanding, labeling, and appropriate expression of affects; exposure to situations that permit the development of emotional and interpersonal solution-focused coping strategies; and, lastly, opportunities to engage with and learn from peers.

Chapter 7

The Neurobiology
of Affect Regulation

This chapter provides an overview of the basic information about neuroanatomy and neurophysiology needed to understand the development of affect regulation. It should be noted at the outset that much of the research in this area to date has been done on animals; the human studies are largely confined to cases of neurological damage. The animal research requires speculation as to equivalences between human and animal behavior and development. In the studies of human neurological insult, the damage is seldom circumscribed—so that conclusions must reflect uncertainty as to whether the functional deficit is a product of damage to the area affected, adjacent tissue, or underlying connections, as well as whether the damage removes function or releases control over another center (see Tucker & Williamson, 1984). Nevertheless, some statements can be made about many of the basic structures involved, their interconnections, and their function in the regulation of affect and the development of psychopathology. Particular emphasis is placed on the amygdala and its connections, as well as on the frontal lobes.

NEUROANATOMY

In this section of the chapter, I have drawn heavily upon Mesulam's text *Behavioral Neurology* (1985), which provides a relatively simple and comprehensible integration of neuroanatomical structure and function. Mesulam (1985) provides a schematic framework for understanding brain structure and function, particularly as they relate to behavior (see Figure 7.1). There are principally five types of cortices, ranging from the most highly specialized primary sensory and motor areas to the limbic structures. In between are association cortices (unimodal and heteromodal) and paralimbic structures. The most specialized layers relate to what Mesulam describes as "extrapersonal space," receiving sensory input from the environment and coordinating actions with the external world. Unimodal cortex connects the more specialized cortical areas to the heteromodal association and paralimbic areas, which provide further elaboration and integration with affective and other mental content. The limbic areas, which are the structures in closest association with the hypothalamus, regulate functions critical to survival of the individual and species: "memory and learning, the modulation of drive, the affective coloring of experience, and the higher control of hormonal balance and autonomic tone" (Mesulam, 1985, p. 9). The hypothalamus controls most aspects of the internal milieu (through its control over the autonomic nervous system) and in this role is highly dependent on its connections with the limbic areas (Smith & DeVito, 1984). Connections between cortical areas are most direct and intense between those areas immediately adjacent on the diagram; the structural findings thus support the functional framework.

Although different structures have been included in the definition of the limbic area, Mesulam defines the *limbic structures* as those cortical structures that have a major hypothalamic input. These are the septal area, the substantia innominata, the amygdala, the piriform cortex, and the hippocampal formation. Although the roles of the septal nuclei and substantia innominata are still relatively speculative, they contain the majority of cholinergic cells and provide the major source of cholinergic innervation for the rest of the cortex. They are strongly connected to the hypothalamus and hippocampus and to other limbic and paralimbic areas; these pathways appear critical for intact memory function. Studies in animals also suggest that these pathways establish connections between external objects and their motivational value for the individual. The piriform cortex, which is the main cortical relay for olfactory information, probably plays a modulating role in some aspects of feeding, sexual, and territorial behaviors, given its rich limbic, paralimbic, and hypothalamic connections. The amygdala, which is extensively connected to the hypothalamus and other limbic regions (e.g., the hippocampus), as well as to uni- and heteromodal cortices and the paralimbic areas, plays a vital role in associating affective tone or valence to experience. In this regard, it is involved in the recognition

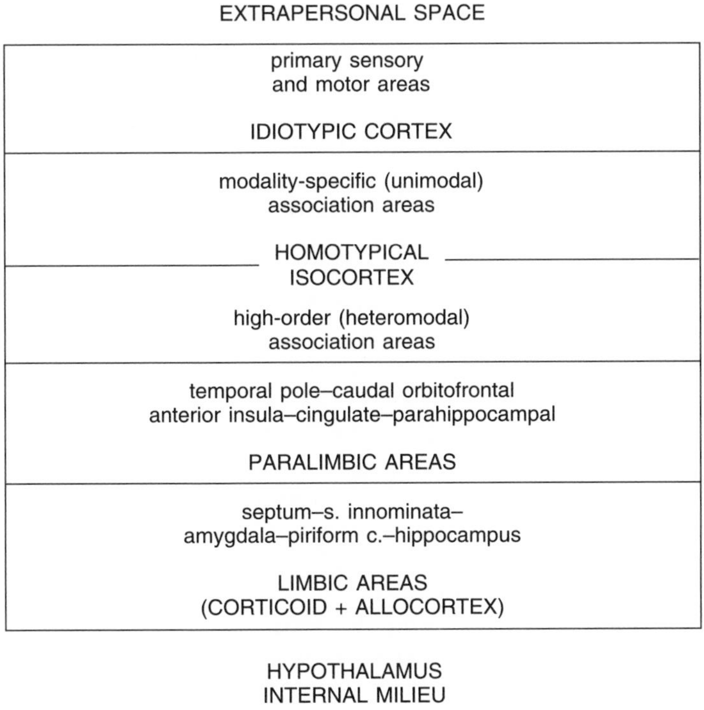

EXTRAPERSONAL SPACE

primary sensory and motor areas IDIOTYPIC CORTEX
modality-specific (unimodal) association areas ———————— HOMOTYPICAL ———————— ISOCORTEX high-order (heteromodal) association areas
temporal pole–caudal orbitofrontal anterior insula–cingulate–parahippocampal PARALIMBIC AREAS
septum–s. innominata– amygdala–piriform c.–hippocampus LIMBIC AREAS (CORTICOID + ALLOCORTEX)

HYPOTHALAMUS
INTERNAL MILIEU

FIGURE 7.1. Cortical zones of the human brain. From Mesulam (1985). Copyright 1985 by Oxford University Press. Reprinted by permission.

of emotional relevance of objects, as well as in displays of emotion. Specifically, and of particular interest to the development of psychopathology, it is involved in fear conditioning and the experience of strong emotional states such as rage (see below). Furthermore, it appears to play a role in connecting emotional states with autonomic, endocrine, and immunological responses. The hippocampal formation, which derives its cortical sensory input largely from paralimbic areas, is extensively connected with the hypothalamus as well as the amygdala and septal areas. Its chief role is in memory and learning, where it appears to regulate the imprinting and rekindling of information.

According to Mesulam (1985), the heteromodal and paralimbic areas provide "a synaptic buffer between external reality and internal urges," and in doing so provide "behavioral flexibility in a way that transforms the rigid stimulus–response bond of lower species into the more adaptive set-goal relationship of higher species" (p. 31). Whereas the heteromodal areas are more involved in perceptual and cognitive associations, the paralimbic areas are more concerned with affective and motivational processes.

Heteromodal association areas provide for integration of input across modalities (including sensory and motor channels), as well as between primary sensory and unimodal association areas and between paralimbic and limbic areas. This integration of input allows mood to influence cognition and vice versa. The temporoparietal heteromodal association areas appear to be important in a variety of perceptual–motor processes, including language and spatial functioning, as well as awareness of the body in space.

The prefrontal heteromodal association areas are particularly important because of their substantial connections with paralimbic structures, including the cingulate, caudal orbitofrontal, and insular regions. These neurons are very sensitive to the behavioral significance of information. These areas participate in the motivational aspects of movement initiation, in the modulation of response inhibition, in attention, and in planning. Mesulam (1985) comments that although it has been difficult to define some of the functions of the frontal lobes in humans from monkey lesioning, it is clear that "the resultant deficits are not confined to any one sensory modality and that many represent a dissolution of purpose, foresight, inhibition and motivation" (p. 30). The orbitomedial frontal cortex appears to be involved in regulating inhibitory and emotional behavior through its connections to the cingulate and anterior temporal lobes. In contrast, the dorsolateral frontal cortex, which has extensive connections with other association cortices, is more involved with sensory integration, planning, and goal-directed behavior (Malloy, Bihrle, Duffy, & Cimino, 1993).

An orbitomedial frontal syndrome has been proposed, characterized by anosmia, amnesia with confabulation, "go–no go" deficits, personality change, and hypersensitivity to pain (Malloy et al., 1993). Schore (1994) has recently proposed a theoretical model placing the orbitofrontal cortex, particularly in the right hemisphere, at the apex of a system of affect regulation. He argues that this cortex is uniquely placed—with dopaminergic and noradrenergic innervation, sensory input from all modalities, and control over sympathetic and parasympathetic output to the hypothalamus—to act as the main cortical regulator of affect. He places his model in a developmental–psychoanalytic framework, proposing that optimal growth of the orbitofrontal cortex occurs in the context of a relationship with the main caregiver in which positive feedback from the caregiver during the infant's first year encourages dopaminergic innervation, with accompanying increases in positive affect. He posits that following this early increase in positive affects, development of noradrenergic innervation results from the caregiver's constraint of the young toddler, which produces muting of affect (often accompanied by the appearance of shame). Schore speculates that the development of internal working models depends on these early interactions, and on the development of the orbitofrontal cortex and its connections with limbic and hypothalamic structures.

Impairment of dorsolateral prefrontal cortical function produces a lack of goal-directed behavior, apathy, and difficulty with working memory—symptoms typical of the negative syndrome in schizophrenia and of severe depression. Indeed, Goldman-Rakic and Selemon (1997) have proposed that a working memory deficit related to dorsolateral prefrontal dysfunction provides a conceptual framework for understanding the behavioral disorganization and negative syndrome in schizophrenia. Dolan et al. (1993), using regional cerebral blood flow in depressed and schizophrenic subjects, showed reductions in dorsolateral prefrontal function correlating with poverty of speech across both groups; these findings suggest that this dysfunction is more symptom-specific than disorder-specific.

The paralimbic areas include the temporal pole, the insula, and the caudal orbitofrontal cortex encircling the olfactory structures, and, encircling the hippocampal formation, the parahippocampal regions, the retrosplenial area, the cingulate gyrus, and the pre- and subcallosal regions. Their connections are primarily with heteromodal cortex on the one side and limbic areas on the other. Their functions include memory and learning, regulation of drive and affect, and higher control of autonomic response. Clearly these functions are carried out in their relationship with higher centers, as well as in connection with limbic structures.

The basal ganglia have two components, the striatum and globus pallidus. The striatum includes the caudate, the putamen, the olfactory tubercle, and the nucleus accumbens. The caudate and putamen, referred to as the *dorsal striatum,* receive dopaminergic input from the pars compacta of the substantia nigra, while the olfactory tubercle and nucleus accumbens receive input largely from limbic structures such as the amygdala and hippocampus, causing them to be labeled the *limbic striatum.* The limbic striatum has a higher turnover of dopamine and greater density of cholinergic cell bodies than does the dorsal striatum. In addition to their role in the automatic execution of behavior, the striatal structures may have specialized roles similar to those of the cortical areas, from which they receive their main input. The head of the caudate is closely connected to dorsolateral prefrontal cortex, and damage to it produces deficits similar to prefrontal cortex lesions. Studies on cats suggest that the nucleus accumbens is important in the channeling of drive and affect, reflecting its limbic connectivity. The globus pallidus receives the outflow from the striatum, sending it to thalamic nuclei, the habenula, and other structures. Although its main function is motor control, this involves substantial sensory–motor integration, including input from the amygdala (probably through the nucleus accumbens).

Because the basal ganglia are part of loop circuits involving prefrontal, thalamic, and amygdalar centers, Graybiel (1997) has proposed that "these dominant patterns of connectivity suggest that iterative patterns could be set up in basal ganglia loop circuits and their affiliated structures and that as a consequence, these basal ganglia circuits could be used for establishing and later expressing behavioral repertoires built up through experience" (p. 462). Although this type of role has been better understood for motor functions, Graybiel postulates analogous pattern generators for cognitive functions. These generators would serve to coordinate cognitive activity; defects in these circuits could account for disordered patterns of thinking. Furthermore, Graybiel suggests that as cognitive planning is central to the development of intention, the infant's sense of self may evolve from the experiencing of intent, action, and consequences, the underlying neural mechanism being the loop circuits involving the basal ganglia. Similarly, she proposes that the development of reality testing also emerges from neural activity in these circuits, as the individual experiences the feedback or consequences of intentions and actions.

The thalamus primarily relays subcortical information to the cortex. Although each part of the thalamus is connected to many cortical areas, most nuclei are preferentially connected to one area. In addition to its connections with primary sensory cortex and unimodal association areas, the thalamus has extensive connections to heteromodal cortex, paralimbic areas, and limbic structures, many of which are reciprocal. Mesulam (1985) speculates that the function of these connections relates to the imprinting of associations and to their reactivation under specific conditions. In response to findings of thalamic pathology in schizophrenia, Jones (1997) has articulated an elegant theory stressing the importance of connections (arising developmentally or as a result of experience)—in this case, primarily thalamic–cortical–subcortical—as sites of pathology and a means of explaining symptoms in schizophrenia. He argues that because of the many reciprocal connections between the thalamus and prefrontal areas, pathology in one area may directly influence connectional patterns and "result in activity-dependent changes in gene expression for molecules involved in the neurotransmission process, with functional consequences" (p. 483). As a result, he postulates that loss of inputs may interfere with the normal oscillation of cell collectives that increases signal-to-noise ratio in transmission. This would result in less effective transmission and possibly account for loss of focus or failure to differentiate relevant from irrelevant stimuli and responses in schizophrenia. According to this theory, early vulnerability factors that have an impact on brain connections can produce later functional disconnections that may relate more directly to psychopathology.

Although he designates a group of cortical structures as *limbic structures* (see above), Mesulam (1985) defines a further grouping called a *limbic system,* comprising (1) the hypothalamus; (2) the limbic structures; (3) the paralimbic cortical belt; (4) the limbic striatum and limbic pallidum, the ventral tegmental area of Tsai, and the habenula; and 5) the limbic and paralimbic thalamic nuclei. He does so based on their anatomical interconnections as well as their common behavioral affiliations—that is, a focus on homeostasis of the internal milieu, memorization, and the channeling of drive and affect, as opposed to sensory–motor processes. Furthermore, these structures share a vulnerability to the herpes simplex virus, suggesting a common membrane antigen. They are also susceptible to the development of independent seizure foci and kindling, and, have a particularly high density of cholinergic innervation and opiate receptors.

Many brain pathways function as channels, such that there is a specificity of function dedicated to a particular column or pathway. When damage occurs along such a path, the deficit is specific to that function (e.g., language or vision). In contrast, there are more diffusely projecting pathways that appear to have a modulating role, affecting the state of the entire cortex. These projections are seen as being capable of affecting the efficiency of cortical processing without affecting the content. Although theorizing in this area is still somewhat speculative, it is presumed that such projections affect arousal, mood, and motivation. Mesulam (1985) refers to these as "state-dependent functions," in contrast to the earlier "channel functions." There are four main pathways contributing to this control of state: cholinergic neurons in the septal area and substantia innominata and in the reticular formation; noradrenergic neurons in the locus coeruleus (LC); serotonergic neurons in the brainstem raphe nucleus; and dopaminergic neurons in substantia nigra and in the ventral tegmental area of Tsai. The specific roles that these neurotransmitters play are addressed below.

In addition to the whole-brain functions noted above, there appears to be a degree of hemispheric specialization. The left hemisphere has primary responsibility for language in right-handed individuals, while the right hemisphere appears more involved in processing nonverbal material. These aspects of right-hemisphere function include face identification, spatial distribution of attention, and the emotional aspects of communication. With respect to the organization of emotions, it has been suggested that the right hemisphere is more specialized than the left, and that the right anterior hemisphere plays a role in the display of emotions while the posterior areas are involved in decoding emotions.

NEUROTRANSMITTERS

Neurotransmitters—the chemical messengers that convey information across neural synapses—have been extensively studied in recent years. They are broadly grouped into the monoamines, the amino acids, and the neuropeptides (and latterly the gases nitric oxide and carbon monoxide, although these are not discussed here). The monoamines have been the most thoroughly studied, partly because of the availability of substances that mimic and block their action, and partly because of their theoretical relevance to various disorders. They include dopamine, norepinephrine (NE), serotonin (5-HT), and acetylcholine. These monoamine neurotransmitters all arise from cell tracts in the reticular core, have extensive subcortical and cortical connections, and arise early in development. Their functions are seen as "modulatory" of neural activity in the cortex, corpus striatum, and limbic system. All appear to play some role in affect regulation, although the specifics of their roles are still somewhat speculative. For much information about these neurotransmitters, as well as the less well-studied transmitters, I have relied on several recent reviews (Harris, 1995; Panksepp, 1993; Ciaranello et al., 1995).

Monoamines

Dopamine

Dopaminergic neurons arise from the substantia nigra and the ventral tegmental area of Tsai, and innervate the corpus striatum (caudate and putamen), forming the nigrostriatal tract; the frontal cortex, forming the mesocortical system; and the limbic system, forming the meso-limbic system. There are several types of dopamine receptors: pre- and postsynaptic, using a variety of second messenger systems (chemical pathways within the cell). There is evidence that the number of dopamine receptors (D1 and D2) declines with age (Seeman et al., 1987).

The dopamine system appears to play a role in facilitating approach behaviors (including those motivated by rewards) and in mediating anticipatory eagerness and positive emotionality (Panksepp, 1993). Recent genetic studies have linked the D4 dopamine receptor gene and the temperamental trait of novelty seeking (Cloninger, Adolfsson, & Svrakic, 1996). Excessive dopaminergic activity has been implicated in hyperactivity, aggression, and psychotic behaviors (both drug-induced behaviors and those associated with schizophrenia), while reduced dopaminergic activity has been associated with lack of motivation and withdrawal. It is presumed that these actions occur through the mesolimbic and mesocortical systems. Reduction of dopaminergic function in the nigrostriatal tract occurs in Parkinson's disorder. Extrapyramidal side effects of antipsychotic medications appear to occur through their effect on the nigrostriatal dopamine system, whereas the positive antipsychotic effects probably occur through the mesocortical and mesolimbic systems. Tourette's syndrome appears to involve an increased sensitivity to dopaminergic neurotransmission (Johnston & Singer, 1982).

More recently, Haber and Fudge (1997) have postulated that excess stimulation in the amygdala could result in enhanced dopamine-mediated firing in midbrain areas. They base this speculation on the extensive connections between the amygdalar system on the one hand and the substantia nigra and ventral tegmental area on the other. Although complicated theoretically by the issue of whether the amygdalonigral connection is largely inhibitory or not and whether tonic or phasic responses are more likely, this model has been used to provide an explanation for altered dopamine function in schizophrenia. Given the wide influence the dopamine system has on the striatum and cortex, these authors suggest that substantia nigra cells "are in a position therefore to use information about reward and motivation to influence the execution of a wide variety of behaviors, including initiation of movement and cognition" (p. 478).

Norepinephrine

Arising from the LC in the floor of the fourth ventricle, noradrenergic neurons innervate essentially the entire cortex and limbic system. Because of their extensive connectivity throughout the early-developing cortex, noradrenergic neurons are assumed to play a role in cortical development (Harris, 1995). With the development of other brain cells, their relative predominance wanes. However, because of their extensive arborization throughout the cortex, they appear to play a major role in enhancing signal-to-noise detection, especially in sensory cortex.

In addition, the LC appears to modulate the level of arousal

through its connections to forebrain areas and to enhance synaptic efficacy in the hippocampus (Berridge, Arnsten, & Foote, 1993). This latter
action appears to occur through the cellular memory mechanism of
long-term potentiation (LTP). As described by Berridge et al. (1993), LTP
"refers to a use-dependent, long-lasting increase in synaptic strength
or efficacy: when excitatory synapses are rapidly and repetitively stimulated for brief periods (tetanic stimulation), the post-synaptic neurons
generate action potentials more readily upon subsequent stimulation"
(p. 559). These authors provide evidence that the LC enhances cognitive function "under 'noisy' conditions where irrelevant stimuli impair
performance" (p. 560). Some of this function occurs in the dorsolateral
prefrontal cortex, mediated by alpha-2-noradrenergic receptors (Berridge et al., 1993). The LC receives input from the periphery via
medullary relays and, given its extensive limbic connectivity, integrates perceptual and emotional information with autonomic responses. Clark et al. (1987a, 1987b) have proposed a model for the
regulation of attention, contrasting the noradrenergic innervation of
sensory cortex with the dopaminergic innervation of motor cortex.
They suggest that the noradrenergic system acts as an input regulator,
whereas the dopaminergic system is an output regulator.

Overactivity of the LC has been implicated in panic attacks (Gorman et al., 1989), hyperactivity (Zametkin & Rapoport, 1987, although
see below), anxiety, and inhibition (Kagan et al., 1987). Underactivity
of the LC has been presumed to play a role in depression, although it is
not clear whether this presumed deficit is the result of earlier overactivity (see Chapter 9). Given its presumed role in cognitive functioning, deficits in this system have been posited in aging, Korsakoff's
amnesia, schizophrenia, and attention-deficit/hyperactivity disorder
(ADHD). This is based on the improved performance on tests of
prefrontal cortical function in these disorders when subjects are given
an alpha-2-adrenergic agonist such as clonidine (Berridge et al., 1993).
Adverse early experiences in primates appear to have long-term sensitizing effects on this system (Rosenblum et al., 1994; see Chapter 5 for a
fuller discussion).

Serotonin

Serotonergic neurons are located in the midbrain raphe nucleus and
innervate most of the cortex, striatum, and limbic system. They also
appear to play a modulatory role, initially in the growth of cells in the
embryonic cortex, and later (in interaction with the other monoamines)
in the general excitability of the cortex. Low levels of 5-HT have been
implicated in aggressive and suicidal behavior, while altered function

has been suggested in depression, schizophrenia, and autism (Harris, 1995) and the paraphilias (Kafka, 1997). Adverse early experiences in primates have an enduring blunting effect on serotonergic function, in contrast to their sensitizing effects on the noradrenergic system (Rosenblum et al., 1994).

Spoont (1992), in a review of serotonergic function in neural information processing, describes the role of 5-HT as one of "signal stabilization." Given its interaction with the two other modulatory monoamines (dopamine and NE), she speculates that 5-HT plays a constraining role, reducing locomotor and exploratory behavior (dopamine-mediated), the intensity of the startle response, aggressive and impulse behaviors, and feeding and sexual behaviors. She suggests that this modulation of arousal occurs through altering signal-to-noise ratios in target regions. She also conceptualizes 5-HT's role in constraining information flow as including (1) preventing overshooting of other elements within the system, and (2) controlling the sensitivity of the system to perturbation by other stimuli. Increased affective instability or stress reactivity is seen as the result of lowered 5-HT activity in limbic circuits. Relating this to psychopathology, Spoont points to the correlation between elevated Psychoticism and Neuroticism scores on the Eysenck Personality Questionnaire and reduced 5-hydroxyindoleacetic acid (5-HIAA, a metabolite of 5-HT) in cerebrospinal fluid (CSF) as suggesting vulnerability to negative affective states and anxiety. The release of 5-HT's modulatory control over the dopamine system would yield greater impulsiveness, which, when combined with negative affective states and anxiety, might explain the correlation between both violence and suicidality and lowered CSF 5-HIAA.

Acetylcholine

Cholinergic neurons arise in the basal forebrain complex and diffusely innervate the cortex, hippocampus, and limbic system. They arise somewhat later in development than the other monoamines and appear to play a role in higher cognitive functions, especially memory. Deficits in acetylcholine have been associated with Down's syndrome and Alzheimer's disease.

Amino Acids

As indicated above, I have relied heavily on recent reviews of neurochemistry, and I have drawn much information about the amino acids from Ciaranello et al. (1995). The amino acids glutamate, aspartate, glycine, and gamma-aminobutyric acid (GABA) are distributed throughout the nervous system. Although important in intracellular metabolic processes, they also act as neurotransmitters. Glutamate and aspartate are generally defined as excitatory transmitters, in contrast to glycine and GABA, which are inhibitory.

Although glutamate acts as a typical excitatory neurotransmitter by opening ion channels, it also acts as a neuromodulator through the N-methyl-D-aspartate (NMDA) receptor. The NMDA receptor exerts an effect only when activated in conjunction with another depolarizing stimulus. Although involved in many areas of the central nervous system, glutamate and aspartate play important excitatory roles in the cerebellum; in the neocortex and its projections to the striatum and thalamus; and within the hippocampus, where it is thought to be involved in associative learning and memory. Currently, one of the most important issues with respect to glutamate is the production of tissue damage and cell death when it is released locally in high concentrations. This can occur as a result of anoxia, hypoglycemia, or high steroid concentrations. A neurotoxic effect of glutamate has been implicated in Huntington's disease and in Parkinson's disease. Because it also exerts a neuromodulatory role with respect to dopamine, reduced glutamergic function has been suggested in schizophrenia (Carlsson & Carlsson, 1990).

While glycine appears mainly active in the spinal cord, GABA is distributed throughout the central nervous system. Within the brain, GABA appears to play an inhibitory role in the cerebellum; in several feedback loops involving the cortex, striatum, thalamus, and substantia nigra, which serve to modulate thalamocortical activity; in cardiovascular pathways in the medulla; and in the brainstem. Clinically, the inhibitory action of GABA appears to underlie the anxiolytic function of many drugs (e.g., the benzodiazepines, which act at the GABA receptors). Dysfunction of the GABA system has also been implicated in Huntington's disease, Parkinson's disease, and the so-called "stiff-man syndrome." The fact that GABAergic striatal neurons are particularly sensitive to glutamate-induced neurotoxicity, which may develop with anoxia or high levels of steroids, suggests that deficits in the GABAergic system may be relevant to the development of psychopathology in cases where etiological factors such as obstetric complications or high levels of stress have been found.

Neuropeptides

Oxytocin and vasopressin, which are synthesized in the hypothalamus and released by the posterior pituitary, have long been understood to be endocrine hormones acting on peripheral organs. More recently, their role as neurotransmitters acting centrally has been better understood. A recent review by Insel (1997) highlights a likely role in mediating social behaviors, such as pair bonding and attachment. Oxytocin appears to mediate affiliative behaviors in females, while vasopressin plays a similar role in males. Although much of the literature on these neuropeptides has been developed from studies in animals, deficits in these neurotransmitters may play a role in such disorders as autism and other instances of so-called "failed attachment." A variety of other peptides, such as the enkephalins and beta-endorphins, are principally involved in pain regulation, where they play a modulatory role.

THE AMYGDALAR SYSTEM
AS AN "EMOTIONAL NETWORK"

The Amygdala and Its Connections

LeDoux (1993) suggests that the amygdala is the central processor of emotional information in the brain, and thus he refers to the amygdalar system as an "emotional network." Because of its extensive input from both subcortical areas and uni- and heteromodal sensory association cortices, as well as closed-loop connections with the hippocampus, LeDoux sees the amygdala as able to respond to a variety of sensory stimuli important in triggering emotional arousal. Because of its extensive connections to frontal cortex and central grey matter and to the hypothalamus, the amygdala, once activated, can then coordinate a variety of responses to emotionally meaningful stimuli. Figure 7.2, from LeDoux (1993), is a schematic illustration of the amygdalar system.

LeDoux (1993) describes two modulatory systems that interact with the amygdalar system. The central modulatory system comprises the structures in the ascending brainstem reticular formation—the four state control pathways described by Mesulam (1985; see above) and specified according to their neurotransmitters. LeDoux suggests that the reticular tracts, which modulate attention to emotionally relevant stimuli, do so after input from the forebrain systems involved in evaluating the emotional significance of stimuli. Activation of the brainstem neurons should then increase the excitability of the forebrain system (including sensory areas, the amygdala, and the other limbic structures). In this way the central modulatory tracts may regulate the intensity and duration of emotional reactions, while the quality of the reaction is determined by the forebrain evaluative system, encompassing the amygdala and other structures. Peripheral modulatory systems include feedback from the autonomic nervous system, the endocrine system, and the sensory system. Of particular importance may be emo-

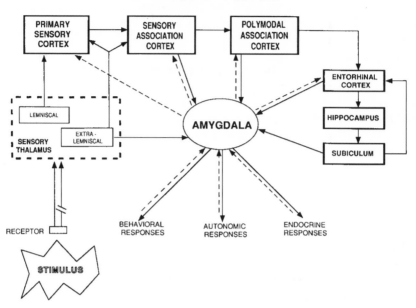

FIGURE 7.2. Proposed model of the role played by the amygdala and its input and output connections in emotional processes. From LeDoux (1993). Copyright 1993 by The Guilford Press. Reprinted by permission.

tional control over release of adrenocorticotropic hormone (ACTH) from the lateral hypothalamus, an important aspect of the stress response (see Chapter 5). Both the amygdala and hippocampus have steroid receptors, which, through their hypothalamic connections, may allow for integration of emotional and cognitive feedback regulation of stress-related release of ACTH. The interconnectivity of the amygdala with prefrontal structures, sensory association cortex, the hippocampus, and the hypothalamus, as well as both central and peripheral modulatory structures, provides an overall system that LeDoux (1993) sees as "wired in such a way as to sustain its own activity" (p. 115). This may be particularly important in understanding the development and maintenance of a variety of emotional states.

LeDoux (1992) describes the connections between the thalamus and the amygdala and between the cortex and the amygdala as responsible for the indelibility of emotional memory. These connections are probably mediated by synaptic plasticity in the amygdala, which in turn is mediated by excitatory amino acids (glutamate and NMDA). It also appears that more intense situations create more intense memories, mediated by noradrenergic influences on the amygdala at the time the memory trace is being stored (McGaugh, 1992). This effect, however, has an inverted-U shape, as both low and high levels of NE interfere with storage. The hippocampus is also responsible for memory, but, in contrast to storage of emotional memories by the amygdala, the hippocampus records spatial and temporal dimensions of stimuli and participates in the categorization of information (a process that is vulnerable to stress).

The role of the amygdala in conditioning is demonstrated well in a report on patients with bilateral brain damage localized to the amygdala, the hippocampus, or both (Bechara et al., 1995). In this study, the patient with damage only to the amygdala showed no conditioned autonomic response to visual or auditory stimuli, but retained knowledge of the facts associated with the stimuli (e.g., color). In contrast, the patient with hippocampal damage acquired conditioned autonomic responses, but showed deficits in memory of the stimuli. The patient with damage to both structures did not condition to the stimuli, nor did he remember the characteristics of the stimuli.

Fear Conditioning and the Amygdala

Ever since "lack of fear" in Kluver–Bucy syndrome was localized to the amygdala (Weiskrantz, 1956), its role in the conditioning of fear and in anxiety states has been presumed. The basomedial nucleus (BM) of the amygdala responds to species-relevant stimuli, such as rats in cats and facial expressions in primates. (See Adamec & Stark-Adamec, 1989, for a discussion of structure and function.) Furthermore, because of its connections with the hippocampus, it is presumed to have the capacity to respond to stimuli that evoke emotional memories (Gloor, 1986).

The most relevant early experimental work in this area has been undertaken by Adamec and Stark-Adamec (1989) in studies of what they call "defensiveness" in cats. They have shown that defensiveness in cats, like a personality trait, is relatively stable, but that the display of defensiveness depends on the situation. Defensive cats do not display defensive behavior in familiar situations or with familiar individuals, but do so in response to a stimulus that is perceived as threatening. They presume that defensive and nondefensive cats are not qualitatively different, but do differ in the extent to which stimuli activate the neural bases for attack and defense or withdrawal. They believe that these neural bases comprise two separate but antagonistic mechanisms in the cat brain—one facilitating approach or attack, and the other facilitating withdrawal. As a way of teasing out the differences between defensive and aggressive substrates, these authors have looked at the development of defensive and aggressive behaviors under a variety of rearing situations, including early exposure to live and dead prey. Starting with animals that from an early age appeared to be naturally defensive, they examined factors that might modify this basic predisposition, assuming that early attack–approach facilitation might reduce defensiveness. Defensiveness was not reduced by early exposure to threatening stimuli such as live prey, but was overridden by "safe" or killed prey later in their development. However, complete lack of exposure to threatening prey produced lifelong defensiveness.

One component of the physiological basis for defensive behaviors resides in a circuit involving the ventromedial hypothalamus (VMH) (and its projections) with a center in the BM that tonically facilitates defensive behavior and inhibits attack. The antagonistic attack circuit involves the lateral hypothalamus with tonic facilitation from the ventral hippocampus (VHP) and lateral amygdala. In a study using evoked potentials, Adamec and Stark-Adamec (1989) found that the more defensive cats exhibited larger evoked potentials in the VMH with pulsed stimulation from the BM. As there were no differences between defensive and nondefensive cats with respect to cellular response in these nuclei, or in threshold to evoke a response, they conclude that the greater response in the VMH in defensive cats is due to greater strength of synaptic transmission from the BM to the VMH. They suggest that in defensive cats, firing of the BM cells in response to normally threatening stimuli renders the VMH cells more excitable, effectively lowering the threshold to subsequent stimuli and thus resulting in an enhanced behavioral reaction. Firing of the BM in aggressive cats actually enhances potentials in the attack circuit through the VHP, whereas in defensive cats there is no increase in potentials in the attack circuit. Thus the same stimulus can provoke different behavioral reactions, with attack being facilitated in aggressive cats and defense in defensive cats.

Kindling of these structures can produce increases in defensiveness and aggressiveness. Seizures that enhance transmission from the BM to the VMH (the substrate for defense) enhance defensiveness, while those which elicit discharges in the VHP (the modulator of attack) enhance aggression. Adamec and Stark-Adamec (1989) conclude that the behavioral differences between defensive and aggressive dispositions are mediated by these differences in excitability in limbic and hypothalamic circuits. They also provide evidence for two neurochemical paths involved in the development of a defensive disposition—one relying on benzodiazepine receptors, and the other relying on NMDA receptors. Finally, they point out the parallels between the defensive disposition in cats and Kagan's concept of inhibition in humans.

THE FRONTAL LOBES AS GUIDES TO BEHAVIOR

Although the amygdala is probably a central processor of emotional stimuli, the frontal lobes appear to guide behavior through their capacity to make complex discriminations and interpretations of situations. There is evidence that infants display greater right frontal activation when approached by a stranger, whereas approach by their mothers elicits greater left frontal activation (Fox & Davidson, 1987). Furthermore, expressions of joy elicit greater left than right activation, in contrast to expressions of sadness or distress, which are connected with greater right than left frontal activation. The relative asymmetry (right > left) between resting right and left frontal activation predicts the likelihood that an infant will cry at maternal separation. Davidson and Fox (1989) interpret these differences as representing a general affective predisposition. This notion is supported as well by the findings that infants (1 and 3 months old) and toddlers of depressed mothers display greater relative right frontal EEG asymmetry (due to reduced left frontal activation) than do infants of nondepressed control mothers (Dawson, Klinger, Panagiotides, Spieker, & Frey, 1992; Field, 1995; Jones, Field, Fox, Lindy, & Davalos, 1997). This is comparable to findings in adults, and as the relative right frontal EEG asymmetry persists during remission, Henriques and Davidson (1990) have suggested that it may constitute a trait marker. Dawson (1994) has shown that although the type of affective response is related to left versus right activation, the intensity of emotional reaction is related to activation of both hemispheres. She has also shown that infants with disorganized attachment relationships exhibit greater frontal activation, both left and right, which suggests greater intensity of reaction or poorer modulation.

Dawson (1994) and others have speculated that the left and right frontal regions are specialized for different types of affect regulation: The left frontal region employs language-based strategies in sequentially organized schemes, while the right reacts to novel situations that interrupt ongoing activity. With development over the first year, the infant learns to attend to relevant stimuli, to inhibit responses, to associate stimuli with internal states, and to plan to meet his or her needs. These developing capacities appear to be recruited in the service of affect regulation, as do gaze and gaze aversion. The development of these functions coincides with increased glucose metabolism (Chugani, 1994) and synaptic connections in frontal cortex (Huttenlocher, 1994).

Given the evidence that affect regulation is affected by experience, interest has begun to focus on how factors such as parenting might influence brain development. The concept of an internal working model implies neural structures that mediate this response expectancy. Edelman (1987) has postulated the development of "cortical maps" (involving the limbic system) that develop from a pattern of stimulation of groups of neurons. Given repetition of experience, these maps become relatively stable neural configurations that may be elicited preferentially in similar situations. Dawson (1994), in exploring the evidence for such neural patterns, examined behavioral responses and frontal activation in infants of depressed mothers. Infants of depressed mothers, during playful interaction, displayed less left frontal brain activation than infants of control mothers; in contrast, during maternal separation, they displayed less distress but greater left frontal activation than infants in the control group. The different frontal activation patterns between children of depressed and control mothers suggests the formation of different neural networks that mediate affect regulation. To what extent these networks are determined by experience as opposed to genetics or other constitutional factors remains a question for future research.

DEVELOPMENTAL ISSUES

The mature brain develops through a process of multiplication of nerve cells in the primitive neural plate, migration of these nerve cells to their eventual anatomical locations, development of synaptic connections, and cell loss or pruning of synaptic connections. Generally, the later-born cells migrate to the more superficial layers of the cortex. Once cells assume their final position, a vigorous growth of connections begins to occur. This process is affected by extracellular chemicals and by the neurotransmitters, such as 5-HT, NE, and dopamine. Loss or pruning of synapses appears to depend on experiences occurring within a so-called "sensitive period" and produces increased facilitation of the remaining synapses. Greenough, Black, and Wallace (1987) have distinguished between *experience-expectant* growth, which is produced through pruning of excessive connections as the maturing organism interacts with species-predictable events, and *experience-dependent* growth, which results from experiences unique to the organism. This process of synaptic elimination continues into adolescence in humans.

There is evidence that activity in postsynaptic neurons is necessary for continued survival of presynaptic neurons. (For a more complete review, see Todd, Swarzenski, Rossi, & Visconti, 1995; for a discussion of models of neural function, see Changeux & Dehaene, 1989.) Studies of brain changes related to experience have focused largely on exposing animals to enriched or depriving situations. These studies have clearly demonstrated changes in brain areas deprived of their normal inputs and of increased cortical growth in animals exposed to enriched environments (Black, Jones, Nelson, & Greenough, 1998). Although similar studies have not been performed on humans, there is no reason to assume that the changes that have been observed in animals do not also occur in humans.

PSYCHOBIOLOGICAL THEORIES
OF PERSONALITY AND TEMPERAMENT

Efforts have been made to relate facets of personality or temperament to brain mechanisms. (For a recent overview, see McBurnett, 1992.) Most of this work has grown out of Eysenck's (1967) theories of extroversion–introversion and neuroticism. According to these theories, an individual high in neuroticism has a highly reactive limbic system, which maintains a tonically high level of arousal in the autonomic system long after a stimulus has passed. An extroverted individual is seen as being low in cortical arousal.

Sensation seeking is a trait that has been related to a variety of behaviors, such as drug use, gambling, and conduct disorder symptoms. Zuckerman (1994) has proposed that this trait is related to low levels of platelet monoamine oxidase activity, resulting in high levels of catecholamines (specifically dopamine and NE) centrally. These increased levels of neurotransmitters are thought to increase brain excitability and activation of behavior. Although there is some evidence for reductions in platelet monoamine oxidase in sensation-seeking individuals, the proposed increase in NE and dopamine goes counter to the theory of underarousal in such individuals.

Gray (1987) has provided a more complicated theoretical model to explain dimensions of personality. Simplistically, he proposes three systems: a *behavioral activation system* (BAS), responding to reward, related to the trait of impulsivity, and mediated by dopamine pathways; a *behavioral inhibition system* (BIS), responding to punishment and novel stimuli, related to anxiety, and mediated by 5-HT pathways; and a *fight–flight system*, the personality aspects of which are less well articulated, mediated by NE. He suggests that the BIS has a particularly important role in regulating the function of the other systems. Quay, Newman, and colleagues (see McBurnett, 1992) have expanded the notion of an overactive BAS and underactive BIS to study of children with ADHD and conduct disorder. Newman and Wallace (1993) see disinhibited individuals as continuing approach behavior despite punishment, but argue that they display an intrinsic deficit in the automatic integration of the BAS and BIS processes (e.g., switching modes in light of salient cues), which contributes to their self-regulatory problems.

As noted briefly in Chapter 3, Cloninger (1987) has provided a more linear conceptual framework, with dimensions of novelty seeking (based on the dopaminergic system), harm avoidance (based on the serotonergic system), and reward dependence (based on the noradrenergic system). Individuals can be high or low on each of these dimensions, and various combinations are seen to underlie the varied personality types. He proposes that these dimensions are altered by experience and may reflect up- or down-regulation of receptors, as well as basal activity levels in these various circuits.

Although all of these models require far more testing before their validity can be assessed, they provide interesting conceptual frameworks within which to think of brain–behavior relationships. What are not adequately addressed by these essentially neurochemical theories are the reciprocal connections with other structures (such as the amygdala, which undoubtedly also play a role in enhancing and inhibiting various action tendencies), although the theories of Gray, Newman, and colleagues do integrate the septohippocampal system into their theories of disinhibition (Newman & Wallace, 1993; Patterson & Newman, 1993).

PSYCHOPATHOLOGY AND BRAIN DYSFUNCTION

Although study in the area of psychopathology and brain dysfunction is still in its infancy, there are many intriguing and suggestive findings. In this section I highlight the findings that are most relevant to the thesis of this book—namely, that psychopathology results from a failure of the organism to regulate affect. This may involve deficits in the development or function of such structures as the amygdala, hippocampus, or prefrontal lobes; of neurotransmitters; or of connections among vital areas.

Initial theorizing in the developmental literature grew from the findings that individuals who have sustained brain damage have elevated rates of psychopathology (Rutter et al., 1970; Max, Robin, et al.,

1997; Max, Smith, et al., 1997). Although some of the earlier studies, such as those on premature infants, suggested that good rearing could overcome many deficits, more recent findings on very-low-birthweight infants suggest enduring difficulties in socioemotional development as well as some aspects of cognitive development (Breslau, 1990; Schothorst & van Engeland, 1996; Sykes et al., 1997), and evidence of brain damage appears to worsen these difficulties (Whitaker et al., 1997). There continues to be evidence that adverse environments exacerbate developmental problems in these infants (Bernstein & Hans, 1994; Breslau, 1990; Raine et al., 1996; Sykes et al., 1997). Many very-low-birthweight infants appear to have difficulty with state regulation, and as a result may have increased difficulty modulating arousal (Sykes et al., 1997). The literature is now clear in showing increases in birth complications in individuals with schizophrenia over controls (Hultman et al., 1997), and, increasingly, similar findings in individuals with other psychotic disorders (Kendell et al., 1996). These findings as a whole do suggest either neurodevelopmental, anoxic/ischemic, or stress-induced dysfunction of limbic structures (probably involving amygdala–hippocampus circuits), possibly caused by glutamatergic toxicity.

Neurological *soft signs* (such as motor coordination difficulties) considered to be indicators of mild neurological dysfunction, are elevated in individuals at risk for schizophrenia, but also appear to predict later internalizing psychopathology (Neumann & Walker, 1996). These soft signs predict socioemotional difficulties (including withdrawal) early in childhood, suggesting the possibility that such children experience problems with modulating arousal. Recently, Pine, Wasserman, Fried, Parides, and Shaffer (1997) reported a relationship between soft signs and both internalizing and externalizing psychopathology in boys. These authors concluded that their findings are suggestive of basal ganglia dysfunction, particularly involving prefrontal connections—a circuit also implicated in a recently defined disorder, pediatric autoimmune neurological disorder associated with streptococcal infection. Allen, Leonard, and Swedo (1995) have proposed that streptococcal antibodies attack these structures, producing obsessive–compulsive disorder (OCD) and tics in children with this disorder. (See also Swedo et al., 1997.)

In a general sense there is some evidence of reduced brain capacity in some subjects with schizophrenia, as measured by the P300 wave in event-related potential studies. Schizophrenic subjects with a small-amplitude P300 wave at recruitment showed poorer coping responses and less evidence of significant severe life events prior to onset of illness than did those with a normal amplitude (Pallanti, Quercioli, & Pazzagli, 1997). The authors interpreted this finding as evidence of reduced brain capacity resulting in poorer coping ability. This may be consistent with the multitude of imaging studies in schizophrenia showing reduced volume of grey matter and enlargement of ventricles in some subjects (see Chapter 11). Based on evidence of thalamic volume reductions in schizophrenia, Andreasen (1997) has speculated that the deficit in schizophrenia involves what she calls "cognitive dysmetria" (poor coordination of learning), facilitated by a dysfunctional thalamic–prefrontal–cerebellar circuit. She cautions, however, that it would be specious to presume a single-deficit model in a disorder as complicated as schizophrenia, and acknowledges that many more structures that interconnect with this circuit may also be involved.

More specifically, postmortem studies of hippocampal size, cell structure, and density have shown changes in subjects with schizophrenia compared to controls (Zaidel, Esiri, & Harrison, 1997). Although there have been conflicting results, Dwork (1997) in a recent review, suggests that results confirm at least secondary changes in the hippocampus in schizophrenia; it is likely that as methods improve, cellular abnormalities will become clearer. The origins of such changes remain unknown, although both perinatal trauma and neurodevelopmental abnormalities have been proposed. Furthermore, as the impact of experience on brain growth and development becomes better understood, such factors as rearing and stress (see Ciaranello et al., 1995, regarding the toxic effect of corticosterone on the hippocampus) will undoubtedly be better understood as laying etiological foundations for the development of disorders. In animal studies, prenatal alcohol exposure, early repeated maternal separation, and artificial rearing all reduce the amplitude of the N1 event-related potential component in the dorsal hippocampus—a finding also associated with inhibited behavior (Kaneko, Riley, & Ehlers, 1993, 1994, 1996–1997).

Neuroimaging studies of subjects with tic disorders and/or OCD suggest abnormalities in the basal ganglia (Baxter et al., 1992; Allen et al., 1995). In addition, deficits in response inhibition but not delayed response in patients with OCD versus controls suggest impairment in orbital prefrontal, rather than dorsolateral prefrontal, connections with striatal areas (Rosenberg, Auerbach, et al., 1997). Given the overlap among tics, OCD, and ADHD, all of which can be conceptualized as involving difficulty in response inhibition, it would seem parsimonious to suspect that deficits in orbital prefrontal–limbic connections will be a common finding across these disorders, as well as in other externalizing disorders besides ADHD.

Given the intimate connections among the hippocampus, the amygdala, and other components of the limbic system, it is reasonable to presume that dysfunction in one area may well produce dysfunction in connected areas. Moreover, our tools for measuring the neurobiological components of affect and of its experience, expression, and regulation are still quite primitive. Studies of brain imaging in which affect is elicited demonstrate diffuse activation of many limbic and para-limbic areas (George et al., 1995). With currently available methodologies, these studies have not differentiated affect elicitation from coping with the affect experienced. Obviously, for most individuals the experience of affect produces some reaction with respect to whether that affect is expressed or suppressed and whether a coping response is needed. The great variability in individual experience and responding, influenced by both genetic and experiential factors, makes measurement of brain changes very complicated and difficult to interpret. This makes definitive proof of primary problems complex and will require extensive research on both animals and humans before we can begin to define "causes."

A NEUROBIOLOGICAL MODEL OF AFFECT DYSREGULATION AND PSYCHOPATHOLOGY

Before I attempt to integrate the above-described findings at the neurobiological level, it is important to discuss a conceptual model to which the neurobiological findings can be applied. My view, like that of LeDoux (1996), is that affects have arisen as a mechanism to alert animals to the salience of situations. Over time and with repetition of experience, an individual develops neural networks that operate in a partially automatic fashion to facilitate responses for coping with threat, uncertainty, and danger. Many of the early response patterns are created through the interaction with the caregiver and can be conceptualized as the laying down of internal working models. Genetic and constitutional factors affect the infant's initial experience of affect, its intensity, and its duration, but also provide limits to the types of coping responses that may develop. The arousal of affect induces a response expectancy in the individual and, depending on how the situation is interpreted, may produce a response. If the situation requires a response, the individual's reaction will depend on genetic and constitutional factors as well as learning. This internal affect system is open to modification by factors that affect the intensity of affect experienced or level of arousal, and/or that change the individual's capacity to respond. Both neurobiological and experiential factors are capable of inducing changes in the individual's experience of affect and in his or her capacity to respond to the affective demands of a situation. Of in-

terest here are both the sensitizing effects of experience on neural networks, and the possible dysfunctions that may interfere with the individual's capacity to regulate affect. Within this framework, the ways in
which neurobiology may be integrated into the mind–brain model of
affects and their dysregulation in psychopathology can be explored.

Although Schore (1994), in his model of a system of affect regulation, argues for a sympathetic versus parasympathetic balancing mechanism as central to affect regulation—a position that appears simplistic
(see Berntson, Cacioppo, & Quigley, 1991 for a discussion of a more
complex view of autonomic nervous system functioning), his place-
ment of the prefrontal cortex at the apex of a system of affect regulation is consistent with the literature and with earlier models (Bradley,
1990). Based on the model of panic disorder articulated by Gorman et
al. (1989), I have proposed a more general model for the development
of affect regulation in which the prefrontal cortex integrates experience
(learning, self-esteem, defensive styles) with input from and output to
other limbic structures and the reticular core (Bradley, 1990). (See
Chapter 1, Figure 1.1.)

Gorman et al. (1989) have proposed a tripartite system to understand panic attacks. They describe the actual panic feelings and the accompanying physiological symptoms as arising from brainstem discharge, predominantly from the LC. Anticipatory anxiety, the second
component, is seen as originating in limbic structures such as the
cingulate and parahippocampal gyri. Phobic avoidance is presumed to
originate in the response of prefrontal structures to the experience of
the attack and accompanying arousal. I believe that the model developed by Gorman et al. (1989) can also serve to explain arousal generally, and with it affect regulation. Given the multitude of interconnections between the brainstem tracts involved in arousal (dopaminergic,
noradrenergic, and serotonergic) and its regulation, it appears premature to propose a single locus for arousal. However, it is clear that the
brainstem initiates arousal, which is interpreted and modulated at
prefrontal and limbic levels. Connections with the autonomic nervous
system among all three levels produce the physiological responses typical of arousal (heart rate elevation, sweating, etc.). The limbic structures play a role in associating the experience and its context with the
arousal emanating from the reticular core; they act to enhance or
dampen the arousal, and at the same time provide it with an affective
valence. The prefrontal areas interpret and attempt to modulate the affects originating in the limbic areas. Because of the rich connections
and interconnections among the prefrontal areas, the amygdala, the
cingulate gyrus, the hippocampus, and the ascending monoaminergic
tracts, it seems reasonable to assume that various patterns become es-

tablished through experience and come to act as relatively automatic affect-regulating mechanisms. Presumably, genetic and experiential mechanisms can exert impacts on many different components of this system.

As Schore (1994) suggests, experience with caretakers presumably interacts with genetic or constitutional factors (strength of monoaminergic transmitter systems or amygdala–hypothalamus–hippocampus connections) to produce neural networks (internal working models or schemata) that function to regulate affect. These neural networks provide the basis for automatic patterning of activity and initially involve little cognitive mediation. As the child develops, these networks should become more controlled by cognitive processes, but presumably retain a framework of automaticity that we think of as unconscious. As cognitive mechanisms mature, the increased capacity for inner dialogue, planning, and insight provides for a higher level of regulation of affect. Clearly, however, the capacity to develop more advanced levels of affect regulation depends on intactness of language and cognition, including the ability to coordinate cognitions (see Graybiel, 1997, regarding cognitive pattern generators in basal ganglia), to maintain normal oscillations in cell collectives (see Jones, 1997, regarding thalamocortical connections and recruitment of cell collectives), and to retain thoughts in working memory (see Goldman-Rakic & Selemon, 1997, regarding dorsolateral prefrontal cortex–hippocampus connections and working memory).

For the purpose of understanding the development of psychopathology, dysregulation of arousal can be presumed to occur through genetic differences in brainstem pathways, such as Kagan has proposed with respect to hypersensitivity of the LC in inhibited individuals; through underarousal of individuals prone to antisocial behavior; or through dopaminergic or serotonergic dysfunction in schizophrenia (Haber & Fudge, 1997; Goldman-Rakic & Selemon, 1997). Furthermore, interference with the development or function of limbic and prefrontal structures (Bechara et al., 1996; Bogerts, 1997; Haber & Fudge, 1997; Goldman-Rakic & Selemon, 1997; Jones, 1997)—as in perinatal traumas (which may produce hippocampal damage), disorganized attachments (which produce maladaptive internal working models), or overwhelming or chronic trauma (which may result in sensitization of the amygdala, hippocampus, and cingulate structures)—will also produce a vulnerability to difficulties regulating affect. Although some individuals may be constitutionally extremely vulnerable, such that minimal stress provokes high levels of arousal, I have presumed that more commonly the interaction of several factors produces psychopathology. To take one example, the development of psychopathology may require that an individual be somewhat constitutionally vulnerable (inhibited, with a sensitized defensive circuit in the amygdala) and insecurely attached (with prefrontal–limbic connections favoring avoidance), and then exposed to a stress that cannot be managed through withdrawal. On the other hand, exposure to manageable levels of arousal, such as that occurring in a variety of stress-inducing (learning) situations, facilitates the development of coping strategies; it will presumably do so through the enhancement of prefrontal–limbic connections enabling the individual to regulate arousal. Lack of exposure may impede the development of such connections, leaving the individual with withdrawal or avoidant strategies as the main arousal-regulating mechanisms. Exposure to overwhelming stress may produce maladaptive connections (amygdala-stored memories) and sensitization of pathways (see below). Although some of these pathways may provide the individual with immediate or short-term relief of arousal (e.g., through dissociation), the failure to develop more adaptive strategies for regulating arousal leaves the individual vulnerable to affect dysregulation when these mechanisms fail. Failure may occur with depletion of resources, both neurochemical and psychological, as a result of the intensity or chronicity of perceived stress.

van der Kolk (1994) proposes that under extreme stress, memories are stored through the amygdala but not the hippocampus; consequently, they have a more primitive, somatic quality and are less available to limbic and frontal control. They are readily activated with stress but poorly controlled. This may provide a way of understanding the intrusive recollections and poor startle modulation of individuals with posttraumtic stress disorder. Furthermore, Kolb (1987) postulates that the repeated arousal interferes with habituation and may produce permanent synaptic changes in higher inhibitory centers (the amygdala and hippocampus), which release the brainstem arousal centers, leaving the individual easily aroused and poorly regulated. High glucocorticoid levels may produce hippocampal cell death, producing further interference with control over arousal.

A poorly understood but commonly observed clinical phenomenon is *sensitivity*, an intensity of perception and sometimes of reaction that often makes children more difficult to raise and may make them more vulnerable to the development of psychopathology. It is possible to speculate that this sensitivity is related to enhanced LC activity, which increases figure–ground discrimination or signal-to-noise ratio. As Clark et al. (1987a, 1987b; see above) have postulated, enhanced noradrenergic activity may increase input sensitivity, whereas enhanced dopaminergic activity may increase output sensitivity. What may be relevant is that individuals with enhanced input sensitivity appear more distressed and more vulnerable to arousal in situations of conflict. Given the possibility of sensitization of circuits with experience, such sensitivity may become self-sustaining, making some individuals increasingly vulnerable to high arousal with a sense of decreasing control—a situation that can lead to high levels of anxiety and depression, as well as to loss of touch with reality.

Coping responses and action tendencies give both personality development and the development of psychopathology their unique character. Because these aspects of development depend on the intactness of neural structures and processes, their expression will vary with many of the factors mentioned above. Here, however, intactness of prefrontal–limbic connections may be critical. The individual who has difficulty inhibiting responses, related to orbital prefrontal dysfunction, is more likely to act out impulsively or aggressively in situations of arousal. Similarly, dysfunction of orbital prefrontal–striatal connections is likely to produce loss of inhibition of motor or cognitive activities under stress. Furthermore, individuals with dorsolateral prefrontal deficits may be impaired in their capacity to use experience to cope under stress. Lastly, Rolls (1992), in discussing the neurophysiology of the primate amygdala, points out how the neural network involving the prefrontal cortex, amygdala, and hippocampus allows mood state to influence cognition. In this theory, context (i.e., mood state), because it is stored in areas contiguous to specific memories, can enhance recall of memories, as "recall of a memory occurs best in such networks when the input key to the memory is nearest to the original input pattern of activity which was stored" (Rolls, 1992, p. 159). This effect of contiguity on processing would account for the distorted perceptions or beliefs seen in depression.

Although most of the discussion to this point has focused on the development of internalizing types of psychopathology, underarousal, as measured by low heart rate, is emerging as a strong predictor variable in the development of externalizing and especially aggressive psychopathology (Raine, Venables, & Mednick, 1997). One can speculate that such individuals, also described as fearless and sensation-seeking, are less responsive to punishment and therefore more likely to become oppositional as children. If raised in an environment in which aggressive responses are tolerated, modeled, or even intermittently reinforced, these individuals will develop conduct-related psychopathology. Those individuals who display heightened arousal (skin conductance and heart rate) appear to be less persistent in their antisocial behavior (Kerr, Tremblay, Pagani, & Vitaro, 1997) or, despite exposure to criminal fathers, less likely to become criminals themselves (Brennan et al., 1997). What is important in externalizing psychopathology is that affect regulation is also impaired, as such individuals fail to develop adaptive strategies for managing anger. Such difficulties regularly reduce their opportunities to develop relationships that could provide other strategies for regulating their affects. This may partially explain why many antisocial girls have high levels of depression and why antisocial boys frequently resort to substance abuse. Girls may react to their isolation from relationships with mood disorder symptoms, whereas boys may choose peer-approved strategies for regulating their affects.

CONCLUSIONS

This brief tour through the neurological bases of affect arousal and its possible relationship to psychopathology has primarily highlighted the areas where future research will provide answers, but a few preliminary conclusions are possible at this point. Clearly, the amygdala and its connections appear to play a role in fear conditioning, and to constitute a neural network related to anxiety and its regulation; its connections with the hippocampus seem to be involved in various emotional memories. The frontal lobes and their connections appear to play a modulatory role with respect to attention, motivation, planning, and regulation of affect. The interconnecting circuits that are now being defined will clarify the various components of these complex processes. Recent developments in the understanding of stress reactivity as it relates to up- and down-regulation of glucocorticoid receptors in limbic areas may eventually clarify how these neural structures, through the multitude of neurotransmitters, produce the various symptoms that we define as mental disorders.

Chapter 8

Therapeutic Considerations

As mentioned in Chapter 1, the outcome literature on various types of psychotherapy consistently shows that most therapies "work" (i.e., lead to positive outcomes for patients/clients), and that there is little real difference among therapies in outcomes. (For recent overviews, see Messer & Warren, 1995; Roth & Fonagy, 1996.) Moreover, the results of psychotherapeutic interventions appear equivalent to those of medication in many instances (Elkin et al., 1989; Roth & Fonagy, 1996). I have suggested that one way (among others) of understanding these common general effects is that all effective interventions influence affect regulation, albeit in different ways. In this chapter I elaborate on this idea. I first summarize the evolution of the three main branches of psychotherapy, and note both their increasing likeness to one another and the similarities in their outcomes. I also discuss how the issue of affect regulation is relevant to interactional psychotherapy—a composite that borrows from all three branches. I then review some of the factors that appear common across psychotherapies and some of the research findings about variables related to outcome, and link these variables to affect regulation. Finally, I take a brief look at psychopharmacological and other biological interventions.

EVOLUTION OF THE PSYCHOTHERAPIES, AND MAIN FACTORS AFFECTING OUTCOMES

Although the first systematic application of a theory of psychotherapy is probably best attributed to Sigmund Freud, many of the principles

139

that we now acknowledge as important in psychotherapy were understood and practiced prior to his seminal contributions. These include such things as warmth, caring, conveying understanding of the patient's suffering, and supporting relief from stresses. Freud, however, forced a paradigm shift with his conceptualization of how unconscious processes influence everyday life, and particularly how an understanding of unconscious processes can clarify manifestations or symptoms of psychopathology. Furthermore, his formulation of defenses as ways of warding off anxiety led to the first clear understanding of the development of characterological traits. These ideas were elaborated by his followers and have stood the test of time, in contrast to some of his other ideas.

I believe that the reason why these two ideas have held up to almost a century of efforts to refine psychotherapy, and why they appear in "new clothes" in the newer psychotherapies, is that they are fundamental to understanding psychopathology and to work in psychotherapy. *Unconscious mental representations,* referred to as *transferences* in psychoanalytic writing, have reemerged as *internal working models* in the attachment literature (Bowlby, 1969, 1973, and 1980), *schemata* in cognitive theories (Beck, 1971), and *schemes* in experiential theories (Greenberg et al., 1993). Similarly, *defenses* have been renamed *coping strategies* or *cognitive distortions* in cognitive theories, *maladaptive emotional responses* in experiential theories, and *emotional heuristics* in information-processing models (Clyman, 1992). Proponents of these various approaches will argue about the differences, but at a conceptual level they appear to have more similarities than differences.

Although each of the major schools of therapy values or emphasizes different components or techniques, there is little evidence that these technical differences contribute significantly to outcome (Lambert, 1992; Roth & Fonagy, 1996). Moreover, although purists have argued that certain kinds of changes (in personality traits) are only possible with deeper-level transference or schema changes, and that efforts to achieve change at the level of mental representations are generally preferable to change at the more "superficial" level of coping strategies (Greenberg et al., 1993; Horowitz, Fridhandler, & Stinson, 1992), there is little literature to support these arguments. In fact, Jacobson et al. (1996) demonstrated equivalent changes for cognitive-behavioral therapies, whether the therapists focused on changing attributions, cognitions, or behaviors. As might be expected, however, there is support for a greater impact of longer therapies on more severe disorders, including character pathologies (Messer & Warren, 1995; Roth & Fonagy, 1996). What has emerged strongly is that the therapeutic alliance is predictive of outcome, as are therapist attributes (as perceived by the client) such as warmth, understanding, and adherence to the goals of therapy (Messer & Warren, 1995; Weinberger, 1993).

Therapies evolve, and this has been particularly true of the three main branches of psychotherapy: psychodynamic, cognitive/cognitive-behavioral, and experiential. This evolution, in my view, has brought them closer together. I describe what appears to be current thinking in each of these areas, and in doing so, begin to speculate how they can have similar outcomes through their impact on affect regulation.

Psychodynamic Therapies

Messer and Warren (1995), in discussing models of brief psychodynamic therapy, define two main schools (the drive/structural and the relational), as well as integrative and eclectic models. Differences between the drive/structural and relational approaches appear to be that the drive/structural model has therapists focus on transference, defenses, and resistance issues in a very direct fashion, in contrast to relational therapists, who focus more on transference in the "here and now" and the experience of a "corrective emotional experience." Relational therapists conceive of the transference less as a projection of a patient's infantile wishes onto the "blank screen" of a neutral therapist and more as a construction of the patient's interpersonal reality formed from experience, which induces complementary feelings in the therapist. Whereas the drive/structural therapists believe in the importance of accurate interpretation in producing insight as the main change factor, relational therapists believe that a patient changes through having a new experience with a therapist who does not reinforce the patient's unconscious mental representations of interactions. Generally, in these newer therapies there is more emphasis placed on the therapist's being supportive, empathetic, and real; the underlying premise appears to be that these qualities are necessary for the patient to feel safe enough to express feelings and to risk exploring painful aspects of his or her life (Weiss, 1990).

Messer and Warren also discuss several integrative or eclectic therapies. Of these, Garfield (1992), whose work was influenced by the thinking of Jerome Frank, has defined several common factors that he believes are responsible for change in therapy. In addition to the therapeutic relationship, he cites interpretation, insight, and understanding; emotional release; reinforcement; desensitization; and confronting one's problems. This list clearly overlaps with Weinberger's (1993) list of common factors for effective psychotherapy, which are exposure, alliance, mastery, and attribution. These factors will recur as I discuss the next two groups.

Although all these therapies differ in their valuing of or emphasis on certain techniques, and to some extent in their belief in what is essential to induce change, the commonalities are more significant than the differences, especially in view of the fact that outcomes across therapies appear the same. To my mind, all current effective psychodynamic theories espouse unconscious mental representations (which have cognitive and affective components) and a system of defenses to deal with unpleasant affects. Although they differ with respect to how best to modify the unconscious mental representations, they all seem to agree that it is important for patients to modify these in some way and to learn to employ more adaptive defenses or coping strategies. Although none of the traditional dynamically oriented psychotherapies explicitly refer to desensitization, exposure, or mastery, all imply that change occurs not only through insight but also through *working through* or *reexperiencing*. Both these terms, in my mind, imply exposure to the situation that induces the painful affect (within the therapeutic relationship or as a corrective emotional experience, possibly even in the context of other significant relationships), which through repetition induces desensitization and ultimately a sense of mastery. Carek (1990) has made a similar argument for individual psychodynamic psychotherapy. I believe that we can make the same argument with respect to cognitive/cognitive-behavioral and experiential therapies.

Cognitive and Cognitive-Behavioral Therapies

In 1971 Aaron Beck, one of the founders of cognitive therapy, wrote:

> The relationship of cognition to affect in normal subjects is similar to that observed in psychopathological states. Among normals the sequence perception–cognition–emotion is dictated largely by the demand character of the stimulus situation. In psychopathological conditions, the reaction to the stimulus situation is determined to a much greater extent by internal processes. The affective response is likely to be excessive or inappropriate because of the idiosyncratic conceptualization of the event. The input from the external situation is molded to conform to the typical schemas activated in these conditions. As a result, interpretations of experience embody arbitrary judgements, overgeneralizations, and distortions. Perseverative conceptualizations relevant to danger, loss, unjustified attack and self-enhancement are typical of anxiety neuroses, depression, paranoid states, and hypomanic states, respectively. (p. 495)

Although the early cognitive and cognitive-behavioral therapists focused largely on teaching clients more adaptive coping strategies (Meichenbaum, 1977) or on confronting irrational beliefs in order to encourage clients to react in less maladaptive ways, cognitive therapies have evolved with a clearer recognition of interpersonal processes and the need to address these in therapy (Safran & Segal, 1990). The cognitive paradigm has had an influence on psychodynamic therapists, as reflected in the eclectic therapy of Garfield (1992), but it has also borrowed from the experiential therapies, as demonstrated in the work of Safran and Segal (1990). Throughout the development of cognitive therapies, cognitive therapists have retained some allegiance to their behavioral and social skills origins, with an emphasis on techniques such as homework and practice, and a belief in exposure, desensitization, and mastery. With some of the newer conceptualizations, however, we see an increased emphasis on reworking maladaptive schemata through a therapeutic relationship that conveys a sense of acceptance of the patient and his or her affects, and through this relationship a "corrective emotional experience" (Heard & Linehan, 1993; Safran & Segal, 1990). The parallels with the common factors in psychodynamic therapy are clear.

Experiential Therapies

The early formulations of experiential therapy by Rogers (1951) and Perls (Perls, Hefferline, & Goodman, 1951) emphasized "being" with the client and allowing the client to "actualize" him- or herself through coming in touch with feelings. In newer conceptualizations of experiential therapy, formulations about the theory and process of change emphasize "facilitation of the client's creation of new emotional meaning" (Greenberg et al., 1993, p. 4). Because Greenberg et al. discuss the role of affect and emotion in therapy so explicitly, I quote from their 1993 book, *Facilitating Emotional Change*, at some length. These authors describe *emotion schemes* as "complex synthesizing structures that integrate cognition . . . and motivation . . . with affect . . . and action" (p. 5). These emotion schemes

> form supraordinate emotional meaning/action structures that determine our wholistic experience of being-in-the-world. It is these emotion structures that also automatically organize and stabilize our initially transient emotional reactions to provide our enduring sense of self-in-the-world. And it is these structures that determine what is personally meaningful to us and lead to our immediate emotional experience of being-in-the-world. It is from our emotional reactions that we

can tell what is important to us, how we are appraising our world and how we are coping with it. (pp. 5–6)

With respect to therapeutic emphasis, Greenberg et al. (1993) state:

> The activation of internal emotion structures, the reprocessing of information and its reencoding, thus ultimately leads to change in emotion structures and the generation of new schemes. The therapist's most active role in facilitating the reorganization of emotion schemes is neither one of interpreting the meaning of the client's experience nor of attempting to modify the scheme or to challenge it. It is to focus the client's attention on some elements of his or her experience, not in current focal awareness, to symbolize it and to thereby activate schemes and further process information. This, in turn, promotes self-reorganization of experience and the construction of a new view of self-in-the-world. (p. 7)

The authors are adamant that the goal of therapy is not to provide insight or to modify cognitions, but to facilitate processes that will lead to new experiences and affective problem solving. Although the authors reject techniques incompatible with the nondirectedness of experiential therapy, such as attempting to change a client's cognitions, their formulation is entirely consistent with the psychodynamic and cognitive approaches in regard to the need to change mental representations that act at an automatic/unconscious level to influence affective problem solving.

Interactional Psychotherapies

Broadly speaking, the interactional psychotherapies, including marital/couple, family, and group interventions, seek to change maladaptive behaviors in order to permit more mutually reinforcing interactions with important others. If this behavior change is brought about, it reduces the tensions and negative affects that are aspects of dissatisfying interactions in important relationships. Presumably, if mutually satisfying interactions can be maintained over time, the interactants' attributions, beliefs, and ultimately schemata will be modified to accommodate to the new interactions and expectations. I use behavioral family intervention, a form of interactional psychotherapy in which I am experienced, to illustrate how changing behavioral interactions among family members is linked to affect regulation. *Behavioral family intervention,* a term coined by Sanders and Markie-Dadds (1992), refers to a broad spectrum of behavioral techniques involving parents and children, and includes but is not limited to parent management training. (For reviews, see Sanders, 1996; Kazdin, 1997.)

Children who present with oppositional behavior are typically engaged in aversive interactions with parents, who themselves resort to an inconsistent variety of harsh, coercive, and generally ineffective parenting strategies (Patterson, 1982). Such children frequently perceive themselves as bad and their parents as angry at them. Parents of such children perceive their children as difficult and themselves as failures as parents. Oppositional children learn to express their frustration in temper tantrums and other oppositional behaviors rather than in words, and fail to develop more adaptive problem-solving strategies to deal with conflicts with others. Their parents feel less and less in control of their children's behavior, and with the expectation that they should be able to control their children, they become very frustrated (Bugental, 1992). For these children, as these patterns become entrenched and reinforced over time through similar dissatisfying relationships and interactions with peers and teachers, their beliefs and attitudes begin to reflect their experience, and they automatically assume hostile intent in a variety of ambiguous situations (Dodge, 1993). Parents often back off and give up in their efforts to relate to their children out of their own demoralization, as well as an avoidance of confrontations that elicit unprovoked rage.

Behavioral family intervention aims to reverse this pattern of interaction by providing parents with strategies that enhance their control of their children's behavior, and that diminish the coercive, aversive strategies of yelling and sometimes physical responses. Intervention with the children may focus on their learning more adaptive problem-solving strategies, anger management, and confrontation of hostile attributions. Although this type of intervention with older conduct-disordered youth is less successful, behavioral family intervention and similar cognitive-behavioral interventions with school-age children are generally as effective as are most other psychotherapies (Kazdin, 1997). Parents who are able to implement strategies to control their children more comfortably, and who can, in doing so, reduce their more aversive interactions, report feeling better and having a sense of enhanced efficacy in their parenting role. Children report a lessening of parental frustration and of their own anger. As parents no longer feel demoralized and avoidant of interactions with their children, they report greater enjoyment of their children and their accomplishments. Children report pride in their ability to manage their frustration in more adaptive ways.

Although this description is simplistic, it illustrates the way in

which particular behavioral interventions, especially in less entrenched situations, can modify clients' attributions and beliefs. The
chronic distress that accompanies these maladaptive interactions is re-
lieved, allowing the resurgence of positive and mutually reinforcing
emotional interactions. Presumably, if these more positive interactions
can be sustained modifications to earlier schemata can be made; such
changes will allow children and parents to develop positive expectancies of each other, which will translate into more optimal long-term
functioning.

SIMILARITIES AMONG THERAPIES:
PROMOTION OF AFFECT REGULATION

What can we conclude from this brief tour of recent developments in
psychotherapy? I believe there is an emerging consensus that therapy
promotes affect regulation. Some therapies seek to do this through the
use of behaviors that will indirectly reduce the intensity of affect, such as
breathing and distracting techniques for various forms of anxiety. In others the emphasis is on encouraging the use of adaptive coping strategies,
such as more positive self-talk, which will allow individuals to confront
situations that have in the past been avoided. The need for individuals to
find ways of exposing themselves to previously avoided situations—
such as, discussing painful affects (psychodynamic theories) or encoun-
tering dirt in cases of compulsive hand washing (cognitive-behavioral
theories)—appears as a consistent theme. This process allows for a desensitizing effect if sustained, and is consistent with the concepts of practice in cognitive-behavioral therapies and of working through in psychodynamic therapies (Carek, 1990). One can speculate that if an individual
succeeds in using more adaptive coping strategies (through whatever
mechanism), and if this permits him or her to engage in relationships
that do not reinforce maladaptive internal representations, the individual will modify these representations over time and thus reduce the likelihood of automatic maladaptive emotional responses. The finding by
Brown and Harris (1978) that women from deprived backgrounds
adapted well if they were successful in finding well-adapted spouses
would support this line of thinking. In their outline of a model for change
in psychotherapy, Stiles et al. (1990) state:

> In successful psychotherapy, problematic experiences (threatening or
> painful thoughts, feelings, memories, etc.) are gradually assimilated
> into schemata that are introduced by the therapist or developed in the
> therapist–client interaction by modification of old schemata. As it is

assimilated, a problematic experience passes through predictable stages. The client moves from being oblivious, to experiencing the content as acutely painful, then as less distressing, merely puzzling, then understood, and finally mastered. (p. 411)

Curiously, even Shapiro, the creator of the somewhat radical eye movement desensitization and reprocessing (EMDR), proposes a similar process (Shapiro & Forrest, 1997). However, she conceptualizes it as occurring at a purely physiological level—that is, within brain and autonomic nervous system networks. (See the discussion of biological interventions, below.)

All of the therapeutic approaches described above, or at least their newer versions, articulate the important role played by unconscious mental representations in the individual's capacity to regulate affect. Although they espouse different ways of modifying these internal representations, there is no doubt about the central importance they accord to this modification in achieving change (Beitman, 1992). However, as Weinberger (1993) argues, because of the reciprocal interaction of various facets (schemata, attributions, defenses, or coping strategies) of emotional functioning, no one component of change should be seen as primary; change in one component has the potential to invoke change in another part of the system.

Drawing on the recent distinction in memory theory between *declarative* and *procedural* knowledge, Clyman (1992) has applied these concepts to a psychodynamic theory of the development of mental representations, such as transference. Declarative knowledge, also referred to as *episodic memory*, is that information resulting from experienced facts or events, stored symbolically as language or mental images, and available to recall. Despite being available to recall, declarative knowledge may be conscious, preconscious, or unconscious. Procedural knowledge, in contrast, is the knowledge arising from skill development and is largely unconscious. Because it is not stored symbolically, it cannot be recalled but can be enacted. Clyman (1992) makes a further distinction between *controlled* and *automatic* procedures. Controlled procedures require "that declarative knowledge be conscious during execution of the procedure. With automatic procedures, all of the information is encoded in procedural ... form" (p. 353). Controlled procedures, which are initially slow and poorly coordinated in contrast to automatic procedures, allow the individual to learn new skills through conscious attention. These procedures may, with practice, become encoded as automatic procedures.

Storage of declarative knowledge is dependent on hippocampal function, which is not fully developed until about age 5. This can account for the difficulty most individuals have in recalling memories prior to that age. Procedural memory, which Clyman (1992) links to Piaget's notion of *sensorimotor* schemata (perceptual–motor–affective procedures), appears to be functional shortly after birth. Clyman suggests that relationship experiences and (perhaps most important for present purposes) the rules with respect to emotional behaviors are encoded procedurally. With repetition of interactions within families and caretaking dyads, these become automatic mental processes that lead to an interpretive framework for subsequent interactions and the development of heuristic (coping) strategies. These processes operate at an unconscious level and may be adaptive or maladaptive, depending on the context. If maladaptive, they will lead to distortions in emotion processing when activated. As Clyman points out, this theory provides an explanation for unconscious emotions. (See also LeDoux, 1996.) Painful affect can be warded off defensively, rendering such feeling unconscious. In addition, as emotional interactions are repeated they move from being controlled to being automatic, and "the conscious feeling no longer needs to be experienced in order to execute the procedure, as conscious attention is no longer required" (Clyman, 1992, p. 361). This automaticity supports rapid, direct responses to emotional situations—responses that, from an evolutionary standpoint, would be highly beneficial. Coping strategies, which may also be seen as characterological underpinnings, emerge as the individual selects those ways of acting that best meet his or her goals.

Change of automatic emotional procedures occurs through interrupting the automatic procedural enactment by making the feelings that trigger the process more conscious, reality testing the beliefs associated with the emotional coping strategy, exploring more adaptive coping responses, and encouraging the use of these more adaptive responses in real-life relationships. Clyman (1992) refers to this process as converting an automatic procedure into a controlled procedure through conscious declarative processing; with practice, this controlled procedure becomes another, more adaptive automatic procedure. He also allows for change to occur without the development of conscious processing, as when individuals try out new strategies, either in the safety of the therapeutic relationship or in new relationships that do not reinforce the distortions of the maladaptive mental representations.

Although Clyman does not propose an anatomical basis for the encoding of emotional representations, Schore's (1994) model with respect to the role of the orbitofrontal cortex, and especially its connections with the amygdala, would suggest that these two structures constitute such a neural network. LeDoux (1996) reviews work on unconscious processing of stimuli, especially affective stimuli, and makes a strong argument for the role of the amygdala in the unconscious processing of emotions.

OUTCOME-RELATED FACTORS IN PSYCHOTHERAPY AND THEIR LINKS TO AFFECT REGULATION

If we accept that there are more common factors among the various schools of psychotherapy than there are differences, a brief examination of outcome-related factors in psychotherapy and their links to affect regulation seems warranted. Lambert (1992) divides factors that have been demonstrated to have an impact on outcome in psychotherapy into four categories. In order of perceived magnitude, these are (1) extratherapeutic factors, comprising many client variables, such as ego strength and support systems; (2) factors common to various schools of therapy, largely therapist variables such as empathy, warmth, and acceptance; (3) expectancy factors, such as a patient's belief that something positive will happen as a result of engaging in a socially sanctioned process for relief of suffering; and (4) specific techniques, such as systematic desensitization for phobias.

Client or Patient Factors

Among the client variables most strongly related to outcome is the capacity for *introspection* or the concept of *psychological-mindedness* (Roth & Fonagy, 1996). Although these terms are defined differently by different authors, implicit in these concepts is the ability to examine feelings and their relationship to situations and behaviors. Truax and Carkhuff (1967) in psychotherapy studies of schizophrenic patients, explored the depth of each patient's intrapersonal exploration in the second interview and concluded that it correlated with the final outcome. Furthermore, they found that this was highly influenced by the therapist's level of empathy and unconditional positive regard for the patient.

Individuals described as *alexithymic* have difficulty describing feelings and seeing connections between their feelings and symptoms. (For a complete discussion of alexithymia and its relation to affect regulation see Taylor et al., 1997.) Alexithymic individuals generally fare poorly in, and are inclined to drop out of, expressive psychotherapies. In fact, Taylor et al. (1997) suggest that some alexithymic individuals may be made worse by the arousal induced in expressive therapies. They surmise that such individuals have a deficit in their capacity to regulate affect, and so are unable to tolerate a therapeutic situation in which affects are discussed and examined. Although my thesis is that good therapy generally promotes improved affect regulation, it must be conceded that some individuals may have structural deficits that make engaging in the process of psychotherapy very difficult. These vulnerabilities may include (among others) such ease of arousal that merely talking about feelings produces marked discomfort and a desire to withdraw. If such individuals are not sufficiently motivated to achieve change, they may easily avoid or quickly withdraw from therapy.

Some individuals have developed ways of coping with their feelings that, although maladaptive, at least allow them to function; the symptoms contain their painful or negative affect. I refer here to gender identity disorder, to some eating disorders, and to various character pathologies. Many individuals with such psychopathology may develop some insight into the role their symptoms serve, but cannot risk being without their defenses, as they have grown to rely on these as their main ways of managing their negative or painful affect. Therapy with such individuals will of necessity be lengthy, and is often less successful than with less vulnerable individuals. Other types of defenses (e.g., splitting), if extreme, also may make therapy more difficult, as these strategies can create automatic and rigid mechanisms for containing affects that patients may be reluctant to risk giving up.

Another patient variable related to outcome is a patient's readiness for therapy. Prochaska, DiClemente, and Norcross (1992) have defined five stages of change in psychotherapy: *precontemplation, contemplation, preparation, action,* and *maintenance.* Individuals who are in the precontemplation stage have no intention to change and are generally unaware of their problems. One could speculate that many individuals in the precontemplation stage resemble patients described as alexithymic, although this has not been examined empirically. These authors also argue for matching types of treatment to the stages patients have reached; they propose that such strategies as consciousness raising and environmental reevaluation are needed for those in the precontemplation and contemplation stages, as opposed to self-liberation in the preparation and action stages. These authors do not discuss affect regulation as a component in readiness for change, but a similar conceptual framework can be applied if it is assumed that once clients have become more aware of how their affects may influence their lives, they may become more prepared to work on addressing ways of managing affects more directly (the action stage).

This sense of being prepared to risk doing something to make changes is also dependent on a sense of self-efficacy. Weinberger

(1993), citing Bandura's work, reports: "The higher the level of self-efficacy, the higher the performance accomplishment and the lower the emotional arousal associated with performance efforts" (p. 51). Self-efficacy in therapy can be seen to develop in the context of seeing oneself able to make changes and implies a move from demoralization to "remoralization"—a critical component in Frank's (1973) seminal book *Persuasion and Healing*.

Therapist Factors

Truax and Carkhuff (1967) provided the first empirical evidence for the importance of the therapist variables of accurate empathy, unconditional positive regard, and genuineness in outcome with schizophrenic patients. They also showed that patients exposed to therapists rated as high on all three variables exhibited a drop in anxiety level, whereas patients exposed to therapists rated as low on these three factors experienced a rise in their anxiety. They provided strong evidence that therapists' levels of empathy did not change with time or with different patients, and that therapists with low levels of empathy, unconditional positive regard, and genuineness actually made their patients worse. These provocative findings have stood the test of time. Lambert (1992) notes that therapist variables in successful outcomes include empathy, warmth, acceptance, and encouragement of risk taking. Roth and Fonagy (1996) also comment on a therapist's capacity to deal with client hostility. Weinberger (1993), however, takes pains to point out that such therapist characteristics are important only as they are perceived by a client.

Parallels between the characteristics of a successful therapist and those of the caregiver of a securely attached child have been noted (Holmes, 1993; Beebe, 1993). Just as the attachment literature has recognized that the attachment system is a system for regulation of affect, therapy can be conceptualized as a similar process. In this view, the therapist not only is a "container" in Bion's (1978) sense, but also provides a mirroring function (Holmes, 1993; Beebe, 1993). Presumably with the "good enough" therapist (to borrow a phrase from Winnicott, 1965), a reenactment of affective–cognitive scenarios can occur, permitting schema shifts and therapeutic change. Implicit in this notion of the "good enough" therapist is the capacity to tolerate and accept those client affects that the client has previously warded off, because they have been perceived as painful or threatening. Weiss (1990) states "that . . . patients bring forth repressed material only after they have unconsciously overcome their worry about the consequences" (p. 105).

Expectancy Factors

Expectancy is almost self-evident with respect to its possible impact on affect regulation. Clients who perceive the therapist as having the capacity to help or relieve their distress will experience some reduction in their distress as part of engaging in any intervention. Like a placebo effect, expectancy is often quite powerful.

Specific Techniques

Specific techniques may be quite varied (including relaxation and systematic desensitization). In the literature on the treatment of anxiety disorders, these techniques are used as strategies for reducing the anxiety that accompanies efforts to deal with an avoided or threatening situation. Clearly these techniques, when employed systematically, do play a role in reducing the client's distress and when practiced become a part of the coping repertoire for managing distress.

PSYCHOPHARMACOLOGICAL AND OTHER BIOLOGICAL INTERVENTIONS

It is beyond the scope of the present chapter to attempt to analyze how other interventions, especially the newer psychopharmacological and other biological interventions, may work. I have indicated in Chapter 1 that I believe there is a common anxiety-relieving component to many psychotropic medications. Some authors have suggested that medications like the selective serotonin reuptake inhibitors may modulate negative affective experience in individuals without diagnosed mental disorders, as well as in those with such disorders (Knutson et al., 1998). The interesting work by Baxter et al. (1992), in which the caudate nucleus abnormalities observed in patients with obsessive–compulsive disorder were improved by either medication or cognitive-behavioral therapy, does show that the brain is capable of modification by both biological and psychotherapeutic interventions. In Chapter 9 I cite work suggesting that many antidepressants may act to enhance the capacity of corticotropin-releasing factor receptors in the hypothalamus and amygdala; this results in an individual's becoming less stress-reactive. Clearly, these biological underpinnings will affect and be affected by an individual's experience, and may facilitate (or interfere with) the capacity to engage in psychotherapy. The recent acceptance of the possibility that many psychotherapy patients may require psychotropics to engage optimally in the process of therapy is illustrative of this point.

I would speculate that some of the new interventions, such as EMDR, may act to desensitize neural networks in a way similar to what I have suggested above for the psychotherapies. It appears to do so at a more unconscious or automatic level, however. Electroconvulsive therapy (ECT) produces changes in a number of neurotransmitters, some similar to and some different from those produced by antidepressants (Sackheim, Devanand, & Nobler, 1995). G proteins are important in transmitting signals from hormone and neurotransmitter membrane receptors to second-messenger systems within cells. They have been implicated in the biochemical mechanisms underlying depression, and their functioning has been shown to be improved both with antidepressant treatment and with ECT (Avissar, Nechamkin, Roitman, & Schreiber, 1998). Specifically, McGowan et al. (1996) found changes in G protein messenger RNA in hippocampal areas in rats exposed to ECT and lithium. This work is of course preliminary, but it illustrates the convergence of the effects of different biological interventions, and it points to the question of whether psychotherapeutic interventions may have similar effects.

CONCLUSIONS

For some readers, the points I have made in this chapter will not be news. However, if I am correct in my speculation about an emerging consensus that differing types of interventions have similar effects, this theoretical framework provides a way of integrating developmental, biological, and psychological factors into a coherent approach to therapy. It allows the purists to continue to pursue those specific features that may make one type of therapy or approach more suitable for specific patients. It does suggest, however, that factors common to various approaches—specifically, their capacity to support improved affect regulation—need to be addressed. It allows for the combined use of medication and psychotherapy, on the assumption that reduction of anxiety or mood pressure may be a prerequisite to some patients' engaging in a therapy that requires them to increase their level of arousal or anxiety in order to explore affects and master them, or simply to function. Finally, it implies that all patients, regardless of how much their illness may be affected by genetic or biological factors, can also be understood and helped by a psychotherapeutic relationship.

PART III

Clinical Syndromes

Chapter 9

Internalizing Disorders: Anxiety, Mood, and Related Disorders

In this chapter I deal with those disorders conceptualized as "internalizing," in contrast to the "externalizing" disorders. The most prominent disorders in this category are the anxiety and mood disorders, and the bulk of this chapter is devoted to these two groups; however, at the end I briefly address some other disorders that I believe are related, such as eating disorders and gender identity disorder. I begin the chapter by outlining the reasons for considering the anxiety and mood disorders together in the present context. I then examine the etiological factors that have been shown to be relevant in anxiety and mood disorders: genetic and constitutional factors (with an emphasis on inherited sensitivity to environmental stress), psychosocial factors (with an emphasis on factors in the familial environment that create or enhance stress reactivity), and neurobiological factors (with an emphasis on the neurological impact of stress). After this, I briefly consider the implications of the various findings for treatment of these disorders. Finally, I present an integration of the various etiological factors, emphasizing the need for attention to and more research on both common and disorder-specific factors.

RELATIONSHIP BETWEEN ANXIETY
AND MOOD DISORDERS

I am addressing the anxiety and mood disorders together because the literature supports a common underlying factor leading to these disorders. This literature includes research on the comorbidity of anxiety and depression in both community and patient-based samples; studies demonstrating increased prevalences of both anxiety and depression in families of probands with either condition (Beidel & Turner, 1997); research showing common responses in anxious and depressed patients to a variety of medications and psychosocial treatments (Hudson & Pope, 1990; Tyrer et al., 1988); and, lastly, recent studies showing a common genetic factor in anxiety and depression in both adults (Kendler, Walters, et al., 1995) and children (Thapar & McGuffin, 1997).

Clark and Watson (1991b) have argued that what is common to anxiety and depression is a factor they called "negative affect" and abbreviate as NA—a relatively stable trait with significant heritability. They see NA as representing "the extent to which a person is feeling upset or unpleasantly engaged rather than peaceful and encompasses various affective states including *upset, angry, guilty, afraid, sad, scornful, disgusted,* and *worried*; such states as *calm* and *relaxed* best represent the lack of NA" (p. 321). They also posit that what differentiates anxiety from depression is the presence of "positive affect" (a factor they abbreviate as PA, which is orthogonal to NA) and physiological arousal. Clark and Watson (1991b) regard PA as "the extent to which a person feels a zest for life and is most clearly defined by such expressions of energy and pleasurable engagement as *active, delighted, interested, enthusiastic* and *proud*; the absence of PA is best captured by terms that reflect fatigue and languor (e.g. *tired* or *sluggish*)" (p. 321). They state that depression involves an absence or reduction of PA in addition to the general distress or NA that it shares with anxiety disorders. They also propose that anxiety can be differentiated from depression by the presence of physiological arousal. The evidence for differences with respect to PA between anxiety and depression appears better than that for the presence of physiological arousal. Arousal may not differentiate the two conditions, perhaps because of the heterogeneity of anxiety disorders on this dimension and the fact that peripheral measures of physiological arousal do not correlate well with one another and may not reflect central arousal (Brown, 1997; Brown, Chorpita, & Barlow, 1998; Hoehn-Saric & McLeod, 1993).

Earlier in this book, I have suggested that a temperamental trait described variously as *sensitivity, emotional reactivity, behavioral inhibi-*

tion, or *neuroticism* may be the common underlying factor linking anxiety and depression. There is general, if not universal, agreement that anxiety appears to be the more basic of the two conditions (Kovacs & Devlin, 1998). This is based on the notion that anxiety is a vulnerability factor in many disorders and typically is evident before the first episode of depression (Brown & Harris, 1993; Brown, 1997). There is also some evidence that depression may develop secondarily to a number of disorders, and that although generalized anxiety disorder (GAD) has the most specific link with later depression, the actual number of preceding disorders is more important than type in predicting subsequent depression (Kessler & Walters, 1998). This relationship between number of anxiety disorders and the development of depression is also consistent with the notion of depression's developing in the context of accumulated stresses or *burnout,* an overwhelming situation that leads an individual to believe that he or she cannot cope or that the situation is hopeless (Maier & Seligman, 1976). In a slightly different vein, Akiskal (1991) argues for what he calls "affective temperaments," which are conditioned by factors such as early loss, heredity, and gender, and which in the presence of stressors give rise to depressive syndromes or states.

Brown et al. (1998) used data from 350 outpatients with anxiety and depression to test several dimensions of mood and anxiety disorders, as well as the three factors of the Clark and Watson (1991b) tripartite model of anxiety and depression. Their results, depicted in Figure 9.1, supported five separable symptom domains: mood disorders, GAD, panic disorder, obsessive–compulsive disorder (OCD), and social phobia. In addition, the best fitting structural model included Clark and Watson's two higher-order factors of PA and NA, relating to the emotional disorders as Clark and Watson predicted. In addition to loading on depression, PA loaded (negatively) on social phobia. The issue with respect to heterogeneity of anxiety disorders and autonomic arousal noted above was evident in Brown et al.'s test of the model, as GAD had a negative loading on autonomic arousal while panic disorder had a positive loading. Despite the discriminant validity of these dimensions, GAD loaded most heavily on NA and correlated highly with depression as well as with the other anxiety disorders, leading Brown et al. (1998) to suggest that GAD could be conceptualized as the basic emotional disorder. They also raise the issue that GAD may be better defined as a trait of nonspecific vulnerability to emotional disorders than as a distinct psychiatric disorder in its own right. The authors caution that their findings require replication on other samples, including inpatients, before being generally accepted.

With respect to environmental risk factors, there is also evidence

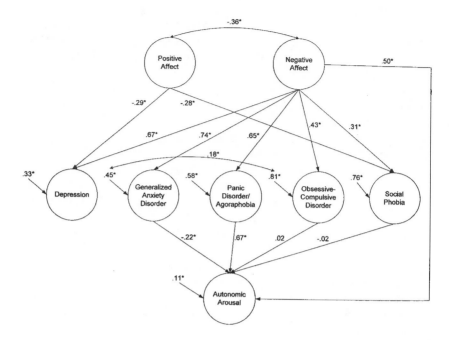

FIGURE 9.1. Completely standardized solution of Brown et al.'s hypothesized structural model—revised. *$p < .01$. From Brown, Chorpita, and Barlow (1998). Copyright 1998 by the American Psychological Association. Reprinted by permission.

of overlap between anxiety and mood disorders. Brown and Harris (1993) have shown that adverse early experiences in childhood and adolescence (including parental indifference, sexual abuse, and physical abuse) raise the risk of both depression and anxiety in adulthood. In a companion paper, Brown et al. (1993) have examined factors appearing to differentiate anxiety and depression. Whereas depression is more closely linked to loss in adulthood as a whole and is more susceptible to deficiencies in social support, anxiety appears more closely linked with early adverse experiences. The authors acknowledge that the onset of both conditions is often provoked by a recent threatening event, interpreted as a "loss" in depression and a "danger" in anxiety.

Finally, on the basis of the common response of a variety of disorders to antidepressant medication, Hudson and Pope (1990) have proposed that major depression, bulimia nervosa, panic disorder, OCD, attention-deficit/hyperactivity disorder (ADHD), cataplexy, migraine, and irritable bowel syndrome share a pathophysiological abnormality. They call this group "affective spectrum disorders" and suggest that if a shared abnormality could be demonstrated, this proposed group would emerge as one of the most prevalent disorder categories affecting humankind.

GENETIC AND CONSTITUTIONAL FACTORS

With the recent studies of large samples of twins, such as the Virginia Twin Registry (females) (Kendler, Neale, Kessler, Heath, & Eaves, 1992a, 1992b, 1992c, 1993) and the Vietnam Era Twin Registry (males) (Lyons et al., 1998), genetic researchers are now beginning to distinguish the relative contributions of genetic and environmental factors to a variety of mental disorders. Genetic factors have been shown to play a significant role in major depression, GAD, agoraphobia, social phobia, specific phobia, and OCD, as well as in alcoholism and bulimia nervosa. In all these studies, despite significant heritability (the amount of the variance due to genetic factors is frequently in the range of 30–50%), unique or nonshared factors in the environment also emerge as etiologically important. These include exposure to stressors on an individual basis, as well as unique aspects of family relationships that are different for each family member. (Shared-environmental or familial-environmental factors, by contrast, are factors in the environment that all family members experience.)

Kendler, Kessler, et al. (1995) prospectively assessed factors related to onset of major depression in twins, and concluded that genetic factors increase the sensitivity of individuals to the depression-inducing effect of stressful life events. This notion is highly consistent with Kagan's work on inhibition as described in Chapter 3, and with the theories of Eysenck, Strelau, Gray, and Cloninger that an increased reactivity or neuroticism underlies these disorders. This view is further supported in an earlier report on the same population by Kendler, Neale, et al. (1993) of a common genetic liability to the personality trait of neuroticism and depression; with Goodyer, Ashby, Altham, Vize, and Cooper's (1993) finding that negative emotionality was the only temperamental predictor of depression, particularly (but not exclusively) in girls, and in siblings of depressed probands (Kelvin, Goodyer, & Altham, 1996); with Hirschfeld et al.'s (1989) report that lowered emotional strength and resiliency differentiated at-risk subjects who developed depression from those who did not; and with a study on personality traits linked to mental disorders, in which stress reaction and negative emotionality were both linked to anxiety and mood disorders (Krueger, Caspi, Moffitt, Silva, & McGee, 1996). It is also consistent with Hudson and Pope's (1990) notion of a common underlying pathophysiology in depression, several anxiety disorders, and several other disorders. Animal studies of a genetically based increased reactivity, and Suomi's (1991a, 1991b) work on animal models of depression (see below), are also consistent with the notion of an increased sensitivity to environmental events as a significant factor in the development of anxious and depressive behavior.

Given the arguments described earlier for a common factor in depression and the anxiety disorders, I propose that the shared genetic liability in all these disorders is a sensitivity to environmental stress. I also argue that this vulnerability may arise as well from environmental factors. Before examining the more specific studies of genetic factors in anxiety and depression, I briefly review the animal studies and studies on childhood inhibition suggesting that reactivity to environmental stressors is a vulnerability factor in depression and anxiety.

Stress Reactivity in Depression and Anxiety

Animal Studies

Suomi (1991a, 1991b) reviews his own and others' work with rhesus monkeys studied longitudinally and provides a useful discussion of monkey–human behavioral similarities, especially with respect to adolescent depression. Mother–offspring social separation, especially at the time of maternal mating, has been used to explore individual differences to this common stressor. All infants and juveniles respond to this separation with behavioral agitation, consisting of increases in locomotor activity and "coo" vocalizations, as well as reductions in exploratory and play behavior. They also exhibit physiological arousal characterized by elevations in adrenocorticotropic hormone (ACTH), cortisol, and heart rate, as well as increased norepinephrine (NE) turnover. Whereas most monkeys gradually show a decrease in signs of distress, some individuals in the monkey colony display more intense and prolonged reactions to this stress. Some of these monkeys become withdrawn and display huddling behavior, which Suomi likens to depression. When these offspring are reunited with their mothers, these intense behavioral and physiological reactions diminish, although they may remain above preseparation levels for some time. These individual reactions are consistent over time, in that a monkey displaying increased reactivity as an infant is also likely to react similarly as a juvenile and as an adult.

Adolescent monkeys display a somewhat different behavioral pattern of reaction to the stress of separation. Although they display behavioral agitation, manifested as stereotypic motor activity and some aggression, they do not typically vocalize their distress or huddle. However, in contrast to younger and older subjects, they show persistent elevations of the serotonin (5-HT) metabolite 5-hydroxyindoleacetic acid (5-HIAA) in cerebrospinal fluid (CSF). As with the younger subjects, these behavioral and physiological reactions in some individuals are more prolonged and intense; these are the same individuals who as infants and juveniles displayed this enhanced reactivity.

The heritability of this enhanced reactivity has been demonstrated through selective breeding and cross-fostering. The reactivity can be reversed by prior treatment with antidepressant medication. Suomi has compared these reactive monkeys to Kagan's inhibited children, as both display fearful or anxious reactions in novel or challenging situations. However, in familiar, stable circumstances, the reactive monkeys cannot be distinguished from other members of the troop. Suomi points out that although these differences are clearly heritable, such intense reactions to separation can also be influenced by rearing situations (which are discussed in greater detail later in this chapter).

Human Studies

As indicated in Chapter 3, the trait of inhibition has been linked to the development of anxiety disorders. Inhibited children are slow to approach strange or novel situations, vocalize less in new social situations, and are more inclined to be fearful and to withdraw in novel or unfamiliar circumstances. These children also display greater physiological reactivity and have been presumed by Kagan et al. (1984) to have a lower threshold for limbic arousal. As noted above, these children have been compared to the reactive monkeys described by Suomi (1991a, 1991b).

Rosenbaum, Biederman, and collaborators have demonstrated that children of parents with panic disorder, agoraphobia, and depression have high rates of inhibition; that parents of inhibited children have elevated levels of anxiety disorders; that children with behavioral inhibition are more likely to develop an anxiety disorder than are noninhibited children (Biederman et al., 1990) and that inhibited children whose parents have an anxiety disorder are at the highest risk of developing an anxiety disorder (Rosenbaum et al., 1992). In a 3-year follow-up of the initial samples, Biederman et al. (1993) showed that inhibited children were more likely than noninhibited children to develop multiple (four or more) psychiatric disorders, multiple (two or more) anxiety disorders, avoidant disorder of childhood, separation anxiety disorder, and agoraphobia. Among inhibited children, the risk for developing multiple anxiety disorders and avoidant disorder increased markedly from baseline. Curiously (I attempt to integrate this below), inhibited children also developed more oppositional defiant disorder over this follow-up period than did the noninhibited children. Moreover, Hirshfeld et al. (1992) demonstrated that those children who continued to manifest the trait of inhibition over the ages from 4 to 7½ years were most vulnerable to developing multiple anxiety disorders. Their parents also had higher rates of multiple childhood anxiety disorders and of continuing anxiety disorder. Lastly, parents of children with behavioral inhibition and anxiety had higher rates of multiple anxiety disorders than did parents of children with behavioral inhibition only or parents of children with neither behavioral inhibition nor anxiety (Rosenbaum et al., 1992).

Although we can only speculate on the relationship among reactivity, inhibition, and neuroticism, it would appear that increased reactivity to stress, as measured by any of these concepts, plays a role in the development of anxiety disorders. The fact that children with inhibition whose parents also have an anxiety disorder are at the highest risk suggests the importance of either additional genetic or psychosocial factors.

Time and Interaction Effects for Genetic Factors

Although the data with respect to genetic factors playing a part in the development or vulnerability to developing an internalizing disorder are clear, studies are now demonstrating that the patterning or interaction of genetic and environmental factors may vary with type of disorder, time of onset, and stability or change of disorder over time. In a study examining genetic contributions to continuity, change, and co-occurrence of antisocial versus depressive symptoms in adolescence, O'Connor, Neiderhiser, Reiss, Hetherington, and Plomin (1998) found that the stability of both antisocial and depressive symptoms was largely accounted for by genetic factors. Genetic factors also accounted for change in antisocial but not depressive symptoms between waves of measurement. The genetic factors that accounted for change in antisocial symptoms differed from those that predicted antisocial symptoms in the first wave. The co-occurrence of antisocial and depressive symptoms was also mediated in part by genetic factors. As in other studies, these authors found that nonshared-environmental factors (i.e., factors unique to the individual) contributed significantly to the stability of antisocial and depressive symptoms. Although shared-environmental effects were moderately important in antisocial behavior, they were relatively unimportant (especially in comparison to nonshared-environmental effects) in depression.

Another study shows that the relative importance of genetic and environmental factors affecting disorders in childhood or adolescence may differ. Although Thapar and McGuffin (1994) found significant genetic effects in predicting depressive symptoms for their whole sample (twin pairs aged 8 to 16), when their sample was divided into younger and older groups, shared-environmental factors emerged as more important in explaining depressive symptoms (according to parental report) in the 8-to-11 age group. Eley, Deater-Deckard, Fombonne, Fulker, and Plomin (1998) used data from the Colorado Adoption Project study depressive symptoms in middle childhood; they found negligible heritability, modest shared environment and substantial nonshared-environmental effects for both sibling adoption and parent–offspring designs. The Eley et al. study used both parent and child reports of depressive symptoms when children were ages 9, 10, 11, and 12. These results contrast with the findings of significant heritability in twin studies. Although these studies suggest a diminished role for genetic factors in childhood disorder, they may also reflect reporting differences between childhood and adolescence, as well as discrepancies between child and parent reports of symptoms. They do, however, point to the complex nature of the genetic–environmental interaction, especially when developmental changes are considered.

In an elegant analysis of the Virginia Twin Registry data, Kendler, Walters, et al. (1995) tested various etiological models combining common and disorder-specific genetic, familial-environmental, and unique-environmental (individual-specific) factors for six major psychiatric disorders in women: phobia, GAD, panic disorder, bulimia nervosa, major depression, and alcoholism. (See Figure 9.2.) The best-fitting model included two genetic factors common to more than one disorder, the first of which loaded heavily on phobia, panic disorder, and bulimia, and the second of which loaded heavily on GAD and major depression. Disorder-specific genetic factors were found for GAD (modest) and alcoholism (heavy). A common familial-environmental factor was found for several disorders, but was most important for bulimia. The common unique-environmental factor was very important in GAD and major depression; important, but to a lesser degree, in phobia, panic disorder, and alcoholism; and unimportant in bulimia. Disorder-specific unique-environmental loadings were relatively high in each disorder.

In a similar modeling of phobias in their sample (female), Kendler et al. (1992b) found a strong effect of the common individual-specific

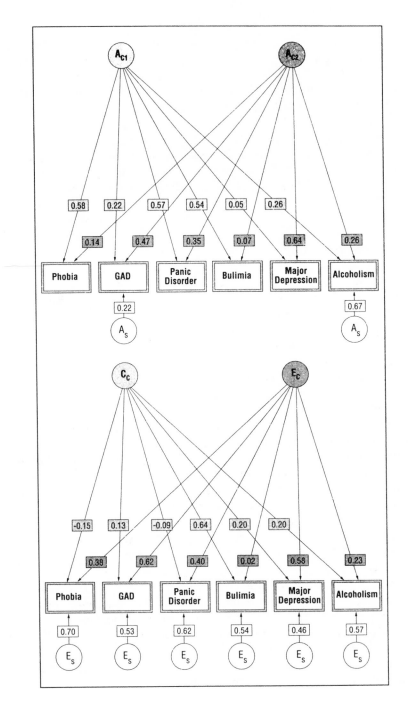

environmental factor in agoraphobia and social phobia, whereas disorder-specific experiences were particularly important in simple phobia (now known as specific phobia); important, but to a lesser extent, in social phobia; and unimportant in agoraphobia. Genetic factors common to all the phobias were most important in animal phobia and least important in agoraphobia. The authors concluded that simple phobia is the result of a modest genetic vulnerability interacting with exposure to phobia-specific traumatic events in childhood. In contrast, agoraphobia and social phobia emerge from the joint effect of a slightly stronger genetic influence (more disorder-specific than common to all phobias) and nonspecific environmental experiences (Kendler et al., 1992b).

Using the same population, Silberg et al. (1990) assessed the etiological bases of self-reported depressive symptoms. They concluded that the most useful model contained one genetic factor, one shared-environmental factor, and four unique-environmental factors. The four unique-environmental factors accounted for the largest proportion of the variance in symptom report and had factor loadings similar to the four factors that emerged from the phenotypic analysis of the scale: a "depressed affect" factor, a "positive affect" factor, a "somatization" factor, and an "interpersonal sensitivity" factor. Again, this study suggests that the genetic factor involved in depression (in common with other disorders) may be vulnerability to stress, whereas the unique-environmental factors may be what contribute the specifics to symptom reporting and presumably to disorders. The shared-environmental factor could be willingness to report symptoms or openness to discussion of feelings.

This type of modeling, which is now being applied to the new

FIGURE 9.2. *Top:* Parameter estimates from the best-fitting multivariate twin model for the genetic common and disorder-specific factors. The model contains two additive genetic common factors (A_{C1} and A_{C2}), which load most strongly on phobia and panic disorder and on generalized anxiety disorder (GAD) and major depression, respectively. Disorder-specific additive genes (A_s) are present for only two disorders, GAD and alcoholism. *Bottom:* Parameter estimates from the best-fitting multivariate twin model for the environmental common and disorder-specific factors. The model contains one familial-environmental common factor (C_C) and one individual-specific or unique-environmental common factor (E_C). No disorder-specific familial-environmental loadings were obtained, whereas every disorder had disorder-specific unique-environmental loadings (E_S). Reprinted from Kendler, Walters, Neale, Kessler, Heath, and Eaves (1995). Copyright 1995 by the American Medical Association. Reprinted by permission.

generation of twin studies, allows us to capture the complexity related to the interaction of common and disorder-specific genetic and environmental risk factors. What such studies indicate is that both common and disorder-specific genetic and environmental factors need to be understood more fully in the development of each disorder. As I have argued above, I believe that the common genetic liability in the internalizing disorders is increased sensitivity to environmental stressors. The common individual-specific environmental factor is most likely a combination of the impact of early experiences conditioning the individual's responses to stress. This could be conceptualized as the development of internal working models and coping responses. An individual who is more vulnerable to reacting physiologically with a heightened stress response (whether this vulnerability has a genetic or an environmental basis) will be more likely to develop a disorder. How that disorder develops, however, depends on both genetic (common and disorder-specific) and environmental (some shared with other family members, but largely unique to the individual) factors and may be different at different developmental stages. Because not all vulnerable individuals exposed to stressors develop disorders, we need to examine other factors that will interact to increase or decrease the likelihood of the development of an anxiety or mood disorder.

Integrating Genetic and Constitutional Factors with Other Factors

Kendler, Kessler, Neale, Heath, and Eaves (1993) have delineated the major risk factors that need to be incorporated into a model to explain the development of an episode of major depression in the women being followed in the Virginia Twin Registry. These are "traumatic experiences," "genetic factors," "temperament," and "interpersonal relations." The best-fitting model using these variables explained 50% of the variance. Genetic effects were both direct (60%) and indirect (40%), through increased risk for prior episodes of depression, increased risk for recent stressful life events, higher levels of neuroticism, and greater risk for lifetime traumas. Early childhood factors such as parental warmth operated indirectly through reduced risk of prior depressive episodes; lower levels of recent difficulties, of lifetime traumas, and of neuroticism; and higher levels of social support. Childhood parental loss had similar indirect effects but in the opposite direction. Similarly, lifetime history of traumas had no direct effect, but operated indirectly through its effect on prior depressive episodes and on higher numbers of recent stressful events and recent difficulties. Neuroticism, like genetic factors, had a large direct effect and an indirect effect on liability to prior depressive episodes, as well as an inverse relationship with social support. Social support exerted its modest effect directly to reduce the likelihood of becoming depressed. The impact of stressful life events was both strong and direct.

The finding that genetic factors can predict both lifetime traumas and recent stressful life events, albeit modestly, has informed Kendler and colleagues' notion of "genetic control of exposure to the environment." What is also important in this work is the finding that early adverse experience affects the vulnerability to depression through several of the same mechanisms that genetic factors do—that is, increased likelihood of neuroticism and recent difficulties. This study provides an appropriate introduction to the examination of the nongenetic factors relevant in anxiety and depression, and to the importance of defining the paths through which this complex array of factors operates.

PSYCHOSOCIAL FACTORS

Adverse Early Experiences

As mentioned above, Brown and Harris (1993) showed clearly that adverse early experiences, such as parental indifference and sexual and physical abuse, predisposed women to the development of anxiety (excluding mild agoraphobia and simple phobia) and depressive disorders in adulthood. (See also Weiss, Longhurst, & Mazure, 1999.) Although early loss of mother was a predictor of later difficulties, its impact was washed out when the effect of childhood adversity was considered. (This sample consisted of inner-city working-class and single women.) This led Brown and Harris to the conclusion, noted earlier in several other studies, that the important factors in loss of a parent are the adverse circumstances accompanying that loss.

In contrast, Kendler et al. (1992c), in an analysis of the larger and less at-risk sample in the Virginia Twin Registry, concluded that early parental loss (before age 17) was related to depression, GAD, panic disorder, and phobias, but not to eating disorders. There were disorder-specific differences with respect to whether the loss was due to death or separation. Depression and GAD were related to history of parental separation but not death, in contrast to panic disorder which was strongly related to death and separation and phobias (which were associated with parental death only). These findings refute the earlier theory that depression is more strongly related to loss than is anxiety. They also suggest that different experiences may have differential impacts in leading to psychopathology.

Although work to elucidate the different psychosocial pathways to the various disorders is just beginning and is generally less well developed in the study of anxiety than it is in depression, Harris et al. (1987) demonstrated that for some women inadequate replacement care following the loss of their mothers related to premarital pregnancies and a subsequent series of events, including remaining in a lower socioeconomic status (SES) and having less intimate and dependable relationships. Although low SES has been a consistent finding relating to higher rates of disorder generally, these authors could show that even within a single SES level, significant variables contributed to the likelihood of psychopathology. Obviously, this pattern was only applicable to some situations and did not apply to middle-class women (where low parental care and early marriage were predictors of depression); however, it illustrates the cascade of factors that tends to develop once an individual's life begins to go off track. This will be a recurring theme.

Current Interpersonal Difficulties

The issue of interpersonal difficulties has emerged in most of the recent studies as being relevant to onset or recurrence of depression (Kendler, Kessler, et al., 1993; Brown et al., 1993; Monck, Graham, Richman, & Dobbs, 1994). In attempting to examine the impact of current adverse experience as opposed to early adverse experience, Brown et al. (1993) reported that depression in a sample of inner-city women was often linked to major loss in adulthood as a whole and particularly to shortcomings in social support, in contrast to anxiety, where early adverse experiences were more critical. In the Kendler, Kessler, et al. (1993) study, interpersonal relations emerged as a strong predictor of major depression. This included parental warmth, social support, and recent difficulties (which the authors noted were largely, although not entirely, interpersonal in nature).

In a study of adolescent depression, Lewinsohn et al. (1994) reported that although conflict with parents was not associated with being depressed, it was associated with prediction of subsequent depression. Monck et al. (1994), in examining factors related to anxiety and depression in a community sample of adolescent girls, found that maternal distress level and the quality of a mother's marriage were independently associated with the presence of both disorders. They also found that the impact of life events was no longer significant when the maternal distress level and marital quality factors were considered. Because factors such as childhood adversity may also be linked to difficulties such as parental psychopathology, marital discord, and divorce, it may be hard to separate out the specific etiological roles of these overlapping factors (Young, Abelson, Curtis, & Nesse, 1997).

However, Brown and Moran (1994), in a population survey of 404 working-class mothers living in an inner-city area of London, found that both childhood adversity and current interpersonal difficulties predicted chronicity of depression. In addition, because they found that childhood adversity also increased the likelihood of interpersonal difficulties, they did a small qualitative study to explore possible paths for these connections. As in studies by others, they found that women with adverse early experiences had a long history of poor support and of difficulty in acquiring or maintaining close relationships; some were isolated, and some who had close ties were involved with undependable persons. These findings about the predictive validity of childhood adversity and current interpersonal difficulties on chronicity of depression in women were replicated in a population of psychiatric patients by Brown, Harris, Hepworth, and Robinson (1994).

Brown et al. (1990) studied another sample of working- and lower-middle-class women and found that depression tended to cluster in a small group of these women, who had both a negative environmental factor (negative interaction with husband or child, or lack of a confiding relationship for single mothers) and a negative psychological factor (negative self-evaluation or chronic subclinical depression). These same background risk factors increased the likelihood that a woman would experience a stressful life event related to the onset of a depressive episode.

In contrast to the studies cited above, Murray, Cox, Chapman, and Jones (1995) found that women with postnatal depression were distinguished from women with nonpostnatal depression by the presence of a poor relationship with their own mothers and not by the other indices of social adversity noted above. They interpreted their findings as evidence that postnatal depression is related to the acute biopsychosocial stress of having a new family member, as opposed to longer-term social adversity.

However one interprets the most relevant etiological factors, on the whole these studies suggest the likelihood that adversity begets adversity and that once lives start going off track, they tend to continue doing so. I believe that what is most important in these adverse experiences is conflict in important relationships, especially conflict that an individual perceives as impossible to resolve or escape. This belief is supported by the literature on expressed emotion in internalizing disorders. Although this literature is discussed more fully in Chapter 4, in summary there is good evidence that a high level of expressed emotion, particularly perceived criticism, is a factor in both onset and maintenance of both internalizing and externalizing disorders (Kavanagh, 1992; Stubbe et al., 1993; Vostanis et al., 1994). Taken together, these studies make it plain that interpersonal relationships, involving issues of conflict and support, need to be considered in building a model to explain these disorders.

Recent Stressful Life Events

Recent life events, particularly situations threatening loss in depression and danger in anxiety, were predictors in the Brown et al. (1993) study. This finding replicates much earlier work, and as noted above, "traumatic experiences" constituted one of the four factors in the model proposed by Kendler, Kessler, et al. (1993) for onset of depression in the Virginia Twin registry study. Pursuing their emphasis on the meaning of stressful life events to the individual, Brown and Moran (1998) report that situations interpreted as entrapment or failure are as salient as loss in the onset of depression. Moreover, when such events occur in a situation with other risk factors (e.g., being unsupported), the risk for depression increases significantly. This notion that the meaning of an event reinforces an individual's sense of chronic demoralization or low self-esteem may be very relevant to the sequence proposed below (in which events are able to elicit a mood that triggers a latent schema and leads to a spiraling into affect dysregulation). However, supportive family relationships may play an important stress-moderating role, as in the adolescent sample studied by Monck et al. (1994), where the effect of life events was overshadowed by a mother's level of distress and the quality of her spousal relationship.

Both the Brown et al. and Kendler et al. studies examined major depression. It is reasonable to assume that the same factors—perhaps in less intense forms, or combined with other factors that ameliorate the depressive reaction—are important in less severe forms of depression. There is some evidence that environmental as opposed to genetic factors may be relatively more important in less severe and in late-onset forms of depression (Lyons et al., 1998).

Time and Interaction Effects for Psychosocial Factors

Although life events and other psychosocial stressors have been identified as etiologically relevant in most studies, an emerging literature has also demonstrated that psychosocial stressors appear to be more important in the first episode of illness than they do in subsequent episodes. Post (1992) reviews this literature and provides a compelling argument that stress-induced brain changes sensitize the individual in such a way that subsequent episodes can be triggered by a relatively minor event. This explains the findings of Kendler, Kessler, et al. (1993) that factors such as early childhood adversity, history of traumas, and history of neuroticism exerted a largely indirect effect through their impact on the risk of prior depressive episodes. Post (1992) describes both induction of chemical changes (through intracellular second- and third-messenger systems, which affect a variety of proteins and neurotransmitters) and neuroanatomical changes (such as changes in synaptic number and density). The importance of these findings for early intervention and treatment of disorders is obvious, but they also point to the importance of preventing early adverse experiences in childhood, as the sensitizing effects of these early experiences appear to provoke a chain of difficulties at the level of brain development as well as at an interpersonal level.

Animal Studies of Psychosocial Factors

This notion that sensitivity can develop after exposure to adverse or stressful events is illustrated in the animal literature. The studies referred to in Chapter 4, show that exposure to atypical rearing situations (surrogate and peer), as well as exposure to mothers experiencing the stress of variable as opposed to secure food supply, sensitize the offspring and make them more stress-reactive (Suomi, 1991a, 1991b, 1995). Follow-up of the subjects exposed to these atypical situations suggests that these effects are long-lasting (Kraemer et al., 1989; Coplan et al., 1998). Coplan, Rosenblum, and Gorman (1995) have proposed that the stress experienced by infant primates whose mothers are exposed to a variable foraging situation may be a good model of anxiety. They base their speculation on the similarity and durability of physiological responses displayed by these offspring monkeys.

The psychosocial factors discussed above—early adversity, current interpersonal difficulties, and recent stressful life events—are broad general factors that need to be more fully addressed and placed in the context of the developing individual. To do so, we need to examine those aspects of the caregiving relationship that may be encompassed under the rubric of early adverse experience, and to relate those issues to the other processes that may interfere with the development of optimal affect regulation.

Relating Familial Psychosocial Factors to Affect Dysregulation

Attachment and the Formation of Internal Working Models

Chapter 4 discusses the notion of the attachment system as a system of affect regulation. The literature reviewed there suggests that insecure attachment in general is a vulnerability factor leading to psychopathology. Although some authors have attempted to argue for specific relationships between avoidant attachment and externalizing disorders, the support for such a specific connection is weak. (See Goldberg, 1997 for a discussion.) A stronger relationship appears to exist for a relationship between a more extreme level of insecurity, disorganized attachment (especially when this is connected with abuse), and later psychopathology. However it is too soon to conclude that even this specific attachment pattern leads to psychopathology: Disorganized attachment is more likely to occur in families with a high number of risk factors, raising issues about the specificity of any one factor versus the combined effects of multiple risk factors. Nevertheless, the early adverse experiences reported in both the Brown and Harris (1993) and Kendler, Kessler, et al. (1993) studies included parental indifference or lack of warmth (as well as both physical and sexual abuse); the perception of parental indifference or lack of warmth is consistent with parental qualities related to avoidant attachment. In more extreme situations, such as maternal depression, marital discord, and abuse, the relative unavailability of the mother or hostility directed at the child may be more intense producing more disorganized or disrupted attachment patterns (Cummings & Davies, 1994).

    In any case, insecure attachment predisposes the developing individual to less comfort with affect, and increases the likelihood that defensive processes will be necessary to sustain the child's relationship with the caregiver. As indicated in Chapter 2, the resort to such defensive processes as withdrawal and oppositionality is likely to make the child appear more difficult in the eyes of the parent (Bates et al., 1985).

Threat-Oriented Family Systems

Bugental (1992) has articulated a model of "threat-oriented family systems," which helps to explain how troubled parent–child interactions may proceed at a cognitive or appraisal level for the parent (see Chapter 4 for a full description). As Chapter 4 notes, this conflicted parent–child relationship may contribute to depression in the parent (Brown et al., 1990), as well as to both internalizing and externalizing disorders in the child (Messer & Gross, 1995; Ge et al., 1996). Family studies of internalizing disorders show that the parents of children who develop internalizing disorders are more likely themselves to have or have had an internalizing disorder than are controls (Last, Hersen, Kazdin, Francis, & Grubb, 1987; Kovacs & Devlin, 1998; Harrington et al., 1997). This predisposes them to the development of threat-oriented schemata and a greater likelihood of automatic reactions to situations they perceive as uncontrollable. If a parent's own internalizing disorder is depression (see below), there is a greater likelihood of insecure attachment to the child, which may predispose the child to more "difficultness" (Cummings & Davies, 1994).

The types of interactions described by Bugental (1992) are commonly seen in the children and families presenting to anxiety disorder clinics. Her formulation also provides a parsimonious way of understanding the comorbidity (particularly of internalizing with externalizing disorders) seen in all childhood disorders (Kovacs & Devlin, 1998). Although children may ultimately be referred for an anxiety disorder, they commonly have comorbid disruptive behaviors (typically more oppositional behaviors than conduct problems) that nearly always precede the onset of the overt anxiety disorder. Whether or not their oppositional behaviors meet formal criteria for a disorder, they are perceived by their parents as sensitive, difficult, and frequently noncompliant. These parental perceptions may arise from the sensitivity and stress reactivity of the inhibited children, from the inhibited children's tendency to withdraw from and to want to control situations of uncertainty or from the developing oppositionality that may arise when the children feel that the parents are less than optimally available (as in maternal depression or stress).

A study by Zahn-Waxler et al. (1990) showed that dysregulated aggression (out-of-control child behavior) at age 2 (which can be presumed to be a consequence of the types of interactions described by Bugental) predicted aggressive behavior at age 5 and child report of internalizing difficulties at age 6. Bugental's formulation is also highly consistent with the findings noted in Chapter 4 concerning the high levels of expressed emotion in both internalizing and externalizing disorders of childhood. Ge et al. (1996), who reported on a longitudinal study of adolescents followed from 7th to 10th grade, found that elevated levels of parental hostility, reduced warmth, and problematic disciplinary skills in the earlier grades predicted both depression and conduct problems in 10th grade. Adolescents with comorbid depression and conduct disorder had parents who scored in the most extreme direction. Messer and Gross (1995), in a small but intensive study of 10 families with a depressed child compared to 10 with a control child, found that depressed children and their parents perceived their lives as more stressful and their parenting practices as more negative than controls did. Family interaction in the families with a depressed child was observed to be less rewarding, more aversive, and more disengaged than in the control families. Kendziora, and O'Leary (1993), in a review of parenting in childhood disorders, concluded that "dysfunctional parenting" was a general factor across various disorders. This factor included coercive interactions between parent and child and ineffective parental discipline—again, a pattern consistent with Bugental's theory.

Maternal Depression

Maternal depression has been related to a variety of childhood psychopathologies (Downey & Coyne, 1990; Wickramaratne & Weissman, 1998). Cummings and Davies (1994) and Beardslee, Versage, and Gladstone (1998) provide recent reviews of this literature. Although maternal depression may have some specificity with respect to the development of childhood depression, there is also a large effect on child maladjustment generally (Beardslee et al., 1998; Downey & Coyne, 1990). These more general problems in adjustment are not qualitatively different from those in offspring of mothers with physical illness, mothers with another (nondepressive) psychiatric condition, or mothers who are under stress. Because there is a less well-developed literature on these more general maternal situations than on maternal depression, I describe the findings for children of depressed mothers here; I would speculate, however, that many of these findings could also apply to children whose mothers are psychologically unavailable for any reason.

Downey and Coyne's (1990) review describes depressed mothers as being less active, showing more constricted affect, using less effortful control strategies, and showing considerable hostility and negativity. Although the genetic link has been established, the *processes* by which maternal depression (presumably through some of these attributes) exerts an effect on the development of child psychopathology, both internalizing and externalizing, are less well understood. Because there is a strong likelihood that an individual who develops an internalizing disorder has, or has had, a parent with an internalizing disorder, and because a substantial portion of the variance in predicting the development of a disorder is explained by nongenetic factors, it is important to examine the ways by which maternal depression may affect vulnerability (nongenetic) to such disorders.

Much of the work on the effect of postpartum depression on the developing child has been carried out by developmental researchers. Field (1995), one of the leading researchers in this area, reports that infants of depressed mothers whose depression continues beyond the infants' sixth month show depressed behavior, decreased cognitive abilities, and decreased growth (weight) at 1 year, as well as increased behavior problems as preschoolers. If a mother's depression clears before an infant's sixth month, there appears to be no significant effect on the infant's behavior. In situations in which infants of depressed mothers are exposed to nondepressed adults, their behavior continues to be abnormal. Moreover, these infants do not react to the still-face paradigm (see Chapter 4), which is very distressing for infants of nondepressed mothers. Field interprets this lack of distress on the part of infants of depressed mothers as due to conditioning, since in this test situation the facial affect of the depressed mothers does not appear to be significantly different from their normal expression. Field also reports that infants of depressed mothers, as newborns, display less orientation to inanimate stimuli, less robustness, increased levels of indeterminate sleep, and higher levels of plasma NE. At 6 months they show lower vagal tone and a pattern of right frontal asymmetry similar to that often found in depressed adults and in inhibited children. Depressed mothers also rate their infants as higher in negative affect, and themselves as less depressed, on rating scales than do independent examiners. This suggests a biased cognitive perception of themselves in relationship to their infants.

Lyons-Ruth (1992) describes her longitudinal study of depressed mother–infant dyads. Security of attachment predicted strongly to later problem behavior with disorganized attachment correlating particularly with hostile–aggressive behavior in kindergarten. As these behaviors also predict to later mood disorders, this provides one possible mediating mechanism. Cummings and Davies (1994) discuss maternal depression and child development more broadly, attempting to ascertain the processes by which a mother's affective state influences a child's behavior. They note that maternal depression is associated with higher rates of parental negativity, distance, and coldness, and with increased parent–child conflict as well as increased marital conflict. Each of these factors has been shown to have an impact on the development of externalizing and internalizing disorders in childhood. They discuss several pathways through which these factors might operate, but do assume that there will be interactions among many of these factors.

One proposed pathway is through increasing levels of arousal in the child and concomitant dysregulation of emotions and behavior. Cummings and Davies see this pathway as arising from the attachment-related difficulties described above. In addition, they posit modeling and reinforcement as ways in which the developing child learns about feelings and their display. Lastly, they propose that the child's internal working models, arising out of the negative parent–child interaction, predispose the child to a negative self-view and attributions about the self in relationship to others that may lead to long-lasting interpersonal difficulties. Again, these various paths are clearly not mutually exclusive, and it is likely that they all operate to a greater or lesser extent in affecting the development of children with a depressed parent.

Hammen (Hammen, Burge, & Stansbury, 1990; Hammen, 1992) has proposed that similar interactional difficulties between depressed parents and vulnerable children can perpetuate generations of depression. She and her coworkers tested her model in a follow-up study of children of mothers with recurrent unipolar depression or bipolar disorder, chronic medical illness, or no disorder. The results supported her thesis that both maternal functioning and child characteristics affected child outcomes. In addition, however, there was a mutually reinforcing negative relationship between parent and child, such that a child's behavior affected a mother's functioning and vice versa. These results applied regardless of diagnostic status, being found in medically ill and highly stressed normal women (Hammen et al., 1990; Hammen, 1992).

Thus far, what can we conclude about the impact of insecure attachment, threat-oriented family systems, and a depressed parent on a developing child, particularly as it relates to the child's capacity to develop adaptive ways of regulating affect? I think it is reasonable to surmise that an insecure attachment relationship predisposes the child to raised levels of negative affect, but less comfort with the experience and expression of negative affect. This creates an increased likelihood that the child will use oppositionality as a way of manifesting his or her discomfort and will be perceived by the parent as difficult. With a highly threat-oriented parent, this is likely to lead to a conflicted parent–child relationship and to inconsistent and often coercive discipline. The result will be that the child perceives the parent as hostile and critical, and the parent perceives the child as noncompliant. The internal working models or schemata that the child develops will incorporate a sense of self as insecure in the relationship with the parent, as bad, or as rejected (depending in part on the intensity of the parent's negative affect), and a sense of the parent as uncaring. In my clinical work with anxious children and their families, most of these parents do not present as uncaring, but as confused and overwhelmed by their children's difficult behavior. However, as this conflicted pattern of interaction continues, and especially when it includes high levels of expressed emotion, it is easy to see how the child can develop more stable perceptions of the parent as uncaring (especially if the parent is extremely emotionally preoccupied) and controlling (the "affectionless control" that has emerged in the retrospective accounts of depressed adults).

It is important to point out that this internalized schema may be counterbalanced by a more positive relationship with the other parent or caregiver, thus muting the impact of the more negative relationship (Mathijssen, Koot, Verhulst, De Bruyn, & Oud, 1998). However, the

child enmeshed in a conflicted relationship with his or her main caregiver will have had reduced opportunities to discuss feelings, to develop an awareness of how to tolerate negative affect, and to learn how
to cope with frustration. The development of adaptive coping strategies will undoubtedly be affected by these interpersonal conflicts.

Coping

Although studies of coping in young children are relatively rare, we
can surmise that children at risk for the development of the internalizing disorders will begin to develop coping strategies known to be associated with these disorders in adolescents and adults. The most common attachment pattern associated with lack of warmth or rejection is
that of avoidance. Avoidance or withdrawal is also the most common
reaction displayed by inhibited or reactive children in situations of
novelty or uncertainty.

Cassidy and Kobak (1988) provide an interesting discussion of the
defensive processes related to an avoidant attachment style. Drawing
from Bowlby's theoretical formulations, these authors discuss avoidance as a defensive strategy in response to parental rejection. Based on
studies showing stability of avoidant attachment from infancy into
middle childhood, they suggest that this defensive style will remain a
part of personality functioning for some children and adults. This
avoidant relationship style is initially adaptive in the parent–child relationship, as it is presumed to prevent the arousal related to the parent's
unresponsiveness to the infant's needs, while at the same time it allows
the infant to stay connected to the parent. Presumably, what the young
child learns in these interactions is that negative affect expression is
not acceptable and that strategies are needed to retain connection to
the caregiver without risking alienation through expressions of anger.
These interactions gradually become elaborated into working models,
which, because they operate at a largely unconscious level, may be
more resistant to change. Cassidy and Kobak regard the avoidant infant's strategy as a masking of negative affect, which may be used in
other situations to reduce conflict. They describe studies showing that
avoidant individuals repress negative affect (particularly anxiety and
anger), dismiss the importance of relationships (appearing to be highly
self-reliant), tend to idealize important relationships (including self-
perceptions as perfect), and are rated as more hostile than securely attached individuals.

Dadds, Rosenthal Gaffney, Kenardy, Oei, and Evans (1993), in a
survey of anger expression in anxious subjects, confirm the difficulty
that individuals with anxiety disorders have with internalized hostil-

ity. Although it is reasonable to presume that other forms of insecure attachment will also make individuals vulnerable to internalizing psychopathology, avoidance of negative affect is common in both anxiety and depression, along with idealizing defenses. If a child does not develop more adaptive defenses for coping with negative affect, it is likely that he or she will encounter interpersonal difficulties—initially with parents, subsequently in relationships with peers, and ultimately in adult intimate or confiding relationships.

This discussion has not yet dealt with the more extreme end of adverse early experiences, such as abuse. It is reasonable to assume that abused children are at more risk of insecure attachments in general and of disorganized ones in particular (Cicchetti & Toth, 1995). If the attachment relationship provides the basis for affect regulation, it is thus reasonable to assume that abused infants and young children are at more risk of requiring defensive strategies to maintain a connection with their caregivers. Behaviors observed in young children with disorganized attachments include mixtures of aggressive behaviors and avoidance. Presumably, these patterns may become more stable or rigid as the children learn the optimal ways of reducing arousal and protecting themselves. Dissociative defenses are common in maltreated children and can be viewed as extreme forms of avoidant behavior, protecting the children from overwhelming levels of arousal. Although at this stage we cannot presume to specify a distinct pattern of coping, we can presume that disorganized attachment patterns contribute to a lack of comfort with affect and the development of maladaptive coping strategies. We can also presume that, especially in situations of trauma or extreme abuse, memories may be laid down in ways that may remove them from conscious recall (see the discussion in Chapter 7 of the theory that amygdala-stored experiences predispose individuals to posttraumatic stress disorder [PTSD]). The brain patterns that develop as ways of coping with these internally generated affective states may also be maladaptive, making an individual's efforts to find an adaptive coping response more problematic.

Consistent with Bowlby's concept of internal working models, cognitive therapists have begun to examine how such cognitive–affective schemata might predispose individuals to the development of various disorders. Hammen et al. (1995) have proposed that in the case of depression, these internal structures sensitize an individual to information in a way that contributes to intensification of affect. These ideas are consistent with those of Ingram, Miranda, and Segal (1998), who discuss the cognitive bases of vulnerability to depression. They propose that internal working models of the self as bad are latent but accessed under stress or in situations that induce a negative mood. The

accessing of these cognitive–affective schemata leads to biased processing of information in a way that confirms the cognitive aspects of
the schemata. This intensifies the mood negativity, leading to a spiraling into a depressive episode. Their theory is supported by the findings that negative cognitive–affective schemata that are accessible in a
depressive episode are less accessible when the depression remits, but
can be accessed in remission through a variety of priming strategies
such as mood induction approaches. Accessibility of these schemata
appears to relate to greater vulnerability to developing a depressive
episode (Ingram et al., 1998).

Shirk, Boergers, Eason, and Van Horn (1998) tested out Hammen
et al.'s (1995) hypothesis in four different community samples of children and adolescents. Consistent with the predictions, they found that
depressed and dysphoric subjects responded in ways indicative of
negative interpersonal schemata and expected more affectionless control than did the nondysphoric group. In addition, they showed that
youngsters with more negative interpersonal schemata displayed selective abstraction of negative events, more rapid endorsement of negative descriptors of people in general, and rapid denial of positive
descriptors. Finally, youngsters scoring highly on the measure of negative interpersonal schemata experienced the transition to high school
as more stressful than did those with more positive schemata. The authors concluded that negative interpersonal schemata amplified the effects of stress on depressive symptoms in adolescents in their transition to high school. Similarly, Hammen et al. (1995) tested these ideas
on a community sample of women recently graduated from high
school and followed over a year. Cognitions, interpersonal events, and
their interaction predicted both depression and other symptoms.

Although we can only measure schemata or internal working
models indirectly, these studies lend support to the idea that adverse
early experience exerts its effect on the development of psychopathology through schemata that bias the individual's perception of experience and pattern of response, making the individual more sensitive to
the effects of stress. This does not exclude the likelihood that other
neural networks, both genetic and learned, may also independently affect sensitivity to stress. Although this is only speculative, we can presume that the internal working models of an individual vulnerable to
anxiety disorder are sensitized to threat or danger, as opposed to that
of an individual predisposed to depression, where sensitivity to loss or
entrapment (Brown & Moran, 1998) is more salient. Furthermore, we
can presume that such schemata are not activated unless the individual is stressed (the stress being interpreted in a manner that activates
the schemata), and that the activated schemata lead to distortions in

perception, increasing affect dysregulation, maladaptive coping behavior, and symptoms.

Although the emphasis in this discussion has been on a child's relationships within the family, which are clearly of critical importance
in early development, peer relationships become of significant importance to most children as they approach adolescence. Harter and
Whitesell (1996) tested their own model of antecedents to depression
(self-perceived competence, both peer- and parent-related and parent
and peer support) in a large sample of adolescents. Adolescents with
positive adjustment perceived themselves as being high on dimensions
of both peer and parent support. In contrast, adolescents with depressive symptoms perceived themselves as being deficient in peer-salient
domains (e.g., appearance, likeability, and athletic competence), as
well as in parent-salient domains (e.g., scholastic competence and
behavioral conduct). The possibility that these perceptions may have
become quite stable is illustrated by the fact that in the depressed
group, support from peers, parents, or both did not buffer the negative
self-perceptions. These findings are also consistent with Dodge's (1993)
model of depression, in which he suggests that depressed children will
attend to the negative aspects of new events and view themselves as
causing adversity in a way that prevents them from benefiting from efforts at support.

Factors affecting the development of adaptive coping have been
more fully discussed in Chapter 6. With respect to the internalizing
disorders, the natural tendency to withdraw can be addressed through
exposure. Kagan et al. (1987) report that those children in their follow-
up study who moved from being inhibited as toddlers to noninhibited
as school-age children had parents who encouraged exposure to the
challenging or unfamiliar situations from which these children would
naturally withdraw. N. A. Fox (personal communication, 1998) has
tested these ideas out empirically in following up samples of highly reactive children. When raised by mothers who are not overprotective,
highly reactive children become less reactive. With respect to learning
coping strategies, we can presume that children exposed to threatening
or unfamiliar situations in a supportive way learn that their discomfort
will abate as they remain in the unfamiliar situation. With time and opportunities for desensitization, their internal working models will be
modified to ones in which the unfamiliar situations can no longer automatically elicit the same arousal.

Furthermore, children whose parents understand their own affects and have developed coping strategies may be taught more formal
cognitive strategies for managing their arousal. When parents understand their children's need for "warming up" slowly, when they them-

selves feel comfortable to support and limit their children, and when they are not immersed in marital conflict or other overwhelming stresses, the negative interactions described above are unlikely to develop. However, any one or all of these factors may intervene to create conflict or tension that interferes with a child's capacity to learn about feelings and to develop adequate coping strategies. In addition, the arousal generated in any of these potential interpersonal conflicts may prevent a child from being able to deploy attention flexibly to experience relief, and so to see anything except the negative aspects of most situations.

This hypothesized failure to develop adequate strategies to manage affect is consistent with my own experience that many children seen in anxiety disorder clinics are uncomfortable discussing feelings (especially negative feelings) and do not have at their disposal a repertoire of adaptive coping responses other than emotion-focused strategies such as withdrawal. If not depressed, they are often demoralized, as are their parents; this further restricts their capacity to explore more adaptive approaches.

Children who do not develop strategies besides withdrawal for regulating their arousal become significantly disadvantaged by the time they enter school and the world of peers. They may experience intense separation anxiety at the time of school entry and have ongoing problems relating to peers. Both of these issues can become points of further conflict with parents and teachers. The more insecure such children feel, the less likely they are to expose themselves to the challenging situations that will help diminish their arousal. Kagan's (1989) observation that inhibition becomes stable by 7½ years, and Hirshfeld et al.'s (1992) finding that those children who were stably inhibited at 4 and 7½ years were most at risk for developing anxiety disorders, appear to support these assertions. Rubin, Stewart, and Coplan (1995), in a follow-up of socially withdrawn children, have found that social withdrawal correlates with felt insecurity, negative self-perceptions, dependence, and social deference. Furthermore, social withdrawal combined with negative self-appraisal predicts internalizing difficulties in late childhood and adolescence.

There appears to be considerable overlap with respect to what may be called distorted cognitions across anxiety and depression, although, as indicated by Brown et al. (1993), there is some specificity with respect to the interpretation of stressful life events (loss in depression and threat in anxiety). This apparent lack of more disorder-specific cognitions may reflect the long-standing use of emotion-focused coping strategies in subjects vulnerable to internalizing disorders, which may result from the difficulty such individuals have had throughout their growing up in finding adaptive ways of managing their arousal. As mentioned above, there is some evidence that depressed individuals have more difficulty accessing positive affect than do anxious individuals, and that depressogenic cognitions predict depressive symptoms (Lewinsohn, Hoberman, & Rosenbaum, 1988). However, we require more to account for the distinguishing features of disorders. In the Kendler, Walters, et al. (1995) study assessing the roles of common and disorder-specific genetic and environmental factors, the importance of disorder-specific genetic and environmental factors was clear. This suggests that "still to be defined" genetic factors will emerge for each disorder and will explain more completely the unique features of each disorder. This will undoubtedly explain a portion of what may be regarded as coping or defensive style. Moreover, because in all the disorders studied there was also a fairly large component explained best by a disorder-specific environmental factor, we can presume that factors such as learning and other experience that is unique to an individual will also contribute to his or her internal working models and thus influence the expression of distress as a specific disorder.

NEUROBIOLOGICAL FACTORS

Any discussion of the neurobiology of anxiety and mood disorders is necessarily speculative. Efforts to develop models have focused largely on neurotransmitters. It is now quite clear that no one neurotransmitter can be responsible for the complexity of interactions that relate to the experience, expression, and regulation of affect (Geracioti et al., 1997; Owens, 1996–1997). As I have noted in Chapter 7, current investigators have turned to neural networks comprising a number of brain areas to begin to understand how affects are stimulated, processed, interpreted, and regulated. This has led to more sophisticated examinations of the results from neuroimaging. Despite this, there are still major difficulties in interpreting the results from neuroimaging studies. In some technologies, such as positron emission tomography (PET), the level of resolution may not be fine enough to allow clear visualization of some of the structures such as the amygdala, which appear to be particularly relevant in the study of the mood and anxiety disorders. In others, many of the findings appear to be relatively nonspecific, such as frontal lobe dysfunction. The study of disorders per se is confounded by the heterogeneity of symptom manifestation, as well as by comorbidity. In studies using affect induction techniques with nonclinical populations, there is reasonable skepticism that the affect induced in a short-lived experiment is equivalent to the experience of someone who has struggled with the experience of negative affect for a period of time. Furthermore, in measuring brain function in any of these situations, it is often difficult to know what is being measured: the affect alone, the reactions that affect may induce because of associations to it, or efforts to cope with the affect—all of which will differ dramatically across individuals.

In spite of all these caveats, some general findings appear to be theoretically consistent and empirically supported. At the end I expand upon the findings on stress reactivity described in Chapter 5, since these offer a way of addressing some of the disparate findings about neurochemistry and brain imaging, and are consistent with the present theory of affect regulation.

Findings from Brain Imaging Studies

EEG techniques, such as spectral analysis, brain electrical activity mapping, and event-related potentials, all have the advantage of being noninvasive, relatively easy to carry out, and relatively inexpensive. For this reason they have been more widely used, especially in studies of children, than have the more invasive, expensive, and restraining techniques such as PET and magnetic resonance imaging (MRI). However, with EEG techniques it is difficult to ascertain exactly which brain areas are most responsible for the electrical activity, and it is not possible to measure activity from deeper structures. Despite such difficulties, these techniques do provide measurement of rapid state changes, and for this reason may be quite relevant in the study of affect and its regulation.

Using EEG techniques on both children and adults over a number of years and with different "at-risk" and diagnostic groups, Davidson and collaborators have amassed impressive results that are theoretically consistent with their notion that the left anterior region (including both frontal and temporal areas) is specialized for approach behavior and positive emotions, while the right anterior region is specialized for withdrawal behavior and negative emotions (see Davidson, 1992, for an overview). Greater activation of right than of left frontal areas is seen with induction of negative emotions, such as disgust. In contrast, greater left frontal activation is seen with the induction of happy feelings.

In collaboration with Fox, Davidson (1992) carried out a series of experiments with infants. Exposure to an actress displaying laughter elicited left-sided (as opposed to right-sided) activation in 10-month-old infants, as did sweet-tasting substances in neonates. In contrast, substances that caused the infants to grimace produced right-sided activation. Furthermore, 10-month-old infants displayed right-sided EEG activation with the approach of a stranger and left-sided activation with the approach of their mothers. The infants in these studies differed greatly with respect to the degree of resting or baseline asymmetry, although they all showed the state-related changes described above. In a study of adults with a 3-week retest of baseline asymmetry, the authors found moderate stability, supporting their belief that this frontal asymmetry reflects a trait-like variable.

Using the same EEG measures with depressed subjects, Davidson and colleagues (see Davidson, 1992) found more relative right-sided frontal activation at rest than in nondepressed subjects. This difference was primarily due to less left-sided activation in the depressed subjects. They also showed that depressed subjects displayed less right-sided posterior (parietal) activation than controls—a finding consistent with spatial deficits in some depressed subjects. In assessing subjects whose depression had remitted versus nondepressed subjects, Davidson and collaborators found a similar reduction in activation in the left frontal region in the previously depressed as opposed to the never-depressed subjects. They concluded cautiously from their findings that this relative frontal asymmetry is a trait marker for depression.

Pursuing these theories further, Davidson's group conducted studies of subjects' resting asymmetry as a predictor of later negative affect on exposure to affect-eliciting film clips. Relative right frontal activation at rest predicted fear responses to the film clips. Their findings suggested that resting anterior asymmetry primarily indexes the relative balance of positive and negative response tendencies for an individual. Studies of infants in a maternal separation paradigm also reinforced their main findings, in that those who cried displayed more right-sided activation in a baseline recording than did those who did not. When these same assessments were applied to toddlers preselected to be inhibited or uninhibited (according to Kagan's approach to categorizing such children), the inhibited children displayed much greater relative right-sided frontal activation than did the uninhibited. The group difference was primarily due to reduced left-sided activation in the inhibited children. In interpreting these findings, Davidson (1992) acknowledges that the relative asymmetry may result from threshold differences in the elicitation of negative affect or in individuals' capacity to regulate negative affect, and that these two positions are not necessarily mutually exclusive. He emphasizes that he views these differences as *vulnerabilities* to positive or negative affect—vulnerabilities that require a situation or event to elicit the affect.

Subsequently, Jones et al. (1997) reported decreased left frontal activity in 1-month-old infants of depressed mothers. This followed a similar report on 3-month-old infants. This EEG asymmetry correlated with sad and precrying behaviors in the infants. It is not yet possible to ascertain whether this relative frontal asymmetry is due to genetic or environmental effects or both, but it does appear to be a relatively stable aspect of brain function related to the response tendency to positive or negative affect. Although such an association is speculative, the findings would be consistent with a neuroticism or emotionality factor—an indicator of vulnerability to internalizing disorders.

Using assessment of cerebral blood flow and metabolism through techniques such as PET and MRI on depressed patients with neurological disorders such as Parkinson's disorder and Huntington's disease, various laboratories have shown abnormalities in the caudate nucleus, the orbitofrontal and inferior prefrontal regions, the inferior parietal cortex, the temporal lobes, the medial prefrontal cortex, and the cingulate cortex. (Kennedy, Javanmard, & Vaccarino, 1997, review these studies.) In patients with major depression, seasonal affective disorder, and bipolar disorder, decreased activity has been found in caudate, anterior cingulate, orbitofrontal, inferior frontal, dorsolateral prefrontal, parietal, and insular regions. Kennedy et al. (1997) report that the results of cognitive activation studies are contradictory, with increases in some areas and decreases in others. Similarly, the results in emotion induction paradigms are inconsistent. Despite these inconsistencies, Kennedy et al. suggest that there is some consistency with respect to the areas involved. These include the prefrontal and orbitofrontal cortices, as well as the cingulate and periamygdalar areas, suggesting the importance of the limbic–paralimbic–frontal networks in affect regulation. In describing pharmacological challenge studies, Kennedy et al. (1997) note the consistent findings of activity in anterior cingulate and anterior temporofrontal regions in paradigms that invoke anxiety. Overall, although the actual studies present inconsistencies with respect to increased or decreased activity, the consistency with respect to the sites involved—the prefrontal cortices, the cingulate gyrus, and the amygdala—is important and in line with the present theorizing about the main pathways involved in affect regulation (see Chapter 7). The difficulty with these studies stems from the issues noted in the introduction to this section. That is, it is very difficult to know what aspect of an individual's experience is responsible for the measured changes— the affect itself, the associations connected to experiencing affect, or the efforts to cope with the affect.

In contrast to measuring brain function in depressed versus non-depressed subjects, one group of British investigators has attempted to bring some clarity to these issues by examining regional brain metabolism and blood flow, and correlating differences with symptom clusters. Bench, Friston, Brown, Frackowiak, and Dolan (1993) assessed regional cerebral blood flow (rCBF) in 40 patients with major depression. Patient symptom ratings were factor-analyzed into three recognizable dimensions of depressive illness and were then correlated with the rCBF findings. The "anxiety" factor correlated positively with rCBF in the posterior cingulate and inferior parietal cortices bilaterally. The "psychomotor retardation and depressed mood" factor correlated negatively with rCBF in the left dorsolateral prefrontal cortex and left angular gyrus. The third factor, "cognitive impairment," correlated with decreased rCBF in the left anterior medial prefrontal cortex.

Although at this time we can only speculate about the pathways involved in the development of anxiety and depression, the fact that most of the deficits demonstrated are left-sided is consistent with Davidson's (1992) theorizing that left-hemisphere activity underlies positive affect and approach behaviors, and so deficits in motivation and mood would be expected to correlate with deficits in left-sided brain function. It is important, however, to point out that Davidson's theory refers to predominantly trait-like or response tendencies, whereas the Bench et al. (1993) study was measuring brain function in the depressed state. Given the expectation that a state of depression would be likely to involve not just response tendencies but actual deficits, and would also involve increased arousal related to stress, we should expect additional findings. The "anxiety" factor that correlated with increased activity bilaterally in posterior cingulate cortex may constitute the "arousal" factor that distinguishes vulnerability from disorder. The abnormalities in the frontal and prefrontal areas related to cognitive difficulties and to depressed mood and retardation, respectively, may well reflect a combination of trait characteristics and structural changes that may arise from the individual's efforts to cope with distress.

Although there is a great deal of overlap between disorders in brain imaging findings, some studies have begun to suggest a degree of specificity with respect to disorders such as OCD, where striatal dysfunction may be more prominent than in other anxiety disorders (P. K. McGuire et al., 1994; Rauch et al., 1994; Rosenberg, Keshavan, et al., 1997). However, given that few studies have compared findings across disorders with sufficiently large numbers of subjects to detect differences, it is still too early to speculate on the specificity of brain changes to disorders. Undoubtedly, findings will emerge that explain symptom differences as in the Bench et al. (1993) study, and these may help us refine our concepts of disorder categories. A recent example of such a study is a report by Dolan et al. (1993), in which they compared rCBF in patients with schizophrenia versus patients with depression.

They subdivided both patient groups into those meeting criteria for "poverty of speech" (a symptom of psychomotor retardation) and those not meeting these criteria. They found a reduction of rCBF in the left dorsolateral prefrontal cortex in patients with "poverty of speech," regardless of diagnosis.

Although I believe that neuroimaging will gradually reveal the brain areas that relate to various functions of affect regulation and symptoms of psychiatric disorders, we are still trying to understand how these functions and dysfunctions arise. Specifically, we need to understand how the various factors discussed earlier in this chapter affect brain development and function. This means attempting to build a developmental model in which aspects of brain function reflect the psychological and behavioral functions with which we are familiar.

Developmental Neurological Dysfunctions

Several areas of research are suggestive in terms of the neurodevelopmental factors that may be relevant to anxiety and depression. These include studies of prenatal stress, pre- and perinatal obstetrical factors (including low birthweight), and neurological soft signs.

Studies in animals have demonstrated that stress during pregnancy can affect the offspring's behavior (Clarke & Schneider, 1993). Although early work in this area applied fairly major physical stressors to gravid females, more recently the stressors used have involved disruption of social bonds, and are thus perhaps more analogous to human stresses that have been posited to be contributory (Schneider & Coe, 1993). Despite contradictions across studies, there is some consistency overall, in that the offspring appear to be more stress-reactive (Black et al., 1998). Furthermore, these effects appear to be partially reversible, depending on the quality of maternal care (Maccari et al., 1995). There is debate in the literature about timing of the stressors, about acute versus chronic stress, and about the mechanism through which maternal stress exerts its effect (Schneider & Coe, 1993). Some of these effects have been replicated through injections of ACTH during mid-pregnancy suggesting that activation of the hypothalamic–pituitary–adrenal (HPA) axis is an important pathway (Schneider et al., 1992). Studies in humans to date have been less clear, but they have also been limited in number. However, a follow-up study of individuals whose mothers endured famine during the second trimester of pregnancy showed an increased risk of psychotic depression in males as compared to individuals from nonstressed pregnancies. The effects for first- and third-trimester exposure were not significant (Brown, Susser, Lin, Neugebauer, & Gorman, 1995).

Low birthweight has been identified as a factor influencing developmental outcomes in children, including IQ, attentional problems, school and learning difficulties, and socioemotional difficulties (Breslau, 1995). Although there is evidence that good caretaking can ameliorate some of these effects, it appears that those at the lowest extreme are at significant risk, regardless of the adequacy of the caretaking environment (Bradley & Casey, 1992; Schothorst & van Engeland, 1996; Sykes et al., 1997). It is assumed that the adverse sequelae of low birthweight result from brain injury, which is more common in these infants than in normal-birthweight infants, although it is also posited that the rearing of these children may pose stresses for parents and thus increase the environmental risks. Whitaker et al. (1997) examined the relation of neonatal cranial ultrasound abnormalities to psychiatric disorder at age 6 in a regional birth cohort of low-birthweight children. They found that lesions affecting white matter, with or without ventricular enlargement, increased the risk for any disorder and particularly for ADHD. However, in children of normal intelligence, such lesions also increased the risk for separation anxiety disorder. These effects were independent of sex and social class.

Soft signs, evidence of mild neuromotor abnormalities, have been associated with both internalizing and externalizing disorders of childhood (Neumann & Walker, 1996). Recently, Pine, Wasserman, et al. (1997) have suggested that these abnormalities are reflective of dysfunction of basal ganglia–frontal connections. Obstetrical complications, which have now been connected not only with schizophrenia but with the internalizing disorders (Gillberg et al., 1989), are presumed to cause ischemic damage and are probably best understood as affecting a child's capacity to regulate arousal or state (Sykes et al., 1997). Given the vulnerability of white matter to ischemic injury and metabolic insult, the results from the Whitaker et al. (1997) study described above might also explain the correlation between obstetrical complications and later emotional and behavioral sequelae. Whatever the explanation, it is clear that there is a connection between various developmental abnormalities and later vulnerability to internalizing disorders. (See Graham, Heim, Goodman, Miller, & Nemeroff, 1999, for a recent overview.) Again, I believe the evidence suggests that these children are less competent in regulating themselves and their affects.

The Neurological Impact of Stress and Its Relation to the Internalizing Disorders

The three major neurotransmitters—NE, 5-HT, and dopamine—have each been implicated in anxiety and depression. Although the earlier theories assumed that deficits in noradrenergic or serotonergic transmission were the primary problems in disorders like depression, theorizing has shifted more recently to conceptualizing deficits in monoamine systems as secondary to glucocorticoids released as part of the stress response (Dinan, 1994). Because this conceptual framework appears more parsimonious and fits theoretically with the central thesis of this book, I explain it in more detail here.

Development of the Stress Response

As discussed in Chapter 5 and illustrated in Figure 5.1, the stress response consists of the release of corticotropin-releasing hormone (CRH) from the paraventricular nucleus of the hypothalamus into the portal venous circulation, followed by release of ACTH from the anterior pituitary. Circulating ACTH stimulates the adrenal cortex to produce glucocorticoids, which act on a number of structures in the central nervous system as well as peripheral organs.

Gunnar (1992) reviews her own and others' work on the reactivity of the HPA axis in infants and young children. Extremely healthy newborns show elevations of cortisol in response to noxious stimulation. Despite equally high levels of HPA activity, healthy newborns show different regulatory behaviors in response to a handling stressor versus a heel-stick blood-sampling stressor. With the heel stick newborns cry, but with handling they show increases in quiescence and other self-regulatory behaviors. With repetitions of these stressors (mock administrations of the heel-stick), these very healthy newborns show habituation to the handling and sensitization to the heel stick. Babies with some obstetrical complications, however, cry in response to both types of stressors and show a breakdown of normal self-regulatory behaviors at high levels of HPA activity. In addition, they fail to show habituation or sensitization to handling or nocioceptive stimulation. Although soothing procedures such as pacifiers can reduce crying in newborns, they do not reduce the HPA response. Procedures that block pain do reduce the HPA response. As infants develop, they show more habituation of the HPA response, gradually approaching the adult pattern.

Rearing and HPA Axis Dysregulation

Separation from caregivers, which has been shown in primates to produce large elevations of cortisol, tends to produce smaller elevations in young children. Gunnar (1992) suggests that the difference may be due to the quality of substitute care. In her laboratory, when a highly sensitive babysitter plays with a young child who has been separated from his or her mother, the HPA response is completely buffered. Gunnar and Barr (1998) cite other studies showing that securely attached infants show a buffering of the HPA response to stressful situations such as medical exams when with their attachment figures (see Chapter 5). Furthermore, studies in rats and monkeys show that enhancement of the quality of maternal behavior results in increased glucocorticoid receptors in the brain, a more efficient HPA response to stress, less fearful behavior, and lower catecholamine responses to stressors. Adverse rearing situations produce the opposite responses.

From animal work, in a reassessment at age 4 of infant primates whose mothers were stressed through a variable-foraging paradigm as opposed to those who had access to a secure food source, Coplan et al. (1998) reported that CSF CRH elevations in the variable-foraging group correlated with elevations of CSF metabolites of 5-HT and dopamine and of somatostatin. Monkey offspring of mothers who must forage for food have previously been described as showing anxiety-like behaviors. Although the mechanism for this effect is not clear (reaction to maternal behavioral changes or exposure to elevated glucocorticoids through the mothers' milk), it is interesting that the effect on the offspring resembles that of prenatal stress in inducing increased stress reactivity. The fact that the "stressor," whatever its nature, has such an enduring impact on both behavior and endocrine variables does suggest that early stress, particularly over a period that may be critical for the development of regulatory structures or functions such as stress control, may have a powerful impact on brain function. A graded exposure to stress that the individual can perceive as tolerable may have the opposite effect—that is, a down-regulation of the HPA axis. This is suggested by the studies cited in the review by Meaney et al. (1996) in Chapter 5.

Control and the Stress Response

Although there is debate about the situations that trigger HPA system activity, there is evidence that having some control over a noxious situation tends to buffer the stress response. Gunnar and Barr (1998) refer to studies with primates carried out by Gunnar in which monkeys were raised in two conditions: The experimental group had control over access to food, drinks, and treats, while the yoked group received whatever the experimental monkeys chose. When observed later, the monkeys raised with some control over their environment were less fearful, were more willing to explore, and showed a smaller HPA response to stress when given drugs to induce anxiety.

Dysregulation of the Stress Response

Although the stress response is generally adaptive, particularly for acute situations, chronic stimulation of this system appears maladaptive. As noted above and described in detail in Chapter 5, the activity and regulation of CRH cells is dependent on the state of regulation of glucocorticoid receptors in the hippocampus and hypothalamus. Type II receptors mediate stress-related cortisol changes, in contrast to Type I receptors, which control mineralocorticoid activity and some (tonic) glucocorticoid activity (De Kloet, 1991). Activation of Type II receptors in the hypothalamus and hippocampus turns off the stress response. In their review of stress and early brain development, Gunnar and Barr (1998) report that although initially increases in glucocorticoid levels in healthy adults produce a sense of increased energy and ability to concentrate, prolonged stimulation of glucocorticoid receptors produces decreases in energy and concentration and feelings of depression. Thus, although brief and moderately intense stresses can organize and promote adaptive functioning, more prolonged or highly intense stresses are likely to be maladaptive. Gunnar and Barr discuss the evidence that adverse early experience may result in an inability to turn off the stress response, resulting in chronically elevated levels of cortisol, such as those found in depression. (See also the discussion in Chapter 5 of the review of Meaney et al., 1996.)

Although the mechanisms for this dysregulation of the stress response are presently speculative, damage to hippocampal cells by chronically elevated cortisol levels may be one factor (O'Brien, 1997). Another possible mechanism for dysregulation of the stress response may be glucocorticoids' induction of activity in CRH-producing cells in the amygdala. Such activity elicits fear behavior, hypervigilance, and increases in central and peripheral catecholamines. Gunnar and Barr (1998) cite studies suggesting that elevations of CRH activity in the amygdala may be a mechanism for explaining the hyperarousal in PTSD. Dinan (1994) suggests that in depression the glucocorticoid receptors appear to have decreased plasticity, resulting in a blunting of HPA responses. This is also true of anxiety disorders (Hoehn-Saric, McLeod, & Hipsley, 1995).

HPA Axis Dysregulation in Depression and Anxiety

HPA axis dysregulation can explain the abnormal response in depressed individuals to an injection of dexamethasone, a synthetic corticosteroid. Nondepressed subjects respond by suppressing cortisol levels for at least 24 hours after an injection of dexamethasone. Many depressed subjects fail to show this suppression. Furthermore, continuing increases in cortisol response to challenge predict relapse (Zobel, Yassouridis, Frieboes, & Holsboer, 1999).

Citing the evidence for both hyperresponsiveness and hyporesponsiveness of the HPA axis, Johnson et al. (1992) have suggested that these two different response biases may underlie melancholic depression and atypical depression. In melancholic depression there is evidence for continuing central arousal, manifested in worry, agitation, and difficulty in sleeping and eating; in contrast, atypical depression is characterized by hypoarousal, manifested in increased sleeping and eating and in lethargy. Johnson et al. also refer to the literature on various metabolic conditions such as Cushing's disease and hypothyroidism, which show dysregulation of the HPA axis and in which depression is a common symptom.

Altemus, Smith, Diep, Aulakh, and Murphy (1994/1995) have provided evidence that dysregulation of the stress response may also be relevant in understanding anxiety. They discuss the fawn-hooded strain of rats, in which there is an impairment of vesicular storage of 5-HT and abnormalities in brain serotonergic function. These rats appear to be hyperaroused: They exhibit more freezing behavior with stress, increased preference for alcohol, hypertension in adulthood, and increased urinary catecholamines, compared with other strains of rats. Altemus et al. found increased messenger RNA for CRH in the central nucleus of the amygdala, and decreased levels in the paraventricular nucleus of the hypothalamus. Although plasma corticosterone levels in this study did not differ from those of the control rats, in other studies when fawn-hooded rats were stressed before sacrifice, corticosterone levels were elevated in contrast to those of controls (see Altemus et al., 1994/1995, for a review). This elevation of corticosterone with exposure to stress can be normalized with antidepressant pretreatment, which is thought to up-regulate glucocorticoid receptors, thus enhancing the control over the stress response.

Other studies provide support for the possible importance of HPA axis dysregulation as a central feature in both anxiety and depression. Abelson and Curtis (1996), in a follow-up of patients treated for panic disorder, reported that mean 24-hour cortisol levels before treatment were the best independent predictor of disability scores at follow-up. They suggest that elevated cortisol levels, presumably reflecting HPA axis dysregulation, may be a vulnerability marker for coping or reactivity with prognostic significance for later disability. Similarly, in a meta-analysis of studies on the dexamethasone suppression test in various categories of depression, Nelson and Davis (1997) found that nonsuppression was significantly higher in psychotic than in non-psychotic depression, suggesting that it may represent a marker of on-going reactivity.

Primary Neurotransmitter Deficit versus HPA Axis Dysfunction

Dinan (1994) raises questions about the primacy of serotonergic or noradrenergic deficits in depression, suggesting instead that deficits in these neurotransmitter systems may be secondary to the effects of circulating glucocorticoids. In support of his argument, he cites work by De Kloet (1991) in rats, which has demonstrated down- and up-regulation of 5-HT1 receptors and alpha-2 (NE) receptors through adrenalectomy and corticosteroid replacement. There is also evidence that increased cortisol increases dopamine levels (De Kloet, 1991). Furthermore, Dinan cites his own and others' work, which suggests that the blunted hormonal responses (growth hormone, prolactin, thyro-tropin) observed in depression can be explained by high glucocorticoid levels. Lastly, he discusses the studies showing that treatment of rats with antidepressants produces an up-regulation of glucocorticoid receptors in the locus coeruleus and raphe nucleus. This up-regulation produces an increased negative feedback and a decrease in overall activity of the HPA axis.

Heuser et al. (1998) report an interesting study that lends support to Dinan's speculations. They administered amitriptyline to depressed and elderly normal subjects, and monitored CSF levels of three neuro-peptides implicated in regulation of the HPA axis: CRH, arginine vasopressin, and somatostatin. In the depressed subjects who improved, amitriptyline produced a decrease in CSF CRH, but not in arginine vasopressin or somatostatin. They concluded that their results supported the notion that antidepressants, although they may affect various components of the HPA axis, have the net effect of reducing HPA axis activity. A similar normalization of HPA axis function has been observed with successful treatment with electroshock therapy (reported in Heuser et al., 1998).

The older notions that there may be primary deficiencies in neurotransmitters such as 5-HT in depression also have to be considered. Certainly, the efficacy of substances that increase 5-HT in the treatment of depression suggest that there are deficiencies in this system, although there is some suggestion that down-regulation of 5-HT receptors may also be the mechanism for efficacy of antidepressants. Because 5-HT has a general inhibitory effect on many systems— including the noradrenergic and dopaminergic systems and the amyg-dala, all of which may be activated in stressful circumstances—a deficit in 5-HT for whatever reason would imply loss of that inhibitory function and increased anxiety or arousal. Spoont (1992) suggests that reduced 5-HT may induce negative affective states as well as impulsivity through reducing the stability of information processing. She argues that the serotonergic system functions to constrain information processing and to prevent overshooting in neural networks. If she is correct in her arguments, the lack of 5-HT modulation of stress-enhanced NE or amygdalar activity would interfere with the dampening down or return to normal of the stress response. This is consistent with the work cited in Spoont's review of enhanced stress reactivity with reduced 5-HT levels. Because there is evidence that the monoaminergic systems have a significant heritable component in animals (Clarke et al., 1995; see also the work with fawn-hooded rats by Altemus et al., 1995), deficiencies in 5-HT's inhibitory function could be presumed to arise on a genetic basis, but could also occur with stress-induced increases in HPA activity (De Kloet, 1991).

Lastly, one of the most thoroughly tested animal models for depression is that of "learned helplessness" (Maier & Seligman, 1976). In this paradigm animals, usually rats, are subjected to uncontrollable or unpredictable severe stress. When removed from the stress, they exhibit "helpless" behavior. Although one can label this as a learned response in a hopeless situation, there is also evidence that depletion of NE and/or of the enzyme controlling its synthesis, tyrosine hydroxylase, also contributes to this reaction. This reaction can be blocked by prior treatment with antidepressants. (Johnson et al., 1992, review these studies.)

Summary of the Findings on HPA Axis Dysregulation

Although the centrality of HPA axis dysregulation in depression and the relevance of the fawn-hooded rat as a model for anxiety must await further testing, HPA dysregulation offers a more parsimonious way of integrating the multitude of neurohormonal findings with the genetic and psychosocial factors discussed earlier in this chapter. It may also provide a way of explaining the gender differences in prevalence of the mood and anxiety disorders. It appears that the HPA axis may be more susceptible to stress-induced dysregulation in females than in males (Weiss et al., 1999). One can speculate that genetic factors as well as adverse early experience can have an impact on the regulation of the HPA axis. Once an individual has been exposed to high levels of glucocorticoids, however, the capacity to regulate their stress response may become dysfunctional. Temperamental predisposition to neuroticism or inhibition may involve overreactivity of the HPA axis or other systems (e.g., amygdala–frontal circuits) that would also increase the individual's stress response. In contrast to the plasticity of the stress response seen in well-functioning individuals, most notably their capacity to return to a normal or baseline level of functioning, stress or perturbations in this easily dysregulated or implastic system may be less likely to be followed by a quick return to baseline or normal function, thus prolonging the dysregulation in the monoaminergic and other endocrine systems. Burnout related to NE depletion or to cognitions of hopelessness may lead to retardation, apathy, and low mood. Internal working models and limited problem-oriented coping strategies may reinforce these reactions conditioned by the neurological substrate. This conceptualization does suggest that interventions that can correct the HPA axis dysregulation should also produce a return to more normal function in the monoaminergic and other endocrine systems, but may not entirely reduce the vulnerability to depression or anxiety unless changes in internal working models and coping strategies also take place. Conversely, treatments that fail to address the HPA axis dysregulation should be relatively ineffective.

TREATMENT CONSIDERATIONS

Although treatment as it relates to the regulation of affect has been covered in Chapter 8, I touch briefly on some of the most salient issues here. Generally, biological and psychosocial interventions appear to be equivalent in their effectiveness as treatments for the mood and anxiety disorders. This has been demonstrated quite clearly in the National Institute of Mental Health Treatment of Depression Collaborative Research Program, where cognitive-behavioral therapy and interpersonal therapy produced outcomes roughly equivalent to those for antidepressant treatment (Elkin et al., 1989). Gould, Buckminster, Pollack, Otto, and Yap (1997) in a meta-analysis of intervention studies in social phobia, highlighted the importance of exposure; otherwise, the different interventions (cognitive-behavioral therapy and antidepressants) did not differ in their effect sizes. Similarly, Ballenger (1998) in a recent review of panic disorder, discusses the fact that there is little difference among cognitive-behavioral treatment, other psychosocial interventions (focused on understanding and regulating affect related to the occurrence of panic attacks), and medication in short- and longer-term outcomes of panic disorder. There is also relatively little difference among tricyclic antidepressants, selective serotonin reuptake inhibitors, and benzodiazepines in the treatment of panic disorder, although side effects differ and contribute to tolerability. What this generalized treatment effect seems to indicate is that the general factor of affect regulation is being addressed in all successful therapies. Clearly, some treatments may be presumed to have a longer-lasting effect if they are able to change the underlying physiology or stress reactivity.

INTEGRATING ETIOLOGICAL FACTORS

Can we integrate the seemingly diverse array of findings presented in this chapter into a coherent narrative? I believe so, through the notion of affect regulation as the central dimension in the development of psychopathology.

It appears that certain factors increase the individual's vulnerability to react more intensely to stress and to have difficulty modulating that reaction. The genetic factor common to anxiety and depression, cited by Kendler, Walters, et al. (1995), as increasing one's vulnerability to stressful life events; the trait of neuroticism (Kendler, Kessler, et al., 1993) or emotionality (Goodyer et al., 1993), which also predicts later internalizing disorders; and the trait of inhibition can all be conceptualized as representing a constitutional or biological vulnerability to difficulty in modulating stress and the accompanying affect. In addition, it appears that perinatal events known to be related to later disorder, such as obstetrical complications or very low birthweight, also impair brain function in a way that contributes to difficulty in regulating state and arousal levels. We can speculate that this damage interferes with neural networks responsible for modulation of the stress response. It is also becoming apparent that stress itself can have an impact on the developing brain that increases the vulnerability of the brain to difficulties with modulating the stress response. Prolonged stress appears to reduce the plasticity of the stress response, making it more likely that the individual will experience chronically elevated levels of glucocorticoids, which may further impair the capacity of the brain to shut off the stress response.

Although I have explained the dysregulation of the stress response in terms of making the individual more vulnerable to further stresses, it is also important to wonder about its impact on other brain structures and on learning. In the studies described by Meaney et al. (1996; see Chapter 5) on rats handled in the first 2 weeks of life, there was an increase in glucocorticoid receptors not only in the hypothalamus, but also in the frontal cortex. It is possible to imagine that this frontal cortex effect may be positive with respect to strengthening coping responses or control mechanisms. Although this connection is speculative, research may begin to elucidate what is happening in the frontal structures, which appear to be particularly affected in depression. Similarly, research will undoubtedly begin to uncover the amygdalar mechanisms that seem pertinent in control over fear conditioning and anxiety, especially in understanding the intense flashback experiences in PTSD (which seem related to amygdalar mechanisms).

It appears that the caregiving environment can buffer the stress response but can also worsen it. The relationship between parents and a constitutionally reactive infant has a higher than average likelihood of becoming conflicted. I am basing this assertion on (1) the infant's being perceived as more difficult; and (2) the increased likelihood of at least one parent's being genetically similar to the infant, and therefore being vulnerable to depression and anxiety and to the parental dilemmas involved in the "threat-oriented family system" of Bugental (1992). As indicated earlier, constitutionally reactive children are very sensitive to affect, concerned about their parents' anger, and conflicted about expressions of their own anger. Their attachment relationship is skewed in the direction of avoidance, which means that they will fail to develop comfort with their negative affect and will not experience their caregivers as supportive. If they use oppositionality as their main way of expressing negative affect, the conflict in the parent–child relationship may worsen and become abusive. Such disruption in their most important support system will produce self-esteem deficits and anger.

Although much literature deals with physical and sexual abuse as etiologically important in the development of psychopathology, these factors constitute the "tip of the iceberg" with respect to dysfunctional and conflicted parent–child interactions. Far more common is the situation in which parents are yelling and emotionally abusive in their frustration. For sensitive, poorly regulated children, this climate feels rejecting and makes them feel bad. It is very difficult for children in such circumstances to learn to regulate their affects without resort to defensive strategies. Many of them fail to learn to talk about feelings so that they can identify their experience. Furthermore, they may try to deal with anger through being very good or "getting things perfect" (the obsessive defenses); may try to deal with sadness through such extreme avoidance that they distort their reality and can appear inappropriately happy; or may become oppositional when they feel uncertain of their control in a situation that appears threatening.

All of these strategies for dealing with their feelings tend to increase these children's interactional difficulties with parents and eventually with peers (Eisenberg et al., 1994). Those children who become quite withdrawn (many of whom may not have the good fortune of a relationship that can buffer their distress) are particularly vulnerable because they are removed from opportunities to learn more adaptive coping strategies. Clearly we can surmise that the internal working models that evolve condition the children to continue to react to persons and events in ways that create less than optimal learning opportunities. If such an individual's self-esteem is sufficiently impaired by this process, and if more adaptive coping strategies are not developed, stresses will cause distress that will be difficult to manage. If this distress is prolonged, the individual may feel trapped, with resulting depression. In anxiety the individual appears to have better self-esteem and, although vulnerable to stress, may be better able to use supports. Some of this difference may be genetic (with respect to degrees of left-hemisphere activation that promote approach behavior), or it may be the result of learning and more supportive early and ongoing relationships. However, anxiety may be a precursor to depression if it is prolonged.

In the Kendler, Walters, et al. (1995) study examining the contributions of common and disorder-specific genetic and environmental factors, the disorder-specific factors were relatively important for several disorders. This suggests that research will define genetic factors that may condition types of reaction to stress, thereby explaining why one individual is more vulnerable to the development of a specific internalizing disorder as compared to another. For example, Rosenberg, Auerbach, et al. (1997) have found evidence of oculomotor response inhibition abnormalities in OCD, which may relate to the findings of striatal dysfunction. The specificity of these findings for OCD is not yet clear. Purcell, Maruff, Kyrios, and Pantelis (1998) report neuropsychological deficits in OCD, but not in depression or panic disorder, on tests of spatial working memory, spatial recognition, and motor initiation and execution. However, in a computer modeling of the symptom of uncertainty in OCD, limbic overdrive produced more uncertainty than did the competing etiological models (Ownby, 1998). This was seen to be supportive of Rapoport and Wise's (1989) theory that excessive drive from the limbic system to the basal ganglia may be important in producing the symptoms of OCD. The other possible etiological mechanisms (e.g., basal ganglia dysfunction) appeared less salient, although there was a trend suggesting their influence. These studies suggest that research will need to focus on ways of measuring contributions from the various brain structures that are presumed to be involved in arousal (limbic and brainstem) and its regulation, including coping behavior (forebrain and striatal), in order to define the uniqueness of disorders.

If the present model is correct, interventions that focus on supporting more adaptive affect regulation would appear to have a greater likelihood of success than nondirected interventions. Because affect regulation can be approached from many different directions (e.g., strengthening coping responses, regulating the dysregulated HPA axis, revising internal working models), there may be many different ways of treating individuals with anxiety and mood disorders. Presumably research will begin to address the factors that must be changed for treatments to be effective or to remain effective in preventing relapse.

RELATED DISORDERS

I believe that the arguments I have laid out above also apply to other disorders. There is evidence from Kendler, Walters, et al.'s (1995) study that bulimia nervosa and alcoholism have some genetic overlap with anxiety disorders and depression. Family history studies of both bulimia nervosa and anorexia nervosa (Lilenfeld, Kaye, & Strober, 1997) also suggest an overlap with the anxiety and mood disorders although the nature of this overlap is not entirely clear. In alcoholism, it is clear that there are strong influences as well from disorder-specific additive genes, but also some overlap with genetic influences for anti-social personality disorder (Cadoret, Yates, Troughton, Woodworth, & Stewart, 1995a). In a recent review, Lilenfeld et al. (1997) suggest that temperamental factors, such as inhibition in anorexia nervosa and impulsivity in bulimia nervosa, may help to explain the differences between these two eating disorders. It is also clear that all these disorders differ in the relative influence of familial-environmental factors versus unique-environmental factors. Kendler, Walters, et al. (1995) found a fairly significant loading for a common familial-environmental factor in bulimia nervosa, which was also present (but to a much lesser extent) in depression and alcoholism. From my clinical experience, the early history and developmental perturbations I have outlined above apply to individuals with eating disorders and to the relatively limited number of adolescents I have seen with alcoholism, which is usually comorbid with another disorder.

In the area of gender identity disorder (GID), with which I am very familiar, the same basic formulation applies. I have argued elsewhere (Zucker & Bradley, 1995) that what makes GID different from anxiety disorders is that there are factors in the family making gender more salient. Specifically, boys with GID appear to believe that they will be more valued by their families or that they will get in less trouble as girls than as boys. These beliefs are related to parents' experiences within their families of origin, especially tendencies on the part of mothers to be frightened by male aggression or to be in need of nurturing, which they perceive as a female characteristic. Girls with GID have a perception of themselves as "protectors," specifically of their mothers but also of other women. They appear to be identifying with the aggressors (often their father, but sometimes with other aggressive males). Beyond these specific dynamics, both boys and girls with GID display the temperament and attachment difficulties I have described above. Their interactions with parents are conflicted, and these children become highly distressed and anxious, with perceptions of themselves as bad and their parents as angry. I conceptualize the symptoms of GID as a child's solution to intolerable affects. This is confirmed by the fact that GID typically has its onset at a time in a child's life when the family has been particularly stressed and the parents are either more angry or less available or both. The GID symptoms, particularly the assumption of the role and behaviors of the opposite sex, act to quench the child's anxiety and to make him or her feel more valued, stronger, or safer.

Although these comments can hardly do justice to the richness and complexity of eating disorders, alcoholism, or GID, I am offering them to suggest the generalizability of this model of affect dysregulation to internalizing disorders besides anxiety and mood disorders. If the present formulation is correct, we should find evidence of dysregulation of the HPA axis in these disorders. Treatments for bulimia nervosa and alcoholism already show significant overlap with treatments for anxiety disorders and depression. Although we have been slow to use antidepressants in young children, anecdotal experience suggests that they may be useful in GID.

CONCLUDING COMMENTS

The literature suggests that stress reactivity, whether genetic or environmental in origin, is a major factor in the development of the internalizing disorders. This vulnerability, in interaction with a caretaking environment that has difficulty responding sensitively to the unique needs of a highly stress-reactive child, will increase the likelihood of an internalizing disorder. The special aspects of each of the internalizing disorders arise out of the multiple and interacting genetic and environmental factors discussed above. Treatment of these disorders should recognize the importance of helping individuals deal with affects and with their vulnerability to enhanced stress reactivity.

Chapter 10

Externalizing Disorders: The Disruptive Behavior Disorders

The broad diagnostic category of *attention-deficit and disruptive behavior disorders* (American Psychiatric Association, 1994)—usually referred to simply as *disruptive behavior disorders* (DBDs) includes oppositional defiant disorder (ODD), conduct disorder (CD), and attention-deficit/hyperactivity disorder (ADHD). By extension, it may also be considered to include adult antisocial personality disorder (ASPD). Despite the discreteness of these categories, there is considerable overlap both among the DBDs themselves and between the DBDs and other disorders (Hewitt et al., 1997; Zoccolillo, 1992). ODD is frequently comorbid with ADHD and over time often leads to CD. CD is the childhood precursor of ASPD; it also co-occurs with anxiety and depression at far more than chance levels (Zoccolillo, 1992). The DBDs are often lumped together as "externalizing," as distinguished from the "internalizing" disorders discussed in Chapter 9. Although the hallmark of the DBDs is behavioral dysregulation, affect dysregulation is also a prominent feature of these disorders, especially dysregulated anger and aggression (Cole & Zahn-Waxler, 1992).

This chapter examines how the development of externalizing behavior in general and the DBDs in particular can be conceptualized in terms of affect dysregulation. I start with an overview of factors related to outcome, and of the course of the DBDs. As in Chapter 9, I then discuss genetic and constitutional factors, psychosocial factors, and neurobiological factors that have been demonstrated or suggested to be involved in the etiology of these disorders. Many of these factors of course differ from those involved in the genesis of the internalizing disorders, but—especially in regard to characteristics of the familial environment—there are also points of similarity.

FACTORS RELATED TO OUTCOME

Although there is general agreement that most significant external-izing behavior problems have their beginnings in early childhood, such problems in preschoolers are not uncommon, and it is important to distinguish those that are likely to be relatively self-limited from those that presage a more enduring course. In a follow-up to an epide-miological study of child development in Britain, Sonuga-Barke, Thompson, Stevenson, and Viney (1997) compared parent ratings of children at age 8 with groups and subgroups of the same children cate-gorized by parent ratings of their behavior at age 3. These included a large group of children rated by their parents as free of problems (36%), a group with minor problems at levels short of clinical signifi-cance ("active," 23%; "timid," 17%; and "naughty," 14%), and a group with severe problems. The severe group comprised two subgroups, "neurotic/CD" (5%) and "hyperactive/CD" (5%). When followed up at age 8, four subgroups (hyperactive/CD, neurotic/CD, naughty, and active) were more likely to be rated as having externalizing problems than were the no-problem controls. The hyperactive/CD group had a mean score four times that of the controls. With respect to internalizing symptoms, the timid and neurotic/CD groups scored higher than the controls. The authors argue that clinically significant problems are more likely to be comorbid with emotion regulation (neurotic) or behavioral regulation (hyperactive) difficulties accompanying conduct problems. Their findings also support the concept of clinical signifi-cance (or initial severity) as a predictor of later problems, as the two se-vere subgroups (neurotic/CD and hyperactive/CD) were most prob-lematic at follow-up. These two subgroups were differentiated by the presence of more difficult circumstances (poor maternal mental health, single-parent status, or unemployed fathers) in the families of the neu-rotic/CD group. Although this study gives some indication of the fac-tors that may distinguish common behavioral difficulties in the pre-school period from more significant problems, it also suggests that there may be a large pool of temperamentally relatively vulnerable children whose outcomes are dependent on the capacity of their caregiving environment to respond appropriately to their needs.

CD that has an onset in early childhood is distinguished from CD that develops in adolescence (Moffitt, Caspi, Dickson, Silva, & Stanton, 1996). Childhood-onset CD is more likely to occur in temperamentally difficult children (some of whom are defined as having ADHD), to be less inclined to remit if it continues into adolescence, and to correlate with more violent behaviors and with ASPD. The childhood- and adolescent-onset varieties of CD are essentially indistinguishable in terms of types and extent of delinquent behavior in adolescence, except for relationship with violent crime (Moffitt et al., 1996). Adolescent-onset CD appears to occur in individuals who have had more "healthy" childhoods and better relationships within their families than is the case with childhood-onset CD. Individuals with adolescent-onset CD are also more likely to stay in school, and appear to have a better capacity for holding jobs and maintaining intimate relationships as they age, than do those with onset in early childhood (Moffitt et al., 1996).

Externalizing behaviors in general are relatively stable over time (Loeber, 1991). In one study, chronicity of family troubles (coercive parenting and poor monitoring) was found to lead to childhood antisocial behavior, which, when accompanied by association with deviant peers, led to early arrest and eventually to chronic offending (Patterson, Forgatch, Yoerger, & Stoolmiller, 1998). Each of the outcomes (childhood antisocial behavior, early arrest, and chronic offending) shared the common processes of disrupted family interactions, frequent family transitions, and social disadvantage. The level of disrupted family interactions and involvement with deviant peers predicted who would follow this trajectory.

In addition to the total number of risk factors, Deater-Deckard, Dodge, Bates, and Pettit (1998) found that the presence of individual risk factors correlated with externalizing behaviors over middle childhood, predicting 36–45% of the variance in outcome. Number of risk factors (cumulative risk status) predicted 19–32% of the variance in externalizing outcomes. The child-specific risk factors were male sex, resistant temperament, and early medical problems, accounting for 7–24% of the variance. Sociocultural risk factors, which accounted for 4–11% of the variance, were low SES, single-parent mother, higher child–adult ratio, teenage pregnancy, unplanned pregnancy, and more stressful life events. Parenting/caregiving variables accounted for 10–20% of the variance. These were more extensive nonmaternal child care, lower paternal involvement in caregiving, higher parental con-

flict, increased exposure to violence, harsher discipline, increased likelihood of physical abuse, lack of positive parenting, and positive
maternal attitudes toward aggression. Lastly, peer rejection in kindergarten also predicted a small but unique proportion of the variance in
externalizing outcomes. These results were specific for the European
American children in the sample; the lack of predictive power for the
parenting/caregiving variable in the sample of African American children raises issues of differences in the meaning of these variables
across cultures.

In a follow-up of children with ODD or ADHD and control children from ages 4 to 9, children who no longer met diagnostic criteria
by age 9 were differentiated from those who did not change by lesser
severity of the variables of family stress, negative maternal control,
and early symptoms at ages 4 and 6 (Campbell et al., 1996). In a 2-year
follow-up of boys in middle childhood who had been identified as
aggressive/rejected, aggressive/nonrejected, nonaggressive/rejected,
and controls, Bierman and Wargo (1995) found that a broad array of
conduct problems, low levels of positive interaction skills, and high
levels of peer dislike and ostracism each made unique contributions to
the stability of social adjustment problems. All of these studies suggest
that the severity of problems (either symptoms or behaviors within the
child, problems within the family, or both) predicts chronicity.

Within the broad domain of DBDs different symptoms or clusters
of behavior have different relative outcomes. Stormshak, Bierman, and
the Conduct Problems Prevention Research Group (1998) compared
differentiated parent ratings of oppositional, aggressive, and hyper-
active/inattentive behaviors in children with DBDs at school entry and
compared them with teacher and peer nomination ratings at the end of
first grade. Aggressive behaviors generalized more readily to the
school setting and were associated with more severe overall dysfunction. More classroom disruption was associated with hyperactive/
inattentive behaviors than with aggressive or oppositional behaviors.
Lastly, the combinations of oppositional/aggressive and hyperactive/
inattentive behaviors were more common than were single behaviors,
and produced a broad level of dysfunction in the social and classroom
milieu.

COURSE

Children with DBDs experience a number of developmental challenges. Their impulsive and aggressive behaviors lead to peer rejection
(Hinshaw & Melnick, 1995; Fabes & Eisenberg, 1992) and, perhaps in

combination with actual language or learning deficits, to academic difficulties (Moffitt, 1993). When these factors are combined with conflict within their relationships with parents and other family members, they often have self-esteem deficits and may feel overtly rejected. They are extremely vulnerable to adolescent difficulties, including association with deviant peers; alcohol and other substance abuse; and ongoing problems with parents, school, and peers (Dishion, French, & Patterson, 1995). Coie, Terry, Lenox, Lochman, and Hyman (1995) found that boys who were both aggressive and rejected in third grade had profiles of increasingly severe internalizing and externalizing problems in adolescence. Because the DBDs, especially CD, may be very difficult to treat once they are long-standing, these individuals are also vulnerable to a number of adult problems, including criminality, substance dependence, poor work performance, and relationship problems. Efforts to prevent this very damaging trajectory have led to an intense interest in the factors that may be more amenable to early intervention. Accordingly, I now examine what is known about risk factors for these disorders in particular and for the onset of externalizing behaviors in general.

GENETIC AND CONSTITUTIONAL FACTORS

Findings from Genetic Studies

As with most other disorders, there is now good evidence that heritable factors influence the development of traits and behaviors central to the DBDs. Heritability has been studied with respect to broad behaviors such as criminal activity (Bohman, 1995) and antisocial traits (Lyons et al., 1995); the disorders ADHD, ODD, and CD (Cadoret et al., 1995b; Eaves, Silberg, Meyer, & Maes, 1997); and externalizing symptoms (Zahn-Waxler et al., 1996), particularly attentional difficulties (Zahn-Waxler et al., 1996), hyperactivity (Thapar et al., 1995), impulsivity, aggressivity (Cadoret et al., 1995b; Schmitz et al., 1995), and novelty seeking (Heath, Cloninger, & Martin, 1994). The trait of novelty seeking has been linked to the dopamine D4 receptor gene (Benjamin et al., 1996; Ebstein et al., 1996; Ekelund, Lichtermann, Jarvelin, & Peltonen, 1999); this is consistent with Cloninger's (1987) theory that the dopamine system mediates approach behaviors, although several studies have failed to replicate these findings. Because many externalizing traits are considered normal traits of personality, it is reasonable to presume that the individuals exhibiting extreme forms of these traits will be most vulnerable to the development of psychopathology. As with traits such as neuroticism, it appears that such traits or factors, acting in combination with environmental risk factors, increase the risk of developing psychopathology (Braungart-Rieker, Rende, Plomin, DeFries, & Fulker, 1995).

In most of the studies showing a heritable component for the DBDs or for traits related to them, there is also a significant contribution from unique-environmental factors. In the Cadoret et al. (1995b) study, adverse family factors in the adoptive home interacted with a biological background of ASPD to increase the risk of aggressivity and CD in adoptees *only* in the presence of the biological background variable. In addition to the influence of unique-environmental factors, there is a significant shared-environmental factor for aggressivity (Schmitz et al., 1995) and externalizing disorders in adolescence (Eaves et al., 1997).

The term *antisocial behavior* covers a heterogeneous group of symptoms and disorders. Silberg et al. (1995) examined the data from the Virginia Twin Study of Adolescent Behavioral Development for the presence of phenotypically and etiologically distinct latent classes. They found four such classes: (1) a nonsymptomatic class, influenced by both genetic and shared-environmental factors; (2) a hyperactivity–conduct disturbance class, accounted for by different types of genetic effects; (3) a "pure" conduct disturbance class, with a very strong shared-environmental component; and (4) a multisymptomatic class explained entirely by additive genetic effects. According to the authors, classes 2 and 4 included those adolescents with the most significant difficulty and worst prognosis, whereas class 3 included many adolescent-onset CD cases (known to have a better prognosis and fewer associated early risk factors, as noted above).

Using the same database, Silberg et al. (1996) found that the covariation between hyperactivity and ODD or CD was almost entirely explainable by common genetic factors in the younger cohort. In the older cohort, by contrast, separate genetic factors for hyperactivity and conduct disturbance appeared to provide a better fit to the model. In contrast to the finding that the same set of genes influenced hyperactivity and CD in early childhood in both males and females, in the older cohort it appeared that different genes influenced the expression of each of these behaviors in boys and girls.

Temperament

Difficult temperament has been associated with externalizing symptoms, with ODD, and with CD in a number of studies. In a longitudinal study of a community sample of children from ages 2 to 8, Kingston and Prior (1995) found that difficult temperament characterized the children with a stable pattern of aggressive behavior, in contrast to those whose aggressive behavior remitted or started later. In a longitudinal study extending into adolescence, Caspi et al. (1995) examined temperament ratings in a population sample from ages 3 to 15. The dimension "lack of control," which comprised ratings of emotional lability, restlessness, short attention span and negativism in early childhood, and irritability and distractibility in middle childhood, predicted externalizing behaviors and lower competence in adolescence. When the same cohort was followed into adulthood (Krueger et al., 1996), comparisons were made between dimensions of personality at age 18 and four types of disorders (mood disorders, anxiety disorders, substance dependence, and CD) assessed at ages 15, 18, and 21. In comparison to the controls, the group with CD was lower on the subfactors called "well-being," "social closeness," "control," "harm avoidance," and "traditionalism," and higher on the subfactors called "social potency," "stress reaction," "alienation," and "aggression." On higher-order factors, the group with CD was lower on "constraint" and "communion," and higher on "negative emotionality." When the groups were separated into subgroups with "pure" versus comorbid disorders, the group with pure CD was higher on the subfactors of alienation and aggression and on the higher-order factor of negative emotionality. Across the sample, amount of symptomatology was associated with extent of personality deviation. Even when effects of time of assessment were controlled for, gender and conceptualization of disorder (pure or comorbid CD) continued to be linked with higher negative emotionality, lower constraint, and lower communion.

Krueger et al. (1996) point out that whereas negative emotionality has previously been linked with mood and anxiety disorders (as it was in this study), it also appears to be quite relevant as a factor in adult CD. In contrast to the mood and anxiety disorders, where the stress reaction subfactor of negative emotionality appears central, in CD the aggression subfactor is more relevant. As these measures of temperament and personality may be influenced by experience, especially as children grow older, this finding of negative emotionality may reflect experience as much as it does a heritable component. However, it does illustrate that difficulty in regulating affect has become a key component of CD at least in early adulthood. The fact that this difficulty relates more closely to aggression may be one factor distinguishing CD from the mood and anxiety disorders. Interestingly, examining temperamental contributions to externalizing behavior and trying to disentangle the effects of withdrawn versus inhibited behavior, Kerr et al. (1997) found a protective effect of inhibition against the development of delinquency. Withdrawal, however, when combined with disruptiveness, appeared to predispose children to delinquency or to delinquency with depression.

Physiological Underarousal

Because individuals vulnerable to externalizing psychopathology may be temperamentally more inclined toward sensation seeking or novelty seeking, physiological underarousal has been theorized as a possible mediating mechanism. This is consistent with the belief that fearlessness or poor fear conditioning may be a factor in their risk-taking behaviors. Raine and coworkers (for a brief review, see Raine, 1997) have undertaken a number of studies examining these issues with respect to aggressive and violent behaviors. Low resting heart rate has been found quite reliably across a number of studies to correlate with antisocial and aggressive behavior. In a large study of children on the island of Mauritius, Raine, Venables, and Mednick (1997) found that low resting heart rate at age 3 predicted increased likelihood of aggressive behavior at age 11. This same group also found that fearlessness, stimulation seeking, and large body size at age 3 predicted childhood aggression at age 11 (Raine, Reynolds, Venables, Mednick, & Farrington, 1998); conversely, they found that high autonomic arousal and electrodermal orienting at age 15 were protective against criminal behavior at age 29 (Raine et al., 1995). Furthermore, in a study of sons of criminal and noncriminal fathers, they found that noncriminal sons of criminal fathers showed higher skin conductance and heart rate orienting reactivity than either (1) criminal sons of criminal or noncriminal fathers or (2) noncriminal sons of noncriminal fathers (Brennan et al., 1997). They argue that these studies support the role of arousal in protecting individuals from engaging in antisocial activity. In his review of this area, Raine cites other studies supporting the role of underarousal as a mediator of disinhibited temperament predisposing individuals to antisocial outcomes, and of high levels of arousal and conditionability as protectors from such outcomes. (See also the description of Kagan's work in Chapter 3.)

Based on the fact that underarousal as a predictor of antisocial behavior appears stronger in higher-SES than in lower-SES samples, Raine (1997) hypothesizes that such psychophysiological correlates may play a more prominent role when other factors conditioning individuals toward antisocial behavior are less dominant. He also raises questions about whether such underarousal may arise as a reaction to the stress of adverse early life experiences. Raine's speculations are partially supported in a study of clinically referred 6- to 13-year-old children with CD. Wootton et al. (1997) found that children high on the trait "callous/unemotional" had a high number of conduct problems, regardless of the quality of parenting they received; in contrast, ineffective parenting was associated with conduct problems in children without this trait. Although there are questions about ceiling effects in this study, it does suggest that in some instances extreme temperamental traits may override the quality of parenting.

Impact of Genetic and Constitutional Factors on Development of Affect Regulation

We can presume that the heritable traits described above will make children with DBDs more difficult to raise. High levels of inattentiveness and hyperactivity make it difficult for such children to listen and comply with parental demands. High levels of sensation seeking, or novelty seeking or other approach-type behaviors will also propel such children toward their own goals, which are often at odds with those of their parents. If these children are physiologically underaroused (which is usually the case), they may be still further hampered in developing age-appropriate affect regulation and coping skills, and still further inclined toward antisocial behavior. As has been articulated in earlier chapters, such traits may make such children very difficult for parents, especially those who are preoccupied or lacking in patience. This sets the stage for conflict and the beginning of coercive relationships. Such children will experience the world and their attempts to cope as frustrating, and their development will go further and further off track. Buffering temperamental traits such as inhibition and arousal may, however, interfere with this negative trajectory.

Given the array of factors presumed to increase vulnerability to DBDs, we should expect a gradual clarification of how each of these factors contributes uniquely or in combination to externalizing behavior. It is important to clarify whether factors act to induce vulnerability to affect regulation difficulties, to impair adaptive coping strategies and executive control, or to make individuals vulnerable to interactional difficulties with caretakers. These effects are not mutually exclusive, but the distinctions among them need to inform our search for mechanisms of action.

PSYCHOSOCIAL FACTORS

Despite the impressive literature with respect to the role of genetic and constitutional factors in the genesis of DBDs, psychosocial factors also play an important role. As with the internalizing disorders, a number of family variables have been found to be relevant with respect to both the onset and maintenance of this group of disorders. Low SES, single-parent status, parental conflict and separation, parental psychiatric and criminal history, and stressful life events have all been identified as contributory. Although some of these variables may operate through unique paths, generally they appear to exert a main effect through compromised parenting (inconsistent and harsh) (Kendziora & O'Leary, 1993) or through parent–child interaction (predominantly negative and critical) (Belsky et al., 1995). This includes an impact on maternal responsiveness and the attachment relationship, as well as in-ept and coercive parenting practices throughout childhood. In late childhood and adolescence, the larger environment (peers and crimi-nal environments) also plays a role. Curiously, genetic factors may be-come more important with age, playing a larger role in adult than in juvenile antisocial traits (Lyons et al., 1995).

The Role of Attachment

Consistent with early theorizing, insecure attachment has been shown to be related to later externalizing behavior problems. This relationship appears stronger for disorganized attachment than for other patterns, but it does not exclude other forms of insecure attachment. Shaw et al. (1996), examining early risk factors and pathways in the development of early disruptive behavior problems in a sample of low-SES families, found that disorganized attachment classification at 12 months and maternal personality risk and child-rearing disagreements during the second year predicted disruptive behavior at age 5. In addition, disor-ganized attachment plus maternal perception of difficult child temper-ament predicted child aggression at age 5. Disorganized attachment, maternal personality risk, and child-rearing disagreements predicted aggression at age 5 as well as aggression at age 3 did. Other forms of insecure attachment also predicted later disruptive behavior, but only if combined with other child or parent risk factors in the second year.

Fagot and Leve (1998) note that not all studies have found a rela-tionship between early attachment classification and later disorder; they also point out that generally the relationship between insecure at-tachment and DBDs appears less strong in low-risk populations. Fagot and Pears (1996) examined variables related to changes in attachment pattern during a child's third year. They found that children who ended up in Crittenden's *coercive* category (a subgroup of insecure at-tachment in Crittenden's system for classifying toddlers and an exten-sion of infant resistant–ambivalent attachment) at age three came largely from the avoidant and resistant categories of infant attachment, but that this change correlated with parenting variables (low SES, fewer instructions, more affect). They also found that a coercive attachment relationship at age 3 predicted both internalizing and externalizing behavior at age 7.

In two separate samples of 4- to 6-year-old clinic-referred children with DBDs, Greenberg, DeKlyen, Speltz, and Endriga (1997) found a disproportionately large number of children with a controlling attachment relationship. (*Controlling* is the preschool equivalent of the infant disorganized attachment rating.) Girls in the clinic-referred group were less likely to be insecure than were the boys. Assessment of separation anxiety revealed that in the clinic group insecure boys had double the distress scores of secure boys, but this anxiety was apparently not identified as an issue by the parents. Mothers' attachment classifications were largely consistent with those of their children.

Although the relationship between attachment classification and externalizing psychopathology is not direct, insecure attachment (particularly disorganized) does appear to make children more vulnerable to later behavior problems. In the Shaw et al. (1996) study, the fact that insecurity of attachment only exerted an effect when combined with later parent or child risk factors suggests either that the factors leading to insecurity in an infant must continue to act and must interact with later variables, or that an insecure attachment makes a child more difficult for many parents (especially those who may be stressed or in conflict, and less than optimally able to set limits and support a toddler). However, the fact that even securely attached children displayed behavior problems suggests that other factors may override the impact of a positive attachment relationship. Lastly, however, security of attachment does change from the first to the second year in some groups—a fact that may be especially relevant for children of depressed mothers and for maltreated toddlers (Field, 1989, 1994). This means that attachment security in the second year may better predict later DBDs. It is also possible that parent–child conflict, which I discuss next, is a better predictor of later externalizing behavior and insecure attachment.

Although the standard approach to the symptoms of ADHD has been to view them as arising from a predominantly constitutional and largely hereditary base (Thapar et al., 1995), work by Sroufe and colleagues suggests that distractibility and hyperactivity may also have their origins in caregiving and contextual factors (Carlson, Jacobvitz, & Sroufe, 1995; Jacobvitz & Sroufe, 1987). In a longitudinal study of a high-risk population of mothers and infants, they found that caregiver variables in early childhood, such as maternal intrusiveness, seductiveness, and overstimulation, predicted distractibility (an early precursor of hyperactivity) better than did biological or temperamental factors. In middle childhood, intrusive caregiving and relationship support at 30 months, along with early distractibility, continued to predict hyperactivity. These authors conclude that there may be several different pathways to ADHD.

Discipline and Parent–Child Conflict

Negative parent–child interaction has been found to be a strong predictor of child behavior problems (Campbell et al., 1996; Fagot & Leve, 1998; Patterson et al., 1998). Patterson and his coworkers at the Oregon Social Learning Center have developed and tested their coercion theory to explain the development and maintenance of antisocial behavior. Patterson proposes that disruptive behavior begins with disrupted parenting practices (inconsistent discipline, poor monitoring, and poor problem solving), reinforced by negative comments. This leads to child behaviors of demandingness and coercion, which are not managed in a way that would contain them. The parents may give in to stop the irritating child behaviors or may allow the children to escape from their demands. The result is that the children continue to engage in aversive behaviors and the parents continue to respond with angry but ineffectual strategies. The children fail to learn many critical social skills, such as delaying gratification, taking turns, or strategies for dealing with frustration in more socially acceptable ways. Because these children and their parents become locked in a conjoint pattern of coercion, they gradually develop negative beliefs about each other, which over time become mutually reinforcing. This coercive pattern of interaction has been found in the majority of studies that have attempted to examine family factors relating to externalizing behavior; it is also supported by intervention studies, which show changes in externalizing behavior that parallel changes in parenting practice or the parent–child relationship (Dishion, French, & Patterson, 1995; Webster-Stratton & Hammond, 1997). Patterson has theorized that although other factors may play a role in the development of disruptive behavior, they do so primarily through their impact on parenting practices.

The other major theoretical approach to understanding parental influences on the development of behavior problems is that of Bugental (1992), whose model of "threat-oriented family systems" has been discussed in greater length in Chapter 4. Bugental's formulation is consistent with Patterson's model, and the results are the same— ineffective discipline and a conflicted parent–child relationship. As noted in Chapters 4 and 9, this conflicted parent–child relationship may contribute to depression in the parent (Brown et al., 1990), as well as to both internalizing and externalizing disorders in the child (Messer & Gross, 1995; Ge et al., 1996). Bugental's model begins to get at intrapsychic variables within a parent that may condition him or her to respond affectively to a child's behavior. I discuss this more fully below.

Attachment insecurity has been posited as a factor in the development of behavior problems. As noted in Chapter 9, Lyons-Ruth (1992) carried out a longitudinal study of depressed mother–infant dyads and found that security of attachment predicted strongly to later problem behavior (disorganized attachment, in particular, predicted hostile–aggressive behavior in kindergarten).

As noted in the literature on high expressed emotion (see Chapter 4), exposure to parental criticism has also been related to externalizing behavior. Research by Vostanis and colleagues (Vostanis et al., 1994; Vostanis & Nicholls, 1995) has linked CD in particular to low maternal warmth and high maternal criticism. However, in other research, the effects of high expressed emotion appear relatively nonspecific across internalizing and externalizing psychopathology (Hibbs et al., 1991). The expressed emotion literature is highly consistent with the models of Patterson and Bugental; moreover, the finding that expressed emotion occurs across internalizing and externalizing disorders does suggest that a common factor in psychopathology is early parent–child conflict, with parental criticism and lack of warmth (perhaps more relevant in externalizing than in internalizing disorders) maintaining the child's sense of rejection and low self-esteem. As indicated in all of these models, the child's coercive or oppositional behaviors complete the vicious circle (Hammen et al., 1990). This is also consistent with an analysis of the comorbidity between CD and mood disorders in a longitudinal sample of a birth cohort in New Zealand, conducted by Fergussson, Lynskey, and Horwood (1996). They found that a substantial amount of the comorbidity between these types of disorders arose from shared variance in risk factors and life pathways. Although their analysis still left a substantial amount of the comorbidity unexplained, I believe that the coercive interactional patterns described above, perhaps together with some overlap of genetic factors, can explain this comorbidity.

As Chapter 4 also notes, there is evidence that children witnessing adult conflict are likely to display an increase in acting-out behaviors (Cummings et al., 1985). This is particularly so for boys and for children rated as aggressive; nonaggressive children are more likely to report distress (Cummings & Cummings, 1988). These authors suggest that the difference between boys and girls may reflect a difference in manner of expressing disturbance rather than in degree of disturbance, with girls tending to react more through withdrawal or anxiety. Gorman-Smith and Tolan (1998) found that exposure to violence was related to increases in aggressive behavior and depression even after previous levels of these variables were controlled for. Ballard et al. (1993), in reviewing this area, have concluded that repeated exposure to anger is associated with heightened emotional and behavioral reactivity to anger. Cummings and Cummings (1988) also acknowledge the possibility of a modeling effect; they specifically cite Bandura's notion that exposure to adult anger acts to disinhibit behavior and enhances the power of modeling. Given that many children at risk for CD live in families where there is an increased likelihood of parental conflict, it is reasonable to assume that children exposed to these angry interactions may become sensitized to anger and more likely to react angrily to frustrations. Furthermore, the highly charged emotional climate in these families may make learning about affect regulation more problematic.

Lazarus and Folkman (1984) have proposed that problem solving or problem-focused coping is difficult when emotional distress is high. Some children may withdraw to deal with their own arousal, and this may become their predominant strategy for managing conflicted interpersonal situations; as emphasized at many points in this book, this prevents opportunities for learning about affects and their regulation, and about strategies for working out conflict. Others may act out their tension in difficult behaviors, further maintaining a high level of arousal but also reducing their chances of developing more adaptive coping strategies. Allen, Hauser, O'Connor, Bell, and Eickholt (1996), in an observational study of parents and their 14-year-old children followed up at age 16, found that those adolescents who at age 14 displayed difficulty discussing disagreements directly with their parents showed increased levels of hostile conflict with parents at age 16. Exposure to hostile parent conflict at age 14 promoted adolescent withdrawal from the hostile parents at age 16. The authors have surmised that those adolescents at age 14 who cannot discuss disagreements openly may need to distance themselves as they try to meet autonomy needs. This pattern, however, also seems to predict ongoing difficulty, as the withdrawal interferes with the development of autonomous relatedness. The idea that early maladaptive behaviors or strategies for managing affect interfere with the development of coping skills is a consistent one. Cummings and Cummings (1988), in their review of children's coping with adult anger, concluded that the relationship with psychopathology is probably mediated by the interference of maladaptive patterns of coping, accumulated stress, or both with the development of adaptive capacities.

Peer Relations

Association with deviant peers has been proposed as both a cause and a consequence of antisocial behavior. It seems clear that children with externalizing behavior are more likely to be rejected, although some aspects of antisocial behavior may actually be valued within the male peer group (Dishion, French, & Patterson, 1995). Patterson et al. (1998) found that involvement with deviant peers, along with the level of disrupted family process, predicted who would follow the trajectory from early antisocial behavior to early arrest. Keenan, Loeber, Zhang, Stouthamer-Loeber, and Van Kammen (1995) found that earlier involvement with deviant peers predicted increased involvement with delinquent activities, but not as strongly as current association with deviant peers. They also propose that this relationship may apply more to adolescent-onset CD than to the childhood-onset variant. That distinction may explain the lack of a relationship between deviant peers and later delinquency in a report by Tremblay, Masse, Vitaro, and Dobkin (1995), who were studying a group predominantly composed of youth with childhood-onset CD. These authors suggest that friends may foster continuity of behavior rather than change, as friends tend to share the same characteristics. Furthermore, these relationships tend to be relatively short-lived and to consist of high levels of coercive interchanges (Dishion, Andrews, & Crosby, 1995). Although this issue may still be open, it is fairly clear that many disruptive children are rejected by their peers, and that this may contribute to further behavioral and emotional difficulties.

Coie et al. (1995) found that boys who were both rejected and aggressive in grade 3 had profiles of increasingly severe internalizing and externalizing problems in adolescence. Similarly, Schwartz, McFadyen-Ketchum, Dodge, Pettit, and Bates (1998) found that victimization in grades 3–4 was associated with externalizing behavior, attention dysregulation, and immature dependent behavior in grades 5–6. Hinshaw and Melnick (1995) examined different possible pathways to peer rejection for boys with ADHD, who were observed (along with comparison boys) in a summer camp setting. Highly aggressive and noncompliant boys (both with and without ADHD) were rejected by peers, as were socially isolated boys with ADHD. Highly aggressive boys with ADHD displayed greater emotional reactivity and less effective affect regulation in frustrating situations. Emotional reactivity and affect regulation correlated with peer status.

Child Maltreatment

Maltreated children can be presumed to be at the negative extreme on all of the risk factors described thus far (Rogosch, Cicchetti, & Aber, 1995). They are more likely to be aggressive and rejected than nonmaltreated children. They have more difficulty understanding negative affect in interpersonal situations, and this impaired understanding appears to act as a mediator between maltreatment in general and later behavioral dysregulation, as well as between physical abuse in particular and later peer rejection. In adolescence, maltreated youth reported more verbal and physical abuse both toward and by their dating partners (Wolfe, Wekerle, Reitzel-Jaffe, & Lefebvre, 1998). They were also seen by teachers as engaging in more acts of aggression and harassment. Clearly, maltreated individuals are at high risk for both internalizing and externalizing difficulties, and some of that risk may be related to difficulties both in understanding negative affect in others and in regulating their own negative affect.

Impact of Psychosocial Factors on Development of Affect Regulation

As indicated in earlier chapters, psychosocial factors can be explored on many different levels with respect to the development of affect regulation. For the sake of simplicity, I briefly examine speculations about internal working models or schemata and coping strategies in individuals with DBDs. First, however, some information about general findings with respect to affect regulation in children with externalizing behaviors is presented to provide a background for these speculations.

Eisenberg et al. (1996) examined the relations of affect regulation and emotionality to problem behavior in elementary school children. In general, low affect regulation, negative emotionality, and general and positive emotional intensity predicted behavior problems. The child's capacity to regulate affect buffered the effect of negative emotionality on problem behaviors, with the effect most significant at higher levels of negative emotionality. Parent- and teacher-rated ego resiliency was also related negatively to problem behaviors. (The construct of *ego resiliency* is felt to tap the capacity of the individual to respond flexibly to the situation; it is contrasted with *ego brittleness*, which reflects an inability to respond to changing demands or to perseverate.) Children with more problem behavior had lower resting heart rates. Also, children who made small, quick gaze aversions during a distressing film sequence had lower levels of problem behaviors. The authors interpreted their findings as consistent with the view that individual differences in children's capacity to regulate attention and behavior, along with the dimension of emotional intensity (combined and separately), predicted childhood externalizing problems. The heart rate and intensity data in this study suggest the importance of constitutional regulation, but the dimensions of negative emotionality and ego resiliency suggest aspects of learned behavior as well.

Internal Working Models

As discussed in earlier chapters, internal working models or schemata provide a way of understanding how early experience continues to exert an impact on behavior. These internalized mental representations of oneself and of others in relationships create expectancies that condition attitudes and beliefs and that ultimately influence coping strategies or defenses. It is generally assumed that these internal structures operate at an unconscious or subconscious level, and that particular working models/schemata (or neural networks) will be more powerful in their influence when the individual is stressed or is experiencing affects that are connected with those models.

There is not a large literature with respect to internal working models in individuals with CD, although much of Bowlby's original theorizing was influenced by his work with juvenile delinquents. Fonagy et al. (1997) have developed a theory using attachment and mentalizing capacity to explain the moral deficit and lack of control over aggression seen in psychopathic individuals (and, by extension, in persons with less severe forms of antisocial behavior). Relying on the notion that lack of connectedness (attachment) to individuals or organizations allows people to break common rules, they suggest that psychopathic individuals have failed to develop any attachment to parents or to significant others that would act to inhibit their behavior. They are driven only by their own wants or needs. In addition, Fonagy and colleagues propose that a correlate of this failed attachment is the lack of the capacity to understand the minds and feelings of others, which they call "mentalizing capacity." They include in this a diminished capacity for self-reflection. They argue that this reduced mentalizing capacity interferes with psychopathic individuals' sense of their own identity and agency, and so they fail to develop a sense of their own responsibility. Their inability to intuit the minds and feelings of others allows them to act with no apparent regard for their victims, treating them as though they were objects standing in the way of a goal.

In a pilot study exploring aspects of this theory, Levinson and Fonagy (cited in Fonagy et al., 1997) compared the Adult Attachment Interviews (AAIs) of a group of prisoners with those of psychiatric inpatients and normal controls; the prisoners and patients were matched for diagnosis, and all groups were matched for age, sex, IQ, and SES. The prisoner and patient groups both had lower rates of secure attachment than the control group. The prisoner group was more likely to have dismissing attachments than the patients, who were more likely to have preoccupied attachments. In addition, the patients were much more likely to be in the unresolved category than the prisoners (82% vs. 36%). There was a much higher history of abuse and neglect among the prisoners than among the patients, where rejection was more common. Both groups reported anger with attachment figures, although this was more current in the patient group and more intense in the prisoner group. Ratings on the Reflective Function scale (a measure of mentalizing capacity) were lowest in the prisoners, intermediate in the patients, and highest in the controls. When violent offenders were compared with nonviolent offenders, the Reflective Function score was lower in the violent offenders.

Although this work is clearly preliminary, it does suggest some support for Fonagy et al.'s (1997) theory. What it also does, if these results can be replicated, is to suggest differences between internalizing and externalizing disorders. Their work suggests that individuals with externalizing psychopathology may have experienced more neglect and abuse than most psychiatric inpatients, and that those experiences may have promoted a style of avoidance or distancing that, at its extreme, allows them to ignore interpersonal issues. Their low reflectiveness also suggests a reduced capacity to be guided by mental introjects or schemata, and an increased likelihood that their anger will be acted out if the situation permits. The high rate of unresolved AAIs in the psychiatric patients, and their current anger at attachment figures, suggest that patients are still connected (albeit ambivalently) with their attachment objects.

Consistent with Fonagy et al.'s (1997) framework, it is reasonable to assume that the internal working models of individuals with CD will reflect their life experience of maltreatment (abuse or neglect), conflict with parents, peers, teachers, failure at school and jobs, involvement with substances as a way of self-soothing, law breaking with and without consequences, failed intimate relationships, and eventually failures with their own children. Their view of the world is understandably hostile and unsupportive. Their view of themselves must contain feelings of being constantly attacked and of being inadequate in most interpersonal spheres, as well as of failing to master other normal challenges. Their understanding of their own feelings is probably limited to general tension or negative emotionality, as they have seldom had adult-supported opportunities to learn about feelings when they were not aroused. Similarly, their opportunities to learn problem-solving approaches to affect regulation have undoubtedly been limited, and they are left with rather primitive physical discharge of distressing affects. Although I agree with Fonagy et al. that at the severe end of this spectrum individuals have probably failed to develop internal structures that inhibit antisocial behavior, I believe that we also need to look more closely at the representations that have developed around management of anger. Some of these individuals have been severely traumatized and presumably have dealt with those experiences through dissociative mechanisms. In those instances where individuals with CD display reactive aggression, it is reasonable to assume that some of this may arise from activation of repressed/dissociated memories or from cognitive–affective schematic representations. This may be different from proactive aggression, which may reflect more distanced and less preoccupied schemata. In this case, individuals may have failed to attach affect to representations or may have dismissed affect as unimportant.

Coping

The coping strategies used by individuals with CD are outgrowths of these internal working models combined with temperamental, neurobiological, and learning factors. As discussed in Chapter 6, temperamental differences in approach style, attentional capacity, and degree of inhibition will affect how an individual perceives the world and responds to it. As indicated above, individuals with CD are more likely to be sensation-seeking, less fearful, and/or less easily aroused. If their CD is comorbid with ADHD, they will also be more impulsive, hyperactive, and/or inattentive. These traits make their behavior more difficult for parents and increase the likelihood of angry interactions. If these interactions are frequent or intense, they will interfere with the development of adaptive coping strategies. As suggested by Eisenberg et al.'s (1996) study, these children may develop more brittle, less resilient strategies, as their conflicted interactions with parents create tension that may interfere with opportunities to discuss feelings and how to manage them. Instead, these children learn through repetition of experience (much of it stressful), with little development of reflection on their own or others' feelings. Because their conflicted pattern of interaction and rejection tends to be repeated with peers and teachers, the scope for change is limited. Withdrawal, coercive interactions, or combinations of the two, provide little opportunity for developing the types of relationships that would permit understanding how others feel and how one's behaviors influence other's feelings. The acting out of angry feelings in coercive interchanges with parents and peers may get others to give in, reinforcing this as a normal way of coping with anger. In addition, the difficulties with control of attention and behavior seen in many individuals with CD (especially those who have comorbid ADHD) may interfere with the early development of strategies to control the intensity of stimuli. The use of brief gaze aversions during a distressing film clip by the nonproblem children in the Eisenberg et al. (1996) study illustrates what appears to be a normative strategy for regulating affect. Limited access to such strategies may force individuals with CD to avoid affect more in order to regulate their experience. In extreme situations where the situation feels overwhelming (traumatic), such individuals may use dissociation or such extreme avoidance that they gradually cut themselves off from feeling (psychopathic lack of concern).

Dodge (1993), in his social information processing model, has described the attributions and cognitive distortions that many children with CD display. Dodge and colleagues have shown that in the first stage of information processing (in which an individual encodes or selects information from the environment), aggressive children use less information and attend more to hostile cues than do nonaggressive children. They also tend to generate fewer response alternatives and more aggressive and ineffective solutions to problem situations. Moreover, they tend to select aggressive solutions with little apparent concern for the negative consequences of their behavior. Such individuals attribute blame to others for their behavior and misinterpret others' intentions, attributing more hostile intent to others than was intended. It is understandable that aggressive individuals develop these ways of thinking, given their repetitive hostile experiences, but their sensitized processing of information appears to reinforce their beliefs, making change difficult. There is some evidence that changing distorted cognitions in such a child, along with improving family behavioral management, reduces externalizing behavior.

NEUROBIOLOGICAL FACTORS

Because a thorough review of all neurobiological mechanisms that may contribute to the development of externalizing behaviors is beyond my scope, I concentrate here on three topics that appear most salient to the neurobiology of aggression: obstetrical complications and neurological soft signs; the hypothesized role of serotonin (5-HT) in modulation of aggression; and some of the brain areas involved in the control of aggression.

Obstetrical Complications and Soft Signs

Obstetrical complications have been implicated in vulnerability to externalizing disorders, as they have been for internalizing disorders

(Allen, Lewinsohn, & Seeley, 1998). Raine, Brennan, and Mednick (1994), in a Danish cohort of 4,269 consecutive live male births, found that birth complications when combined with maternal rejection predicted violent offending in adulthood. Neither variable alone was significant in predicting later violent offending. Obstetrical complications may cause brain damage, which makes it harder for an individual to control arousal or state regulation, as has been proposed for very-low-birthweight infants (Sykes et al., 1997). As noted in Chapter 9, this may make such a child appear more difficult in the eyes of stressed parents and lead to parent–child conflict. Furthermore, these deficits by themselves, or in combination with a conflictual parent–child relationship, may interfere with the development of affect regulation skills.

Soft signs also appear to be more prevalent in boys with ADHD or CD than in controls (Szatmari, Offord, Siegel, Finlayson, & Tuff, 1990), although the specificity of these findings for externalizing disorders is unclear (Pine, Wasserman, et al., 1997). Pine, Wasserman, et al. (1997) speculate that such signs may represent dysfunction in subcortical motor circuits, specifically those involving basal ganglia–prefrontal cortical loops, but also raise the issue that abnormalities in dopaminergic or serotonergic pathways may be involved. Using the same Danish cohort referred to above, Raine et al. (1996) found that a biosocial group (with early neuromotor deficits and unstable family environment) had twice the adult violence, theft, and total crime rates of the other two groups (one with obstetrical complications only, and the other with poverty only).

Although the mechanisms connecting obstetrical complications, soft signs, or neuromotor deficits to later DBDs are not known, Moffitt (1993) has argued that neuropsychological deficits affecting executive control, which appear to be more common in individuals who have both ADHD and CD, may be relevant in both the development and maintenance of externalizing behaviors. Deficits in response inhibition on a "stop signal" paradigm have become fairly well established in assessments of children with ADHD (Schachar & Logan, 1990). More recently, Oosterlaan, Logan, and Sergeant (1998) compared data from eight studies employing this task in groups of children with various childhood disorders. They found that deficits in response inhibition were present in children with ADHD, ADHD and CD, and CD alone. It is not clear whether this shared difficulty with response inhibition reflects a common underlying impairment in executive function or arises from different underlying causes. Moffitt also points to her own finding of a verbal/language deficit in boys with ADHD and CD, which she believes contributes to frustration in academic settings and which (in combination with attentional and impulse control problems) makes

them ill prepared to cope with school demands. She also acknowledges that the nature and causal mechanisms of these deficits are
poorly understood and are not likely in themselves to cause CD, but
do appear to make children vulnerable to the interactional difficulties
with parents, peers, and teachers mentioned above. Fergusson and
Lynskey (1997) found that when the association between reading difficulties and CD were adjusted for confounding factors, such as attentional and early behavioral difficulties, the association was no longer
significant. This supports the argument that reading difficulties do not
cause CD; however, it still allows for reading difficulties to contribute,
as Moffitt has suggested, to frustration in academic settings and school
failure—further stressors in the life of a child with CD.

Serotonin

The role of 5-HT in predisposing individuals to suicidal and violent
behavior has been mentioned in Chapter 7. Constantino, Morris, and
Murphy (1997) examined leftover cerebrospinal fluid (CSF) in 193 neu-
rologically healthy newborns for levels of 5-hydroxyindoleacetic acid
(5HIAA), the main 5-HT metabolite. They found that CSF 5-HIAA was
lower in infants with family histories of ASPD than in infants without
such family histories. This finding in infants is consistent with studies
in adults, but is the inverse of that found in children. Pine, Coplan, et
al. (1997) measured prolactin responses to a fenfluramine challenge in
brothers of youth charged with juvenile delinquency. They found a
correlation between aggressivity and prolactin response (an indicator
of central serotonergic activity), but also a positive correlation between
adverse rearing and prolactin response that was independent of aggressivity. These authors raise questions about the possibility of a developmental change in the relationship between 5-HT and aggression.
It is also possible that chronic elevation of 5-HT activity may lead to
modification in receptor activity over time, resulting in lower levels in
adulthood. This does not, however, explain the finding of the low levels in infants of families with histories of ASPD. These relations are
clearly complex, as they appear to involve initial predisposing variables that may be modified with experience, yielding results that are
difficult to interpret.

Spoont (1992) has reviewed the modulatory role of 5-HT in information processing, and suggests ways in which 5-HT depletion may
contribute to psychopathology. 5-HT containing cells arise principally
in the midbrain raphe nuclei and project widely throughout the cortex,
limbic, and forebrain areas. Generally, 5-HT activity inhibits and 5-HT
depletions facilitate a variety of functions, including locomotor activity

(when dopamine activity is also stimulated), switching to alternate behaviors, punishment-induced behavioral suppression, and the amplitude of the startle response. Spoont theorizes that 5-HT acts to constrain information flow, reducing interference from irrelevant stimuli
and from sensitization to potentially threatening stimuli. Although primate studies show that 5-HT facilitates social behavior (increases in
approach behavior; decreases in avoidance, vigilance, and social soli-
tude), the relationship with changes in 5-HT is not altogether direct.
Spoont speculates that depletions of 5-HT may change an animal's sensitivity to signals that normally suppress social behavior, resulting in
inappropriate social behaviors. This combination of removal of behavioral suppression with respect to locomotor activity and social constraint is suggestive of the child with ADHD. Temperamental traits
such as sensation seeking (which may be dopamine-based), along with
release of punishment-induced suppression, could describe the child
vulnerable to CD. With respect to aggression, the relationship between
5-HT activity and the inhibition of aggression occurs largely in nonaggressive strains of rodents, suggesting genetic differences in 5-HT's
modulation of aggression. Because there is evidence in primates that
the monoamines have a significant heritable component in their expression (Clarke et al., 1995), this would suggest that one aspect of the
genetic liability to aggression may be genetic control over aspects of
the serotonergic system.

Alterations in monoamines can occur secondarily to stress, as discussed in Chapter 9 (De Kloet, 1991). Spoont (1992) also cites studies
showing that deprived rearing situations in rodents produce irritable
aggression in those animals that exhibit reduced 5-HT activity.

Spoont (1992) goes on to speculate that reduced 5-HT may influence the development of aggressive behavior by altering the signal-to-
noise ratio, producing an exaggerated response to a signal. She fur-
thers her argument through reference to the human studies that have
demonstrated negative correlations between CSF 5-HIAA and traits of
hostility, impulsivity, and negative affectivity. She suggests that a propensity for aggression may result from exaggerated reactivity to signals that elicit aggression, combined with an insensitivity to cues that
would normally suppress this behavior. She also emphasizes the contribution of a lack not only of behavioral constraint but also of affective
constraint. These speculations receive support from a study by Knutson et al. (1998), who administered a selective 5-HT reuptake inhibitor
or a placebo to normal volunteers, and assessed personality and social
variables at baseline and during medication. They reported that ad-
ministration of the active drug reduced dimensions of hostility
through a general decrease in negative affect but also increased social

affiliation. These changes were related to plasma levels of the drug at the end of the study.

Brain Areas Involved in Control of Aggression

The brain areas that have been implicated in aggression and its regulation include the hypothalamus, the amygdala, the periaqueductal grey area, the septum, and the frontotemporal lobes. Weiger and Bear (1988), in a review of the neurology of aggression, point out how lesions at various levels of the nervous system produce aggressive behaviors with differing levels of responsiveness to environmental stimuli. Aggressive behavior related to brainstem lesions will be more stereotyped and independent of a person's learning or past history. In contrast, limbic system lesions (where association of relevance of stimulus to response is mediated) may provoke changes in response according to type of stimulus or in intensity of response. Frontal lesions may produce aggressive behavior in which consequences or social conventions are ignored. Thus, in a study where demented patients with frontotemporal dysfunction (demonstrated through single-photon emission computed tomography) were compared to those with Alzheimer's disease, the former showed elevated levels of antisocial behaviors, including assault, indecent exposure, shoplifting, and hit-and-run driving (Miller, Darby, Benson, Cummings, & Miller, 1997). The lateral hypothalamus has been shown to mediate predatory or instrumental aggression, in contrast to the ventromedial hypothalamus, which is largely associated with affective or reactive aggression.

Acetylcholine appears to be the primary neurotransmitter involved in aggression (Weiger & Bear, 1988) but 5-HT appears to play a modulatory role in the hypothalamus and the amygdala, as well as in the periaqueductal gray area, where aggression and escape behaviors appear to be organized (Spoont, 1992). The amygdala can act to facilitate or inhibit aggression through its effects on the hypothalamus. Removal of the amygdala, as in Kluver–Bucy syndrome, produces inappropriate aggressive behavior but also an overall decrease in aggressive behavior. Because the amygdala is prone to kindling, overactivation of amygdala neurons (as may occur in interictal episodes of temporal lobe epilepsy) may account for the heightened emotional responses seen in this disorder. Weiger and Bear (1988) describe such patients as quick to anger, paranoid (secondary to enhanced fearfulness), prone to misinterpret others' actions as personally threatening, and easily aroused. Spoont (1992) points out that the central nucleus of the amygdala and the dorsal raphe nucleus (5-HT pathway) are reciprocally organized, and that these structures are interconnected. Lesions of the central nucleus of the amygdala block fear conditioning and release punishment-induced behavioral suppression. The septum also plays a role in inhibiting aggression probably through its connections to the lateral hypothalamus.

Although these pathways are complex, one can speculate that some aggressive behaviors arise from inadequate modulatory control of hypothalamic centers through decreased 5-HT input from the amygdala or septal nuclei. Conversely, stimulation of hypothalamic centers from irritable foci in the amygdala, as in the situation of kindling, may also induce inappropriate or excessive aggression. If these mechanisms are combined with enhanced stress reactivity, as suggested by Spoont (1992), such individuals may experience high levels of negative affect and may have reduced resources for coping with this tension in constructive ways. Obviously, learning can act to reinforce these mechanisms. Intact frontal–limbic circuits can be presumed to act to inhibit aggressive behavior through attention to consequences and facilitation of verbally and cognitively mediated strategies.

CONCLUSION

Externalizing behavior arises from a complex interaction of genetic and constitutional, psychosocial, and neurobiological factors. Individuals vulnerable to the DBDs appear to have a propensity to aggressive responding to frustration. They grow up in an environment that reinforces this propensity through lack of warmth and through hostile and critical responses to these temperamentally challenging children. The parents of these vulnerable children are likely to be genetically or temperamentally similar to their offspring and to have experienced less than optimal parenting themselves, which may make it very hard for them to marshal the resources or patience to respond positively to these children, whom they perceive as difficult. This conflicted parent–child interaction leads to coercive behaviors in the children that generalize to school and peers, culminating in academic underachievement and peer rejection. Their poor understanding of affect (both their own and others') results in ongoing conflicted interactions, with aggressive acting out and withdrawal becoming the main strategies for managing conflict.

These demoralized children gravitate to other marginalized peers, and together they may act out their hostility and sense of being wronged through more intense antisocial behavior. They may turn to substance use and abuse for purposes of both self-soothing and risk taking. Throughout their development, they experience the world as highly stressful and may from an early age attempt to shut themselves off from painful affects. Those who have been abused may need dissociative strategies to cope. Brain changes may involve hippocampal damage (from ongoing stress; see Chapter 9), kindling of amygdala–hypothalamus circuits, and reduced 5-HT (which allows increased aggressive responding). Their view of the world is one of unpredictable threats, and so they cannot trust others to help them change their pattern of behavior. Finally, they are likely to seek intimate partners from a similar background and to repeat the cycle with their own children. Prevention or early intervention to interrupt this devastating cycle is clearly needed.

Chapter 11

Psychotic Disorders

In this chapter I examine how the theory of affect dysregulation and psychopathology can be applied to schizophrenia and the other psychotic disorders (schizoaffective disorder, schizophreniform disorder, etc.). I address these disorders as a group, since I believe that despite their varied nature and etiologies, they are characterized by common malfunctions in neural networks necessary for affect regulation. Most of the research to date has been done on schizophrenia, so the primary focus here is on that disorder (or group of disorders); moreover, much of the discussion is necessarily speculative, as definitive work on the neural networks involved has yet to be done.

The format for this chapter departs from that for Chapters 9 and 10. I begin by considering two basic issues in the definition of the psychotic disorders: First, are they disorders of cognition or of affect; and, second, are they related to mood (and anxiety) disorders? I then consider various recent conceptualizations of the core symptoms of schizophrenia and other psychotic disorders, as well as factors related to outcome in these disorders. Next, I discuss risk factors grouped according to whether they are *early precursors* (i.e., genetic, prenatal/ perinatal, or early childhood factors in etiology) or *late precursors* (i.e., behaviors and traits in later childhood and adolescence that relate to the development of psychosis). A detailed discussion of neurobiology follows.

BASIC DEFINITIONAL ISSUES

Are the Psychotic Disorders
Disturbances of Cognition or of Affect?

There is much debate about whether the psychotic disorders, especially schizophrenia, are primarily disorders of cognition or of affect. In keeping with a diathesis–stress model, I regard schizophrenia and other psychotic disorders as arising in a situation in which a sensitive and vulnerable individual is easily overwhelmed by stresses for which he or she lacks effective coping strategies. I also believe that such an individual has defects in neural networks that control sensory gating, attention, and working memory, such that the individual may be quickly overwhelmed, may have difficulty differentiating internal from external messages, and may have trouble attending to appropriate as opposed to inappropriate or irrelevant cues. The resulting distortions of perceptions and beliefs will affect the development and deployment of the individual's coping strategies. As I have argued for other types of disorders, a developmental perspective is necessary to understand how one vulnerable individual may become psychotic while another may be simply retiring or highly creative.

Schizophrenia, the most well-studied of the psychotic disorders, is generally regarded as a heterogeneous grouping of disorders (Beiser & Iacono, 1990). Although it was originally conceptualized as a disorder with progressive decline in cognitive function, recent follow-up studies have demonstrated that a significant proportion of patients show little decline in cognitive function (Rund, 1998). It does appear, however, that there may well be a *subgroup* of individuals with a neurodegenerative disorder, marked by a gradually deteriorating course, progressive enlargement of brain ventricles, accelerating loss of brain tissue, and progressive delays in treatment response (Knoll et al, 1998). This group appears to differ from other groups that do not display progressive deterioration and in which dysfunction may be more related to a functionally hyperactive dopamine system or early neurodevelopmental pathology.

Such a conceptualization is also consistent with the idea of different developmental paths to schizophrenia, as described by Walker et al. (1996). Using cluster analysis, these authors examined the variation in trajectories from childhood through adolescence to schizophrenia in adulthood. They found that one group showed more behavior problems, a more rapid escalation of behavior problems, and more obstetrical complications than the other group. While acknowledging that these differences may simply reflect severity, Walker et al. suggest that they may also reflect differing courses. The notion that there may be several different pathways to a similar outcome (psychosis, in this case) has been labeled *equifinality* and is a concept enjoying considerable attention in developmental psychopathology (Cicchetti & Rogosch, 1996). It does suggest the need to explore a variety of etiological factors, mechanisms, and their interactions to understand some of the ways in which individuals become psychotic.

Before beginning this exploration, I briefly describe the sources of evidence for the position that psychotic behavior arises, at least in part, from a failure in regulation of affect. In monozygotic twins discordant for schizophrenia, the sick twin displays greater stress reactivity and higher levels of neuroticism (DiLalla & Gottesman, 1995). Measures of anxiety correlate with level of reality distortion and positive symptoms (Norman, Malla, Cortese, & Diaz, 1998). Affect-decoding difficulties in schizophrenia appear to be more specific for negative affect, and individuals with schizophrenia appear to be highly sensitive to the negative emotions of fear and anger in particular (Mandal, Pandey, & Prasad, 1998). Social anhedonia, a factor thought to be characteristic of individuals with schizophrenia, appears related to social anxiety, decreased positive affect, and increased negative affect (Blanchard, Mueser, & Bellack, 1998). Lastly, high expressed emotion (EE), poor empathy, and critical attitudes in the relatives of individuals with schizophrenia are related to poorer outcomes and relapse (Giron & Gomez-Beneyto, 1998; Vaughan & Leff, 1976; Linszen et al., 1997).

In addition to the strong findings of cognitive dysfunction in schizophrenia, there may be several other reasons why there has been a tendency to think of this and other psychotic disorders as cognitive rather than affective in nature. These include the difficulty that most schizophrenic individuals have in expressing affect and in recounting their earlier affective experience; the perception that the stresses that may precipitate a psychotic episode seem relatively less clear than they do in mood and anxiety disorders; and the slow onset, which in many cases may obscure the factors involved in individuals' perception of what has been stressful. In my view, however, none of these factors is necessarily a reason for discounting the importance of affect dysregulation in the psychoses, and the first one may actually provide further support for it: The difficulty in expressing affect may itself be an aspect of the affect disturbance.

Are Psychotic Disorders Related to Mood (and Anxiety) Disorders?

In addition to the debate as to whether the psychotic disorders are largely affective or cognitive disorders, there has been a debate as to whether the psychotic disorders and mood disorders are related. This has been supported by findings of increased rates of mood disorders in relatives of schizophrenic probands with a family history of schizophrenic-spectrum illness, and an increased risk of schizophrenia and related disorders among the same probands with family histories of major mood disorders (Baron & Gruen, 1991). Furthermore, in the high-risk offspring of parents with schizophrenia, there is an elevated risk for mood disorders in the offspring (Mirsky, 1996).

Schizotypal personality disorder or personality traits, thought originally to reflect vulnerability to schizophrenia, have also been found in some (but not all) studies to be elevated in families of individuals with mood disorders. Kendler, McGuire, Gruenberg, and Walsh (1995), examining the factor structure of schizotypal symptoms and signs in an Irish cohort involving subjects with schizophrenia, mood disorders, and no psychiatric diagnosis and their families, found that negative schizotypy and avoidant symptoms distinguished relatives of probands with schizophrenia from relatives of probands with non-psychotic mood disorders. However, they also found evidence for nonspecificity of schizotypal traits, which led them to conclude that this apparent vulnerability factor (schizotypy) is neither highly specific nor nonspecific for schizophrenia. This would suggest an area of overlap between these two types of disorders, which could be related to genetic and/or environmental factors and which has the capacity to influence vulnerability to development of major psychiatric disturbance, as Mirsky (1996) has suggested.

Crow (1986) has argued that the mood disorders and schizophrenia are on a genetically determined continuum. He bases his argument on the overlap of mood and psychotic symptoms in patients; the overlap of schizoaffective disorder diagnoses in relatives; and his notion that there is an observed continuum of severity of psychosis and other deficits from unipolar depression through bipolar disorder to schizoaffective disorder and schizophrenia. This position is also consistent with findings by Coryell, Keller, Lavori, and Endicott (1990a, 1990b) of more morbidity in patients with schizoaffective mania and depression (especially if chronic) than of patients with pure mania and pure depression. Furthermore, depression has been a common finding in individuals with schizophrenia (Koreen et al., 1993)—as have "panic-like" symptoms (Cutler & Siris, 1991) and obsessive–compulsive symptoms (Tibbo & Warneke, 1999).

In the earlier psychodynamic literature, symptoms of schizophrenia were conceptualized as an individual's way of dealing with extreme levels of anxiety. Cutler and Siris (1991) point out, however, that for various reasons anxiety has received little systematic attention in the study of schizophrenia. I believe that this ignoring of the importance of anxiety is partly a backlash by biologically oriented researchers at the analytic community's tendency to overgeneralize its theories. Unfortunately, this risks the proverbial "throwing out the baby with the bathwater." Although the evidence for these issues is still arguable, there does appear to be enough overlap to suggest that psychotic, mood, and anxiety disorders may at least have mechanisms in common. I argue that some of the overlap arises from difficulties in affect regulation and stress reactivity, but also that differences in sensitivity and coping do distinguish these types of disorders from one another (Wiedl & Schottner, 1991).

CONCEPTUALIZATIONS OF SYMPTOMATOLOGY

For years investigators have struggled with defining the core symptoms of the psychotic disorders, particularly schizophrenia. The two basic sets of processes proposed by Crow (1980) and others, *positive* and *negative* symptoms, have provided a framework for much productive investigation (McGlashan & Fenton, 1992). However, the causes or underlying mechanisms for these two groupings, particularly negative symptoms, have not been well defined. Positive symptoms appear to represent the acute stress reaction and are commonly regarded as resulting from a hyperdopaminergic mechanism in mesolimbic pathways. Negative symptoms have at times been regarded as the result of the neurological deficits (principally affecting frontal–limbic circuits) that are presumed to be core features of schizophrenia, but they have also been seen as resulting from withdrawal and depression. The fact that positive symptoms remit with acute treatment and negative symptoms appear more stable has reinforced this view (Carpenter, Heinrichs, & Wagman, 1988). More recently (and particularly with the newer neuroleptics), there is evidence that negative symptoms can improve, albeit less dramatically than do positive symptoms (Czobor & Volavka, 1996).

McGlashan and Fenton (1992), in their review of the positive–negative distinction in schizophrenia, conclude that negative symptoms correlate robustly with poor premorbid social functioning, may relate to lower intelligence, have a strong association with neurological abnormalities, are relatively independent of positive symptoms, and predict poor outcomes across multiple dimensions more strongly with time. Speaking to the variability across studies, McGlashan and Fenton (1992) point out that although positive and negative symptom dimensions can be measured reliably, they may not have been assessed reliably in the studies these authors surveyed. Furthermore, there has been some inconsistency across studies in terms of which items have been included predominantly in positive or negative symptom domains. Because flat affect and poverty of speech were considered negative symptoms in all of the assessment systems reviewed, McGlashan and Fenton (1992) suggest that they become core defining criteria along with the positive symptoms: delusions, hallucinations, thought disorder, and disorganized behavior.

A number of authors have struggled with the failure of the positive–negative distinction to capture the core features of schizophrenia adequately. This effort to subdivide symptoms has led to a number of factor-analytic studies with different proposals for splitting and lumping. Andreasen, Arndt, Alliger, Miller, and Flaum (1995) have proposed that positive symptoms be subdivided into what they call "psychotic" and "disorganized" dimensions. Using their framework, this group (Arndt, Andreasen, Flaum, Miller, & Nopoulos, 1995) followed a relatively young, predominantly neuroleptically naive population with diagnoses of schizophrenia or schizophreniform disorder from time of admission for 2 years. They found that negative symptoms already prominent at time of initial assessment remained relatively stable, in contrast to the psychotic and disorganized positive symptoms, which declined over the follow-up period and were generally less stable.

Currently there is general acceptance of a three-factor solution, but not about the content or labels of the three factors. Lenzenweger, Dworkin, and Wethington (1991), following earlier work by Strauss, have reported support for the positive–negative distinction plus a third distinct factor, which they call "premorbid personal–social relationships." A three-factor model proposed by Liddle in the 1980s has now been well replicated (Liddle et al., 1992). These factors are defined as follows: "psychomotor poverty" (poverty of speech, flatness of affect, decreased spontaneous movement), "disorganization" (disorder of thought content and process, inappropriate affect), and "reality distortion" (hallucinations and delusions). This framework has led to models linking specific brain regions to symptom clusters (Liddle et al., 1992; O'Donnell & Grace, 1998), and it promises to yield new insights into the mechanisms underlying symptoms in schizophrenia and psychoses more generally.

Efforts have been made to relate the factor structure of schizotypy to the main symptom clusters in schizophrenia. To date this has been only partially successful: Relative overlap has been found between negative symptoms (psychomotor poverty) and negative schizotypy and between positive symptoms (reality distortion) and positive schizotypy, but there is less agreement with respect to overlap with the third factor, disorganization (Bergman et al., 1996; Vollema & van den Bosch, 1995). To some extent, this may also reflect differences in instruments and methods used to measure schizotypy (Kendler, Thacker, & Walsh, 1996) but may also reflect state specific aspects of schizophrenia.

TIMING OF ONSET AND OTHER FACTORS RELATED TO OUTCOME

The continuity among childhood, adolescent, and adult forms of schizophrenia now appears to be established, with the neurobiological and neuropsychological factors being similar (Jacobsen & Rapoport, 1998; Tompson, Asarnow, Goldstein, & Miklowitz, 1990). Comparing individuals with childhood-onset versus adolescent-onset schizophrenia, Hollis (1995) found a greater prevalence of language and speech impairments in the childhood-onset group. Both groups differed from age-matched nonpsychotic psychiatric controls with respect to premorbid social, motor, and language impairment. Childhood-onset cases do appear to have a more insidious onset and more progressive deterioration than do adult-onset cases (Jacobsen & Rapoport, 1998). Insidious onset appears to be related to more chronic outcome in both childhood and adulthood (Eggers & Bunk, 1997). Eggers and Bunk followed up childhood-onset cases into middle age and reported that 25% showed complete recovery, 25% a partial recovery, and 50% a chronic outcome. In a 2- to 12-year follow-up of a population of chronically ill schizophrenic patients hospitalized at the National Institute of Mental Health, Breier, Schreiber, Dyer, and Pickar (1991) found that 78% of the sample had suffered a relapse, 38% had attempted suicide, and 24% had had episodes of major mood disorders. Response to optimal neuroleptic treatment during the index hospitalization predicted outcome, but initial (drug-free) levels of positive and negative symptoms did not.

In addition to initial treatment response, the recovery rate in adult-onset cases varies, depending on a number of demographic and illness variables. Poor premorbid social functioning is one of the strongest predictors of poor outcomes in both child and adult populations (Erikson, Beiser, Iacono, Fleming, & Lin, 1989; Johnstone, MacMillan, Frith, Benn, & Crow, 1990; Werry & McClellan, 1992). Individuals who return to a family environment marked by high EE, or who spend significant time with high-EE relatives, tend to have higher relapse rates (Vaughan & Leff, 1976). Females tend to have a better (less chronic) course than males (Breier et al., 1991), and to come into contact with the mental health system an average of 4–5 years later than males do. (Beiser & Iacono, 1990, discuss the factors that may influence the perception of a later age of onset in females.) Individuals in developing countries also show a more benign course (Beiser & Iacono, 1990). Schizophreniform disorder generally has more positive symptoms than negative symptoms, and has a better outcome than schizophrenia does (Kendler & Walsh, 1995).

Based on their own follow-up of individuals with chronic schizophrenia and on the literature in general, Breier et al. (1991) have proposed a model to describe the course of chronic schizophrenia. The initial deteriorating phase takes place from midadolescence to about age 30. The stabilization phase, which may go on for another 10–20 years, is followed by a final phase in which there may be modest improvement.

RISK FACTORS: THE CONCEPT OF EARLY VERSUS LATE PRECURSORS

In a recent review of risk factors in psychosis, Olin and Mednick (1996) subdivided risk factors into *early precursors* (i.e., genetic, *in utero*/perinatal, or early childhood factors of etiological interest) and *late precursors* (i.e., factors in somewhat older individuals that predispose them to, or that signal, future psychosis). Under the early precursors, these authors included family psychiatric history, obstetrical complications, neurological abnormalities in early childhood, and early separation and institutionalization. With respect to late precursors, their focus was largely on behaviors and personality traits in late childhood and adolescence that have been shown to relate to the later development of psychotic behavior.

Although this is a large literature, a reasonable consensus about early and late precursors is emerging from studies of high-risk populations. In these studies, children of parents with schizophrenia have been compared with children of parents with other psychiatric disorders (e.g., parents with mood disorders, in the New York High-Risk Project; Erlenmeyer-Kimling et al., 1995) and nonpsychiatric controls. Those at-risk individuals who develop schizophrenia have been compared with those who develop other disorders or who remain well; the effects of different rearing conditions (kibbutz vs. parents, adoptive/foster parents vs. biological parents) have also been examined. Olin and Mednick (1996) provide a table outlining the control groups in the various studies.

A word on the treatment of family factors in the high-risk studies and in other research on the psychoses is in order here. Because many of the parents in the high-risk samples have been severely ill, their children have in some situations been exposed to rather disrupted upbringings; these are not typical of the majority of individuals who develop schizophrenia or other psychoses, the majority of whom have been raised in their own homes by nonpsychotic parents. In contrast to the large literature on family factors in the mood and anxiety disorders, demonstrating the presence of adverse rearing situations, the family literature in schizophrenia has focused largely on communication deviance and EE. Because there is less literature bearing directly on family developmental factors, but because many of the studies suggest an interaction between suboptimal rearing environments and individual vulnerability, I speculate that some of the familial psychosocial factors discussed in Chapter 9 are also relevant here.

In the next two sections, I discuss early and late precursors of psychotic disorders in more detail. Under early precursors, I include genetic and constitutional factors, obstetrical complications, early neuromotor and attentional deficits, and adverse rearing experiences. Under late precursors, I consider behavioral indicators, psychosis proneness, attentional dysfunction in older individuals, and other markers.

Early Precursors

Genetic and Constitutional Factors

As in other mental disorders, the importance of a genetic component in schizophrenia is quite clear. Family history studies reviewed by Prescott and Gottesman (1993) show that approximately 12% of first-degree relatives of an individual with schizophrenia develop the illness; this contrasts with a prevalence of 1% in the general population. When Prescott and Gottesman pooled the results from newer twin studies, they found a concordance rate of 39% in monozygotic twins versus 10% in dizygotic twins, leading them to conclude that the shared family resemblance is due entirely to a shared-gene effect. Adopted-away offspring of biological mothers with schizophrenia have a higher incidence of psychotic and other severe disorders than do matched adopted-away offspring of biological parents with no history of schizophrenia (Tienari, 1991). Prescott and Gottesman (1993) also cite earlier work by Gottesman and Bertelson examining offspring of twins discordant for schizophrenia, where the risk of developing schizophrenia was similar in the offspring of affected and unaffected monozygotic twins (17%), but significantly different from that of offspring of an unaffected dizygotic twin (2%). This difference provides clear support for the presence of a genetic factor that can be transmitted despite the lack of its expression in the parent, and suggests the importance of another factor necessary for its expression. Prescott and Gottesman (1993) conclude that the evidence from genetic studies to date is most consistent with a multifactorial model, in which liability comes from the combined influence of multiple genes and multiple environmental factors. They also propose that this liability has a continuous distribution in the population, with increased levels of these factors leading to increased likelihood of the development of schizophrenia.

Schizotypal traits and schizotypal personality disorder have become objects of study in themselves, as they are presumed to represent vulnerability factors. Interest in these traits emerged from the first family studies of relatives of individuals with schizophrenia, where it was noted that many relatives displayed abnormalities in their behavior or functioning that could be construed as subthreshold variants of schizophrenia. Consistent with this, most of the high-risk studies have found increased numbers of high-risk offspring with schizotypal or paranoid personality disorders or schizophrenic-spectrum disorders (Olin & Mednick, 1996). An exception occurred in the New York High-Risk Project: When offspring of schizophrenic parents were compared with offspring of parents with affective disorders, the latter offspring had a higher rate of schizoaffective disorder than did the former. There was also no difference in the rates of psychosis as a whole or of all schizophrenia-related psychosis (schizophrenia; schizoaffective disorder, mainly schizophrenic; and unspecified psychosis) between the two groups. However, schizophrenia and unspecified psychosis occurred only in the offspring at high risk for schizophrenia (Erlenmeyer-Kimling et al., 1995). The authors concluded that the familial liability to narrowly defined schizophrenia is not shared by families with a history of mood disorders, but that there is overlap in the liability to schizoaffective disorder and schizotypal personality disorder.

In the follow-up of the Israeli High-Risk Study of offspring of probands with schizophrenia, Mirsky, Kugelmass, et al. (1995) found a higher than expected incidence of mood disorders in the high-risk offspring raised on the kibbutz. As the incidence of other psychiatric disorders was also higher in the kibbutz-raised high-risk children, they concluded that kibbutz rearing in vulnerable children increases the risk of severe forms of psychiatric disturbance generally. These findings and those of the New York High-Risk Project do, however, suggest that there may be several different types of vulnerability inherent in schizophrenia and/or the factors that contribute to this broad group of disorders.

Torgersen, Onstad, Skre, Edvardsen, and Kringlen (1993) examined the type and nature of personality disorder among biological relatives of individuals with schizophrenia versus relatives of subjects with mood disorders. They found that the prevalence of schizotypal personality disorder was greater in the former group of relatives than in the latter group, and that the negative criteria for this disorder (odd speech, inappropriate affect, and odd behavior) as well as excessive social anxiety were also higher in the former than in the latter group. However, several of the other criteria (such as ideas of reference, recurrent illusions, social isolation and suspiciousness) were just as high in the relatives of subjects with mood disorders. The authors concluded that the criteria for schizotypal personality disorder contain a "true" subcomponent related to schizophrenia, but also a nonspecific subcomponent shared by schizophrenia and mood disorders. This may account for the apparently weak genetic link between schizophrenia and true schizotypal personality disorder, as well as for the discrepant findings with respect to prevalence of schizotypal pathology in relatives of subjects with schizophrenia and/or relatives of individuals with mood disorders. Because of the high level of social anxiety in the relatives of the schizophrenic probands, Torgersen et al. raised the possibility that excessive social anxiety may be a marker of the genetic link between schizophrenia and schizotypal personality disorder.

As indicated earlier, Kendler, McGuire et al. (1995), in a factor analysis of schizotypal signs and symptoms, compared first-degree relatives of subjects with schizophrenia to relatives of subjects with mood disorders and other control groups. They found that odd speech, social dysfunction, and negative schizotypy (poor rapport, aloofness, guardedness, and odd behavior) strongly distinguished the relatives of schizophrenic probands from controls; suspicious behavior, avoidant behavior, and positive schizotypy (illusions, ideas of reference, magical thinking), although weaker, were also significant. Although some aspects of schizotypal personality disorder appear relatively nonspecific to schizophrenia, the Kendler, McGuire, et al. study does suggest that certain aspects such as odd speech, social dysfunction, and odd behavior may be part of a specific vulnerability to schizophrenia. The authors state that these same factors have emerged most strongly in other similar studies, in contrast to the weaker findings, for which evidence from other studies has been less consistent.

Using a subsample of twins from the Virginia Twin Registry, Kendler, Ochs, et al. (1991) compared correlations between positive and negative symptom schizotypy on the one hand, and with attentional measures and smooth-pursuit eye-tracking function on the other. They found significant correlations between negative symptom schizotypy and trait anhedonia, attentional dysfunction, and eye-tracking error. Positive symptom schizotypy did not correlate with either the attentional or eye-tracking measures. Except for eye-tracking dysfunction, Kendler, Ochs, et al. concluded that their results were more consistent with a dimensional than with a categorical or "disease" model of schizotypy. Generally, these findings and others suggest that one or more components (probably genetically mediated) producing attentional dysfunction, eye-tracking dysfunction, odd behavior, odd speech, and social dysfunction may be distinguishable vulnerability factors for schizophrenia.

Obstetrical Complications

That obstetrical complications contribute to the development of schizophrenia is now reasonably well established (Olin & Mednick, 1996). In Mednick, Parnas, and Schulsinger's (1987) report of the Copenhagen High-Risk Project, those high-risk subjects who later developed schizophrenia had more and more severe perinatal complications. A later analysis of these data by Cannon et al. (1993) showed that this connection between delivery complications and schizophrenia held *only* for the high-risk subjects and was correlated with periventricular damage.

Two recent, methodologically more sophisticated studies with reasonably large samples have confirmed the relationship between obstetrical complications and psychosis. Kendell et al. (1996) surveyed Scottish standardized birth records for 115 schizophrenic–control pairs born between 1971 and 1974 and found a highly significant increase in birth complications of both pregnancy and delivery in the schizophrenic subjects. Hultman et al. (1997) surveyed prospectively recorded birth records of 107 subjects admitted with a diagnosis of psychosis (82 with schizophrenia, 25 with other psychotic disorders) and compared them to 214 controls matched for gender, time, and place of birth. They found a high nonoptimality score (7 or more complications out of a possible 34) for the total patient group, with an odds ratio of 4.58. Even those with 2–6 complications experienced some increased risk compared to controls, and an odds ratio of 1.67. There was no difference between the subjects with schizophrenia and those with other psychotic disorders. Specific risk factors for the total patient group were older maternal age, early rupture of membranes, a small head circumference, and disproportionate (both high and low) body weight for body length. The females in this sample who developed schizophrenia were significantly smaller at birth than the males (remarkably more so than the controls), this difference being most evident in head circumference. These findings suggest that some of the pregnancy complications are related to growth retardation *in utero*, whereas others may reflect difficulties at the time of birth, probably producing anoxic damage to the infant. These speculations are supported by several recent reports.

Bracha, Torrey, Gottesman, Bigelow, and Cunniff (1992) examined fingertip dermal ridges of 30 pairs of monozygotic twins, 23 of whom were discordant for schizophrenia and 7 of whom were normal. They found greater differences on total finger ridge counts between the twin pairs discordant for schizophrenia than for the normal twins, suggesting perturbations during the second trimester for the twin who developed schizophrenia. In a similar vein, Davis, Phelps, and Bracha (1995) found that monozygotic twins concordant for schizophrenia were more likely to have shared a placenta, whereas monozygotic twins discordant for schizophrenia were more likely to have had separate placentas. Because twins sharing a placenta also share fetal blood circulation, this lends support to the possibility that toxic factors such as infections may constitute a mechanism that increases vulnerability to psychosis. Olin and Mednick (1996) provide a brief review of the studies on maternal influenza during the second trimester; they conclude that the initial studies have been replicated, and cite further work that ties the effect of maternal influenza to later defects in habituation and visual attention processes. Arnold (1999) and Cannon, Rosso, Bearden, Sanchez, and Hadley (1999) provide recent overviews of neurodevelopmental abnormalities in schizophrenia.

Examining time trends in schizophrenia and changes in obstetrical risk factors with industrialization, Warner (1995) has observed shifts in prevalence between upper and lower classes and changes over time that appear to correlate with changes in nutrition and birth complications. He suggests that some of these trends can be accounted for by increases in birth complications secondary to cephalopelvic disproportion (which itself results from improved nutrition of infants in mothers who themselves have been less well nourished), and from improvements in obstetrical and neonatal care that increase the survival rates of infants who have sustained some impairment.

Although we still need to define the specifics of both the *in utero* effects and the birth complications, the evidence would suggest that at least two separate factors probably contribute to vulnerability: one that arises during development *in utero* and may account for the findings on small head circumference, low body weight, and dermal ridge type (see also Fish et al., 1992, and the discussion below), and another that may result from anoxic injury at the time of birth. Whether these are simply additive in their effects or interact in producing vulnerability needs to be further explored.

Neuromotor and Attentional Abnormalities

In the mid-1970s, Fish (for a review, see Fish et al., 1992) coined the term *pandysmaturation* (PDM) to describe the early features of the neurointegrative defect that has been presumed to underlie the various attentional and perceptual–motor deficits found in schizophrenia. The notion of PDM grew out of earlier work by Bender (1947) in her studies of childhood schizophrenia. Criteria for PDM as provided by Fish et al. (1992) are a transient retardation of gross motor and/or visual–motor development; an abnormal profile of functions on developmental testing (intratest scatter as opposed to overall delay); and a retardation in skeletal growth that parallels the transient lag and abnormal profile. In their report (Fish et al., 1992), they survey the findings from the high-risk studies for evidence of PDM; they conclude that the 12 studies provide evidence for delayed development in infants of schizophrenic patients and in preschizophrenic subjects, and that PDM in these studies was related to schizotypal personality disorder and to cognitive and motor neurointegrative deficits at 10 years. PDM was not related to obstetrical complications. They did identify, however, a small subgroup of offspring of schizophrenic subjects whose most severe motor deficits appeared related to obstetrical complications, PDM, and low birthweight. In trying to understand the various birth complications that have been noted and to relate these to PDM, Fish et al. argue that the low head circumference and low birthweight are most likely manifestations of PDM *in utero*.

Consistent with these findings on neuromotor abnormalities, Walker and Lewine (1990) have demonstrated that preschizophrenic youngsters can be differentiated from their healthy siblings. Using home movies of subjects with adult-onset schizophrenia when they were children, raters who were unaware of the children's later outcomes scored their interpersonal and/or motor characteristics. The raters noted less responsiveness, eye contact, and positive affect, as well as poorer fine and gross motor coordination, in the preschizophrenic children. On the basis of their own work and the literature linking soft signs with later psychopathology, Neumann and Walker (1996) conclude that the evidence is strongest for a relationship between neuromotor abnormalities and signs of internalizing psychopathology, particularly in late childhood and early adolescence. These relationships are strongest for at-risk children and seem almost nonexistent for healthy sibling comparison groups. They also note that most follow-up studies of children with soft signs have shown that these signs diminish with age and are much harder to detect in adolescence. In their follow-up of children with soft signs in comparison to controls, Gillberg et al. (1989) found that a measure of reaction time was the only significant difference between the groups at an assessment in adolescence.

Neumann and Walker (1996) do note that there is a correlation between early neuromotor difficulties and attentional difficulties in early childhood. Relating patterns of central nervous system maturation to the development of psychopathology, these authors speculate that these neuromotor abnormalities are related to maturational abnormalities, with early dysfunction of basal ganglia and later effects on limbic–frontal circuits. (See Walker, Lewis, Loewy, & Palyo, 1999, for a recent review.) Early basal ganglia dysfunction would account for the neuromotor abnormalities and attentional difficulties manifested in childhood, whereas socioemotional dysfunction would result from the later difficulties in frontal–limbic circuits, which are also later-maturing. Although these authors allow for the influence of environmental factors in the development of psychopathology, their model implies a psychopathological process that unfolds with maturation of the various brain areas. It is also plausible to argue—as I have done in previous chapters—that children with attentional difficulties pose challenges for their caregivers, which can be manifested in conflicted patterns of interaction and in later psychopathology (internalizing, externalizing, and/or psychotic).

Attentional difficulties have been common and long-standing findings in studies of subjects with schizophrenia. There is now good evidence that neuromotor and attentional difficulties precede the onset of schizophrenia: Such problems were detectable in high-risk subjects in childhood in the Israeli (Mirsky, Ingraham, & Kugelmass, 1995), Jerusalem (Marcus, Hans, Auerbach, & Auerbach, 1993), New York (Erlenmeyer-Kimling & Cornblatt, 1987), and Copenhagen studies. (See Olin & Mednick, 1996 and Cornblatt, Obuchowski, Roberts, Pollack, & Erlenmeyer-Kimling, 1999 for an overview.) In the New York High-Risk Project, childhood attentional dysfunctions predicted social deficits even in high-risk subjects who did not develop schizophrenia (Cornblatt, Lenzenweger, Dworkin, & Erlenmeyer-Kimling, 1992). These social deficits are described as a relative insensitivity to other individuals, an indifference to their feelings, and an avoidance of interpersonal interactions. Although these authors describe these characteristics as indicating insensitivity, I believe it is possible and clinically more comprehensible to understand this apparent insensitivity as a defense against feelings of discomfort and lack of social skills in persons who may be highly sensitive. However the attention deficits arise,

Cornblatt et al. (1992) indicate that they are detectable from an early age. These deficits appear relatively stable, although some deficits may be exacerbated at the time of acute illness (Rund, 1998).

Mirsky (1996) compared the attentional findings on three samples of schizophrenic subjects and their first-degree relatives. He found deficits both in the schizophrenic subjects and (to a lesser extent) in their relatives, in comparison to controls. Attention scores were subdivided into a "focus–execute" factor, tapping perceptual–motor speed or focusing; a "shift" factor, derived largely from the Wisconsin Card Sorting Test; a "sustain" factor, which loaded heavily on a continuous-performance test; and an "encode" factor, which taps registration, recall, and mental manipulation of numerical information. The deficits in the schizophrenic subjects were primarily in "focus–execute" and "sustain" rather than "encode" or "shift" functions, and were more obvious on the auditory processing task. Mirsky speculates that these deficits may be related to observed abnormalities in the superior temporal gyrus, thalamus, and reticular formation. He also suggests that damage to the superior colliculus or superior olive, regions particularly vulnerable to asphyxic insult (as is likely to occur in perinatal complications) and involved in auditory processing, may provide an answer as to how early brain insult can result in auditory attentional processing difficulties in schizophrenic subjects.

Because language and auditory processing difficulties, as well as neuromotor abnormalities, are common findings in children referred to psychiatric clinics (Cohen, 1996; Neumann & Walker, 1996), research will have to clarify whether these deficits act as a general factor interfering with affect regulation or have specificity with respect to the development of schizophrenia (Beitchman, Brownlie, & Wilson, 1996; Caplan, 1996). As noted earlier, Hollis (1995), studying childhood- and adolescent-onset schizophrenia, found that premorbid social, motor, and language impairments did differentiate schizophrenic from nonpsychotic psychiatric controls. This, however, may have been a function of severity of illness. In a review of precursors to schizophrenia, Tarrant and Jones (1999) conclude that in both clinical samples and general population birth cohorts, delays in developmental milestones, abnormalities in social functioning, and cognitive deficits are elevated in preschizophrenic individuals; however, none of these factors has high specificity for the disorder.

Adverse Rearing Experiences

High-risk subjects separated from their mothers during the first year of life appear to have an increased risk for schizophrenia (Barr et al., cited in Olin & Mednick, 1996). This contrasts with the finding from the same study that low-risk subjects with very early separation were found to be at risk for nonpsychotic disorders. Olin and Mednick (1996) also cite studies by Walker et al. and Gutkind and Mednick in which high-risk boys placed in institutional care were shown to be at enhanced risk for schizophrenia; by contrast, foster care appeared to reduce the vulnerability to later schizophrenia.

The importance of supportive rearing in reducing vulnerability to later psychopathogy has been made clear in the high-risk studies of schizophrenia, as it has been in the literature on other disorders. In the Finnish Adoptive Family Study, Wahlberg et al. (1997) found that the interaction between genetic vulnerability and rearing environment was what appeared to induce vulnerability to thought disorder. Adopted-away offspring of schizophrenic mothers exposed to high levels of communication deviance in their adopted parents showed evidence of thought disorder. Parental communication deviance seemed to have little impact on the low-risk adopted offspring. Surprisingly, high-risk offspring in families low in communication deviance appeared to be less vulnerable than even the low-risk offspring. The findings from the Israeli High-Risk Study are also consistent with the increased risk to vulnerable offspring in adverse rearing situations. Presence of all psychiatric disorders was increased in the kibbutz-reared children, leading the authors to conclude that kibbutz rearing increases the level of severe psychopathology generally in vulnerable children (Mirsky, Kugelmass, et al., 1995). Olin and Mednick (1996) cite similar findings from the Copenhagen High-Risk Project and other studies.

As indicated earlier, the literature on EE has clearly indicated the deleterious impact of high levels of negative, critical, and hostile comments from caregivers on vulnerability to relapse in schizophrenia (Bebbington & Kuipers, 1994). This finding is not specific to schizophrenia, however, and appears to indicate that vulnerable individuals have more difficulty responding to or dealing with negative interactions than do the less vulnerable. Wuerker (1996) examined transactional patterns in high- and low-EE families of patients with schizophrenia and bipolar disorder. She found that, regardless of patients' diagnosis, members of high-EE families engaged in a highly competitive interaction that escalated quickly. Low-EE families, in contrast, appeared to avoid battles. Interestingly, high-EE families were also more responsive. This style of interaction is consistent with interactions described in families of children with either mood disorders or conduct disorder. Wuerker discusses possible ways of understanding her findings, but concludes that a high-EE family system combines over-responsiveness with conflict about "who's in charge." She also suggests that high EE occurs more frequently in a family where a child's withdrawal or negativism is believed to be willful behavior rather than part of the child's psychiatric illness. However, given that many individuals who are not psychiatrically ill use withdrawal or negativism as their main way of expressing their frustration or coping with stressful situations, the parents in a high-EE family may be reacting to their intuitive sense that some of this behavior is under the child's control as well. It is also important to note that in Wuerker's study the patients participated in the conflict with their parents. Clearly, this pattern is highly complex. I would speculate that these patterns of interaction are long-standing.

Interestingly, in a follow-up study of patients with schizophrenia and schizoaffective disorder, Doering et al. (1998) examined factors predictive of relapse and found that childhood factors (traumatic experiences and psychiatric or developmental disturbances) were important, along with other, more expected outcomes (e.g., medication compliance).

Late Precursors

Although there is some overlap between early precursors and late precursors, the literature linking these two sets of factors is just beginning. Presumably, the neurointegrative defect described above should bear some resemblance to some aspects of schizotypal personality or traits, as suggested by Fish et al. (1992). As noted earlier, the study of schizotypy has been a part of the developing understanding of the genetics of schizophrenia, where (as noted by Kendler, McGuire, et al., 1995), it is neither specific nor nonspecific. Here I look at schizotypal traits as they appear to relate to the onset or development of psychotic disorders.

Behavioral Indicators

Older preschizophrenic children have been noted by both parents and teachers to display signs of their difficulty (Done, Crow, Johnstone, & Sacker, 1994; Olin & Mednick, 1996). In comparison with normal controls, preschizophrenic boys have been described as having disciplinary problems, disturbing classmates with inappropriate behavior, rejected by peers, high-strung, and easily excited or irritated. Girls, in contrast, appear nervous. When preschizophrenic children are compared with children with nonpsychotic disorders, girls are described as lonely and rejected by peers, nervous, uneasy about criticism, and passive; boys are seen as lonely and rejected by peers, passive, and high-strung. These behaviors appear to worsen in adolescence, with preschizophrenic boys becoming more antisocial, and girls more passive and withdrawn. Even in one study comparing the at-risk offspring of schizophrenic parents to the offspring of parents with mood disorders, deficits in social competence differentiated the adolescents at risk for schizophrenia from those at risk for mood disorders. Both at-risk groups score higher on a scale assessing positive thought disorder than did normal controls (Dworkin et al., 1990). As I have indicated above, it is not clear whether these behavioral difficulties are predominantly manifestations of the underlying neurobiological dysfunction, as Neumann and Walker (1996) suggest, or results of the conflicted interaction that develops frequently in families with temperamentally challenging children, or (as is most likely) a mixture of both.

Psychosis Proneness

Vulnerability to psychotic experiences predisposes individuals to later psychosis. Chapman and Chapman (1996), using a rating system for psychotic-like experiences and their Psychosis Proneness Scale on a large sample of college students, have demonstrated that high scores on the subscales Perceptual Aberration and Magical Ideation, as well as reports of psychotic-like experiences, predict psychosis 10 years later. Although this scale was originally developed to detect specific vulnerability to schizophrenia, it predicted the broader notion of psychosis better. The capacity to predict psychosis as opposed to schizophrenia per se was also true for the risk factor "attentional deviance" in the New York High-Risk Project (Erlenmeyer-Kimling et al., 1993).

Attentional Dysfunction

As indicated above, attentional/information-processing difficulties have been almost universal findings in individuals with schizophrenia (Saykin et al., 1991). There is, however, still little consensus on the nature or meaning of these deficits (Rund, 1998). Efforts to clarify whether these deficits constitute trait (or vulnerability) factors or state markers have contributed to a large and growing literature. Generally, there is reasonable evidence that some indicators of attentional dysfunction are more likely to be trait factors, as they have been found disproportionately in high-risk subjects and in relatives of individuals with schizophrenia (Erlenmeyer-Kimling et al., 1993). Many of these deficits also appear relatively stable, with those subjects with the highest level of negative symptoms showing the greatest cognitive impairment (Braff et al., 1991; Buchanan, Strauss, Breier, Kirkpatrick, & Carpenter, 1997; Rund, 1998). It is important to note, however, that perhaps as many as 30% of patients with schizophrenia do *not* show any cognitive impairment (Rund, 1998). Furthermore, some aspects of the attentional dysfunction do improve with medication and/or time, suggesting a state component to the dysfunction (Rund, 1998; Spohn, 1996). According to Rund (1998), the more stable deficits include those in verbal skills, memory, and preattentional information processing; the less stable deficits are found in complex attention and concentration, response shift, and attention span. As anxiety or high levels of arousal can interfere with attention generally, reduction of anxiety or arousal can be presumed to improve some aspects of attention and information processing. Because there is also evidence of attentional dysfunction in other disorders, such as severe mood disorders with psychotic features, the specificity of these traits for schizophrenia has been questioned (Nelson, Sax, & Strakowski, 1998; Rund, Orbeck, & Landro, 1992).

These findings suggest that individuals who develop schizophrenia and possibly other psychotic disorders may have trait-related attentional difficulties that contribute to their vulnerability to developing a disorder, but that the illness itself may also contribute to attentional difficulties. Although the persistence of a marker beyond the acute stage and its presence in relatives logically suggest a trait, it is also possible to conceive of this as an indicator of vulnerability to developing symptoms, which may also reflect lingering psychopathology. Thus some measures might better be thought of as markers of the severity of vulnerability to becoming symptomatic than as markers for schizophrenia or other psychotic disorders. Moreover, given current thinking about the deleterious impact of prolonged stress or of an unremitted episode of a disorder on brain function, it may be very difficult to discern what is "primary" without long-term follow-up studies with sophisticated methodologies.

Smooth-pursuit eye-tracking difficulties, which are found in roughly half of the relatives of individuals with schizophrenia, may be a marker of the trait type of attentional difficulties (Levy, Holzman, Matthysse, & Mendell, 1993). Lencz et al. (1993) also found higher levels of qualitative ratings of smooth-pursuit eye-tracking abnormalities in undergraduates with schizotypal personality disorder than in controls. Although these abnormalities were also found in acutely ill individuals with psychotic mood disorders in one study, they dissipated with symptom recovery in these subjects (but not in schizophrenic subjects) and were no more prevalent in relatives of the subjects with mood disorder than in controls (Beiser & Iacono, 1990). Ross, Buchanan, Medoff, Lahti, and Thaker (1998) found a high correlation between poor sensory integration scores in subjects with schizophrenia and eye-tracking dysfunction.

Other Markers

Other abnormalities that have been examined as trait or state indicators of psychosis include electrodermal activity, sensory gating, and event-related potentials. Dawson (1990) has reviewed the literature on electrodermal activity in schizophrenia. He points out that roughly 50% of individuals with schizophrenia are "nonresponders"; that is, they show few nonspecific skin conductance responses, a low skin conductance level, and an absence of orienting responses to novel stimuli. The remaining subjects are at least normally responsive if not hyperresponsive; they exhibit many nonspecific skin conductance responses, have a relatively high tonic skin conductance level, and show orienting responses to novel stimuli. When Dawson and colleagues (see Dawson, 1990) followed up schizophrenic subjects with a recent-onset disorder through remission and bouts of relapse, the electrodermal activity varied with the symptomatic state of the patients. During relapse the schizophrenic subjects showed delayed habituation, considered to represent heightened electrodermal activity and reactivity. When three patients were followed with weekly testing increases in skin conductance level preceded clinical relapse. Dawson and colleagues concluded that this component of electrodermal activity represents a state marker. When Dawson and colleagues (Dawson, 1990) carried out positron emission tomography (PET) brain imaging studies on three responders, three nonresponders (as measured by skin conductance responses), and normal controls, the absolute metabolic rates were higher in the responders than in the nonresponders, with little overlap of the two groups in half of the brain areas examined. The controls had metabolic rates intermediate between those of the other two groups. Based on the relative absence of overlap in the responders versus nonresponders, Dawson (1990) concludes that these groups represent distinct subgroups likely with different attentional and cognitive deficits and brain functioning.

The suggestion from the nonresponder PET studies that some individuals with schizophrenia may have brain metabolic reductions reflecting their withdrawal or deficit state is borne out in the event-related potential studies. The P300 wave is a late component in an event-related potential on the EEG scalp recording; it is thought to reflect processing of unexpected, novel, or behaviorally salient events. Numerous studies of subjects with schizophrenia have shown a reduction in amplitude in this component, primarily over the left temporal areas. Pfefferbaum, Ford, White, and Roth (1989) showed a reduction in P300 amplitude that correlated with negative symptoms in both medicated and unmedicated subjects with schizophrenia. Squires-Wheeler, Friedman, Skodol, and Erlenmeyer-Kimling (1993), however, showed in a follow-up of subjects in the New York High-Risk Project that reduced amplitude was relatively nonspecific and correlated more highly with a global measure of personality impairment across subjects at risk for schizophrenia, mood disorders, or no disorders. Examining an even earlier component in information processing, Javitt, Doneshka, Grochowski, and Ritter (1995) found deficits in mismatch negativity generation, thought to reflect an automatic alerting mechanism designed to stimulate individuals to explore unexpected environmental events. In animal studies, such deficits have been associated with deficits in the N-methyl-D-aspartate (NMDA) receptor. Thus an overall deficit in NMDA receptor neurotransmission could possibly account for the withdrawal and psychomotor poverty observed in negative symptoms (Olney & Farber, 1997).

Consistent with the theory that schizophrenic subjects have a deficit in gating of stimuli that causes them to be easily overloaded, studies measuring inhibition of startle reflexes have shown impairments in individuals with schizophrenia (Braff, Grillon, & Geyer, 1992). Failure of shorter-term habituation, which may relate to greater sensitization in schizophrenic subjects, was also seen. Raine, Benishay, Lencz, and Scarpa (1997) have shown deficits in habituation in university students meeting criteria for schizotypal personality disorder. Increased distractibility, as measured via event-related potentials, is also seen in schizophrenic subjects (Grillon, Courchesne, Ameli, Geyer, & Braff, 1990). These authors interpreted their results as showing that individuals with schizophrenia direct their attention disproportionately to task-irrelevant stimuli.

Drawing on Frith's (1979) theory that schizophrenia represents a failure of inhibitory mechanisms controlling the contents of consciousness, Williams (1996) used priming methodology to examine subgroups of subjects with schizophrenia. This approach involves measuring speed of response to a stimulus preceded by a related or an unrelated stimulus. Typically, subjects respond more quickly to a stimulus preceded by a related stimulus. The theory is that material is stored in association networks, which, when stimulated by a "like" preceding stimulus, are more easily activated (facilitating the response) by the second "like" stimulus. Priming is believed to tap preattentive processing. By contrast, when a previously ignored stimulus (the dissimilar probe) becomes a target, there is an increase in the latency to respond, presumably because the active process of inhibition (which was used to ignore the stimulus originally) interferes with the response. Schizophrenic subjects subgrouped according to whether their predominant symptom pattern was reality distortion, disorganization, or psychomotor poverty showed different responses. The reality distortion and disorganization groups showed a reduced or reversed negative priming effect, which suggested a weakening of inhibitory processes. In contrast, the psychomotor poverty group did not. According to Williams (1996), the results support the notion that weakened cognitive inhibitory processes may play a part in positive but not negative symptoms of schizophrenia. Consistent with greater activation of association networks (reduced inhibition) in subjects with schizophrenia, Maher (1996) has shown that schizophrenic subjects with thought disorder have a shorter latency to respond in priming tasks in which they are required to identify an associated target as opposed to a nonassociated target, in comparison with subjects with mood disorders and schizophrenic subjects without thought disorder.

Spohn (1996) has speculated as to what constitutes a trait or state factor according to what changes with neuroleptic treatment. Thought disorder and distraction improve with medication and are thus thought to be state factors. In contrast, eye-tracking dysfunction, reaction time crossover effect, and skin conductance orienting response dysfunction are not substantially improved by medication and are thus believed to be trait components. Spohn theorizes that thought disorder represents a generalized impairment in interpretation of events or stimuli in the external environment, or in the attributional information value of stimuli. In contrast, eye-tracking dysfunction and other factors not responding to medication indicate impairment in orienting to the perceived occurrence of significant events and perceived changes in the environment. Although changes with medication may be a way of discriminating state from trait variables, it is not clear whether the lack of improvement of some variables necessarily reflects a preexisting "trait" variable, as opposed to a deficit in performance that may also result from a process that began very early and is simply less responsive to intervention.

Efforts to relate specific aspects of neuropsychological performance to core aspects of symptomatology are just beginning. Norman et al. (1997) found a correlation between reality distortion and verbal memory, which they concluded reflected left temporal lobe dysfunction. They could not find associations between psychomotor poverty and tests of dorsolateral prefrontal functioning, or between disorganization and tests of medial basal prefrontal function. As the authors point out, this undertaking is made more difficult by the likelihood that many tests rely on neural networks and cannot be presumed to tap only a single brain region. Furthermore, there is evidence that the deficits that best distinguish schizophrenic subjects from controls involve the capacity to process complex information, as opposed to simple responding or memory tasks (Morice & Delahunty, 1996).

NEUROBIOLOGY

Neueroanatomical and Neuroimaging Findings

As is true for most other aspects of the psychotic disorders, a discussion of their neurobiology is largely a description of work on schizophrenia. Moreover, Buchanan and Carpenter (1997) point out in their essay on methodological issues in the study of the neuroanatomy of schizophrenia that despite interesting findings, we are still far from understanding the significance of these findings. Stevens (1997) also notes that "no morphological or microscopic abnormality has been found that is either necessary or sufficient for the diagnosis" (p. 373). Some of the difficulty is related to methodological issues, which are gradually being addressed in the newer studies. These include the heterogeneity of the disorder, the need to separate state from trait findings, and problems in determining which components are primary versus secondary pathology.

The recent three-factor model comprising negative symptoms, reality distortion, and disorganization holds promise as a better conceptual model for relating symptoms to neuroanatomical and brain imaging findings (Liddle et al., 1992; O'Donnell & Grace, 1998). Furthermore, with recent advances in cellular assessment of postmortem tissue and imaging of neural networks when subjects are required to perform tasks, investigators are beginning to piece together cellular and functional abnormalities. This research and its extensions will undoubtedly provide us with a working model of the brain both in normal subjects and in those with a variety of psychopathological conditions. Currently we can only engage in speculation about the meaning of the findings, the nature of which, although somewhat clearer, remains controversial because of the inconsistency across studies. Andreasen et al. (1997) have neatly summarized this area in their conclusion to a recent study on PET imaging in schizophrenia by saying that schizophrenia involves dysfunctions both in local regions and in circuits distributed throughout the brain.

The most widely replicated finding in neuroanatomical studies of schizophrenia has been enlargement of the lateral and third ventricles (Chua & McKenna, 1995; Sharma et al., 1998; Stevens, 1997). However, this occurs in fewer than a third of individuals with schizophrenia and is not specific to schizophrenia; it is found in a variety of other disorders, including mood disorders. In Sharma et al.'s (1998) study, "presumed obligate carriers" (unaffected parents with a family history of schizophrenia) also demonstrated enlargement of lateral ventricles. Stevens (1997) points out that ventricular enlargement has not been shown reliably to correlate with any of the premorbid risk factors, and that although some studies have shown an association with poor outcome, this has not been a consistent finding.

In her review, Stevens discusses the findings regarding tissue loss that might account for the ventricular enlargement. She indicates that cortical atrophy largely affecting frontal and temporal gyri, which has been found in 5–15% of individuals with schizophrenia, has been postulated to be the result of a neurodevelopmental process because of the apparent lack of scarring or gliosis (Woods, 1998). However, the lack of a difference in cranial volume and head size raises questions about how an early neurodevelopmental process could result in loss of tissue without also affecting these other parameters of brain development. Furthermore, there has been a question about whether there are in fact gliotic (scarring) changes in the brains of schizophrenic subjects (Dwork, 1997). Reduction in the size of medial temporal and subcortical structures (hippocampus, amygdala, globus pallidus, and entorhinal cortex) has also been found, but, again, not in all subjects with schizophrenia. Stevens (1997) contrasts these findings with those from epilepsy, where the neuroanatomical lesions in these same structures are more gross and yet do not produce schizophrenia. Attempting to find some way of explaining these diverse findings, Stevens cites a study by Henn (1994) demonstrating that schizophrenic subjects showed abnormal bilateral activation of many areas in a simple manual task, in contrast to normal subjects, who showed delimited activation of the contralateral cortex. She speculates that this may suggest a combination of inappropriate inhibition of some and aberrant activation of other brain areas. She also raises the possibility that some of this dysfunction may result from "a genetically determined compensatory proliferative response of axons, dendrites or receptors . . . to diverse brain insults" (p. 379).

Dwork (1997) has reviewed the postmortem studies of the hippocampus in schizophrenia and concluded that despite the consistency in findings of ventricular enlargement, there is no consistency in these studies with respect to deficits in hippocampal size, cell orientation, structure, or density. He notes that we may just be beginning to use sufficiently sophisticated tools to detect what are obviously subtle abnormalities. He points out the findings with respect to abnormalities in neuronal immunoreactivity for microtubule-associated proteins 2 and

5 in the hippocampal subfields. Although the meaning of this abnormality is not yet clear and it is not specific for schizophrenia, it may indicate an abnormality in dendritic processes in the hippocampal area that could contribute to abnormal communication between the hippocampus and the cerebral cortex.

Heckers (1997) has examined the evidence for neuropathological changes in the cortex, thalamus, basal ganglia, and neurotransmitter-specific projection systems. He concludes that the most robust finding in the prefrontal cortex (PFC) is the lack of gliosis. He notes that while there may be changes in specific subsets of neurons, such as those containing gamma-aminobutyric acid (GABA), the results in general have been inconsistent with respect to cell number and density. He cites other studies such as those of Benes (1998), who reported a loss of small cortical neurons in the anterior cingulate cortex as interesting but requiring replication. Similarly, the studies by Akbarian et al. (1995) showing decreases in messenger RNA for glutamic acid decarboxylase, the key enzyme in GABA synthesis, in the dorsolateral PFC (with no evidence of cell loss), are suggestive of dysfunction of the GABA inhibitory cells but again require replication. The studies that have shown a reduction in the left superior temporal gyrus, theoretically related to auditory hallucinations, have also not been consistently replicated but are suggestive and require comparison of a larger sample of subjects with and without hallucinations. With respect to thalamic abnormalities, Pakkenberg's (1990) finding of reductions of neuronal and glial cells in the mediodorsal thalamic nucleus appears compelling but likewise needs independent confirmation. Heckers (1997) regards the studies reporting abnormalities in the basal ganglia of schizophrenic subjects as few in number and equivocal in interpretation. He suggests that recent magnetic resonance imaging studies showing increases in basal ganglia volume are best understood as related to the effect of neuroleptics. In contrast, Kung, Conley, Chute, Smialek, and Roberts (1998) found anomalies in symmetric synaptic profiles affecting caudate as opposed to putamen in schizophrenic autopsy tissue; because of the greater caudate than putamen involvement, they suggest that these anomalies are less likely to be drug-related.

In contrast to the equivocal findings about actual morphological changes in the postmortem studies, there appears to be greater agreement about the inability of many subjects with schizophrenia to increase frontal activity in response to task demands (Carter et al., 1998; Weinberger, Berman, & Zec, 1986). (See also Buchsbaum & Hazlett, 1998, for a review of PET studies.) Hypofrontality itself is not unique to schizophrenia, being found as well in subjects with mood disorders (Ketter, George, Kimbrell, Benson, & Post, 1996). Buchsbaum and

Hazlett (1998) suggest that hypofrontality appears more closely related to negative than to positive symptoms. Successful treatment of schizophrenia, which normalizes this reduction in frontal function, also leads to a normalizing of the metabolic abnormalities in basal ganglia. Interestingly, these reviewers point out that the hypofrontality in schizophrenia contrasts with hyperfrontality in obsessive–compulsive disorder (OCD). Successful treatment of OCD also normalizes the metabolic abnormalities in basal ganglia, but in the opposite direction (rates are increased in schizophrenia and decreased in OCD). These studies illustrate the importance of functional networks, with dysfunction in one area being related to dysfunction in another.

Buchsbaum and Hazlett (1998) conclude that the most common finding in studies of the basal ganglia in schizophrenia is reduction of metabolic rate in the putamen. As indicated above, neuroleptics tend to increase metabolic rate in the basal ganglia, whereas dopamine agonists reduce it. With respect to abnormalities of the temporal lobes, these authors conclude that there is probably an overall reduction in activity in the temporal lobes, with left-sided activity greater than right-sided. Thalamic function has variously been found to be reduced, unchanged, and increased in schizophrenia. However, in research using network models, interregional metabolic correlations have been suggestive of dysfunctions in brain circuitry between dorsomedial thalamus and limbic structures, and between anterior thalamus and the frontal cortex.

As mentioned above, Liddle et al. (1992) have been examining correlations between various aspects of brain function (measured with PET) and the three symptom patterns of psychomotor poverty, disorganization, and reality distortion in schizophrenia. They found that increased syndrome scores on psychomotor poverty correlated with decreased perfusion in dorsolateral PFC, medial PFC, and anterior cingulate. Although left-sided reductions appeared greater, they concluded that this was more a matter of degree. They concluded that their findings were consistent with the difficulty (noted above) that schizophrenic subjects have in increasing activity in prefrontal areas with task demands for internal generation of action.

With respect to the disorganization syndrome, Liddle et al. (1992) found relative hypoperfusion in the right ventral PFC and a positive correlation between syndrome score and regional cerebral blood flow (rCBF) in the right medial PFC, anterior cingulate, and dorsomedial thalamic nuclei. Hypoperfusion of the parietal cortices bilaterally was also apparent in this syndrome, as was relative hypoperfusion in Broca's area, which they saw as consistent with the theoretical connection of thought disorder and a disturbance of language. They related the findings in the ventral PFC and anterior cingulate to the difficulties that schizophrenic subjects experience in control of attention and inhibition of irrelevant information.

The reality distortion syndrome scores in Liddle et al.'s (1992) subjects correlated with increased rCBF in the left parahippocampal area, consistent with malfunction in the medial temporal lobe and with the theory of Frith and Done (1988) that hallucinations and delusions result from a failure to distinguish internally generated from externally generated material. Similarly, Bogerts (1997) has argued for the importance of temporal lobe pathology (largely involving hippocampal and parahippocampal areas) as important in positive symptoms in schizophrenia. Liddle et al. propose that schizophrenic subjects with reality distortion have a deficit in the connections between medial temporal structures and prefrontal areas, in what they theorize is an internal monitoring system that guides action. This is also the conclusion of a word recall study of schizophrenic subjects by Nestor et al. (1998), in which subjects were required to remember words that had different degrees of connectivity and network size. These authors interpreted the lack of effect of the network size on the performance of the schizophrenic subjects compared to controls as evidence of faulty modulation of associative links within a putative lexicon thought to be distributed across frontal and temporal lobes.

Despite the lack of consistent findings, which can in part be explained by differences in sample sizes, patient characteristics, and methodology, there is some consensus that there is dysfunction in prefrontal, temporal, limbic, basal ganglia, anterior cingulate and thalamic areas. The intense interconnectivity among these areas will produce secondary changes following loss of function in any one area. Thus it is impossible at present to suggest that neuropathology arises primarily from dysfunction in any one area. Instead, much of the theoretical focus has been on understanding ways in which the symptoms of schizophrenia may arise from disturbances in various circuits. I present several of the current ways of trying to grapple with this complexity.

Neurobiological Models

We have moved from a simplistic understanding of neurochemical and neuroanatomical functioning in schizophrenia to highly complex models. These models involve numerous interactions between brain regions; up- and down-regulation of receptors; growth and loss of synapses and dendrites; and, most recently, at the molecular biology level, factors affecting the expression of RNA and its products. In contrast to older notions of dopamine and serotonin (5-HT) as being largely stimulatory or inhibitory, it is now clear that these neurotransmitters can have very different effects, depending on which cell they are affecting and where on the cell the synapse is placed.

Much interest in schizophrenia research has focused on dopamine and its influence on the PFC, basal ganglia, anterior cingulate cortex, and nucleus accumbens. Reviewing the functional and neuroanatomical aspects of prefrontal pathology in schizophrenia, Goldman-Rakic and Selemon (1997) argue that deficits in working memory are central to this disorder. They acknowledge that a working memory deficit is probably neither necessary nor sufficient to explain all symptoms. However, they provide evidence from their own work and that of others to support their idea that PFC dysfunction necessarily involves dysfunctions within the larger network involving the basal ganglia, thalamus, limbic areas, and cingulate and temporal cortices. Recently these authors have found an increase in neuronal density and a decrease in cortical thickness in several prefrontal areas; they suggest that these findings represent a reduction in the neuropil, the meshwork of axonal and dendritic processes in which neurons are embedded (Selemon, Rajkowska, & Goldman-Rakic, 1995). They propose that this reduction may be caused by dystrophy of neurons and their processes, as opposed to cell loss. This idea is consistent with recent findings of changes in receptor proteins and messenger RNA in various brain areas. If these findings are replicated, they should lead to a more concerted investigation into the neurochemical interactions between various cells in the areas that have been found to be functionally impaired in schizophrenia.

With respect to the PFC and working memory, Goldman-Rakic and Selemon (1997) point out the localization of specific functions in discrete areas. Visual–spatial processing involves the dorsolateral PFC; features of objects or faces are processed in more lateral and inferior regions; and semantic encoding and retrieval and other verbal processes engage more inferior, insular, and anterior PFC. Although most work in schizophrenia has focused on the dorsolateral PFC and the visual–spatial defect, work is beginning to emerge suggesting deficits in other areas of working memory, presumably involving these other anatomical areas.

Dopamine appears to modulate pyramidal cell excitability. Although its effect appears to be primarily inhibitory, this may vary with high and low levels of dopamine. The dopamine effect occurs partly through direct contact of dopamine axons with pyramidal neurons and partly through feedforward inhibition from nonpyramidal interneurons in local circuits. These interneurons in the PFC are largely GABAergic and appear to be innervated to a significant degree by the dopamine family of receptors (D2, including the D4 member of this family). Goldman-Rakic and Selemon raise the possibility that dopamine antagonists may work directly through D4 receptors on pyramidal calls to increase excitation and through local-circuit neurons to reduce inhibition and decrease the threshold of pyramidal cell excitability.

Although Goldman-Rakic and Selemon (1997) focus less on 5-HT, they cite work suggesting that 5-HT has direct modulatory (inhibitory) effects on pyramidal cells, as well as effects on local-circuit interneurons. They conclude that these local circuits formed by pyramidal and nonpyramidal neurons provide the information-processing architecture necessary for working memory. Specifically, the modulation of these networks by glutamate, GABA, 5-HT, and dopamine, if disturbed, could disrupt information processing necessary for holding material in working memory. They emphasize that similar dysfunctions could occur in other brain areas and neural networks.

In a similar vein, O'Donnell and Grace (1998) have proposed that the nucleus accumbens, which acts as a modulator of information flow, may be affected by decreases in hippocampal and local-circuit neuronal modulation of its output to the thalamus, which would ultimately produce reduction in neuronal activity in the PFC. Benes (1998) has proposed a similar model involving dysfunction of the GABAergic interneurons within the cingulate cortex.

Focusing on the rich network of connections among the substantia nigra, the striatum and the amygdala, Haber and Fudge (1997) postulate that excessive stimulation of amygdaloid neurons, because of their extensive connections through the dopamine system (including its extensions into the striatum and frontal cortex), could easily disrupt dopamine levels. It is assumed that one part of the amygdala projection to the substantia nigra is inhibitory, and that enhanced firing of this component would reduce dopamine tone in the system. Other components of the dopamine system that can respond to reduced tone by decreased synthesis of D2 autoreceptor and dopamine transporter would result in increased dopamine available at each firing. Although obviously speculative, this model illustrates ways in which changes in amygdala function that may result from stresses or emotional reactions may influence broad areas of the brain. It could account for both lack of motivation (reduced dopamine tone) and sensitivity to stress (enhanced dopamine available with each firing), both of which are central to the symptomatology in schizophrenia.

Jones (1997) has proposed that disintegration of thought processes may be the result of a functional disconnection syndrome between thalamus and PFC. This proposed dysfunction, which could be primary or secondary to other neurological deficits, relates to findings of cell loss in the mediodorsal nucleus of the thalamus (Pakkenberg, 1993) and volume reductions in the thalamus (Staal, Hulshoff Pol, Schnack, van der Schot, & Kahn, 1998). Jones reports that under optimal conditions, thalamic processing that uses large numbers of neurons (as in perception, cognition, and planning of motor strategies) involves oscillations of cells in a loop between the thalamus and PFC. These oscillations appear to bind neural populations together and permit rapid switching to other collectives. The result is more effective transmission between thalamus and cortex. Jones speculates that difficulties in focusing and paying attention to relevant information, which are typical of thought disorder in schizophrenic subjects, could be related to a failure to bind together these large neural groups into their collective oscillations and a difficulty in switching between collectives. Such a defect would interfere with the PFC's holding representations in mind while planning action. This rather elegant formulation of thought disorder does not exclude pathology in other areas, but does provide a plausible rationale for thought disorder. Andreasen, Paradiso, and O'Leary (1998) have proposed a somewhat similar model linking dysfunction in cortical–subcortical–cerebellar circuitry, which they call "cognitive dysmetria."

Using the anology of a cognitive pattern generator, Graybiel (1997) has proposed a theoretical role for the basal ganglia in schizophrenia. The basal ganglia have long been understood as playing a role in coordination of motor behavior, and Graybiel suggests that the evidence supports a role for them in coordinating motivated behavior and cognition. She cites the extensive connections among basal ganglia, frontal areas, the thalamus, limbic areas, and the midbrain neurotransmitter systems, and the fact that many of these connections are loops that would permit ongoing feedback and regulation of activity. She also suggests that as the infant's developing sense of self is dependent on the differentiation of actively initiated versus passively initiated behavior, the iterative nature of many basal-ganglia-related circuits may play a part in learning what the self does, and so in developing self-awareness. With respect to explaining symptoms of schizophrenia, she suggests that negative symptoms may represent a failure of the circuits that control motivated goal-directed behavior. Lesions of the caudate nucleus produce *abulia,* a lack of motivation and drive. With respect to positive symptoms, dysfunctions of the circuits that connect the basal ganglia to the thalamus, cingulate cortex, and midbrain neurotransmitters may produce attentional dysfunction. Similarly, dysfunction of circuits connecting to limbic areas such as the amygdala or hippocampus may produce interference in distinguishing real from not-real or inner-generated from outer-generated information. Although this theory is quite speculative, it provides an explanation of the apparent lack of coordination of cognitive behavior seen in schizophrenia, and possibly of how a distortion of the sense of self can develop.

Several studies have begun to focus on the ultrastructural and neurotransmitter level of analysis. Olney and Farber (1997) have developed a theory that may explain many of the subtle, diverse, and widespread changes seen in postmortem and imaging studies of schizophrenic subjects. The NMDA receptor is a glutamate receptor often found on GABAergic cells. Drugs that have been known to produce a psychotic reaction in humans, such as phencyclidine and ketamine, block the NMDA receptor; such drugs also kill or injure pyramidal cells in rat brain. Assuming the importance of the GABAergic interneurons in modulating activity in many brain areas, Olney and Farber have proposed that the symptoms of schizophrenia may result from defective filtering by these inhibitory cells as a result of NMDA receptor hypofunction, but apparently only in adult brains. In keeping with the notion that schizophrenia is a neurodevelopmental disorder, Olney and Farber have thus proposed that a genetic or environmental event may trigger NMDA receptor hypofunction, but that its effect does not become manifest until adulthood. These authors cite their own work showing that many classes of drugs useful in alleviating the symptoms of schizophrenia also abort the mechanism by which NMDA receptor hypofunction damages the brain. Because GABAergic modulation appears to occur in many of the prefrontal and limbic areas implicated in schizophrenia, this elegant theory may provide a way of unifying some of the diverse findings.

Another model that cuts across brain areas is that of Adler et al. (1998), who propose that the sensory gating deficits observed in schizophrenic subjects can be explained through a deficit in nicotinic receptors—specifically, the alpha-7-nicotinic receptor. Although they focus on the role of this receptor in the hippocampus, these receptors are also found in the thalamus, where they may be involved in the flow of information to the hippocampus. This sensory gating deficit can be reversed with smoking (which may partially explain the high levels of smoking in patients with schizophrenia), but the effect is not long-lasting, presumably due to desensitization of the receptor. The fact that the alpha-7-nicotinic receptor may be genetically linked to band q14 on chromosome 15 may permit more fine-grained genetic studies of this particular vulnerability. Adler et al. also cite studies relating hippocampal volume to a deficit in the alpha-7-nicotinic receptor. Hippocampal volume changes may then be instrumental in the development of psychosis through impaired learning.

Working from an integrated developmental perspective, Walker et al. (1996) describe a model that assumes an interaction between stress and individual vulnerability. Using the information on factors affecting stress reactivity and hypothalamic–pituitary–adrenal (HPA) axis activation (which may be genetic or related to *in utero* maternal stress, perinatal factors, etc., as described in Chapter 5), they suggest that there is evidence for abnormal HPA axis activation in schizophrenia. In support of their argument, they cite drug studies in which the same drugs that worsen the symptoms of schizophrenia also increase cortisol levels. Moreover, cortisol levels in nonmedicated subjects with schizophrenia are often elevated and correlate with levels of symptoms. Like patients with mood disorders, patients with schizophrenia show a lack of suppression of cortisol to a dexamethasone injection. Neuroleptic drugs reduce HPA activity and lead to a reduction in cortisol levels. Lastly, Walker et al. report their own findings that salivary cortisol is elevated in subjects with schizotypal personality disorder versus controls. They suggest that all of these findings are consistent with the postmortem findings of hippocampal damage in schizophrenic subjects.

Walker et al.'s (1996) newer model expands their earlier model, which postulated a dopamine hyperactivation of striatal–thalamic–cortical circuits as responsible for movement abnormalities, and a later-developing limbic system defect based on abnormalities in the mesolimbic dopamine projections as responsible for the thought abnormalities. They now postulate that these striatal abnormalities reflect a heightened sensitivity to dopamine related to dopamine receptor abnormalities in schizophrenia and schizophrenic-spectrum disorders. Given the increase in dopamine associated with stress (and cortisol release), and the possible modification of dopamine receptor sensitivity with HPA activity, they propose that dopamine may mediate the relationship between stress and symptoms of schizophrenia. They also suggest that there may be a synergism, in that dopamine may increase cortisol.

Clearly, the mechanisms of these interesting postulates require elucidation and proof of direction, but Walker et al.'s theory is consistent with the findings and provides a parsimonious way of understanding how stress may act on an already vulnerable system to enhance HPA axis activation and symptoms. The important concept in stress activation is the capacity to limit the response. This theory would also suggest (as I have done in Chapter 9 for the internalizing disorders) that individuals with this diathesis have difficulty turning off the HPA axis response and so may continue to experience stress, which may exacerbate their condition.

CONCLUSIONS

Although we are still a long way from a definitive understanding of schizophrenia and the other psychotic disorders (or of psychotic behavior generally), many leads suggest that arousal modulation plays a major role in schizophrenia, as it appears to do in other emotional disorders. Walker et al.'s (1996) conceptualization, along with the other frameworks noted above, suggests several aspects to the vulnerability seen in individuals with schizophrenia. Stress reactivity, which may be more acute in such individuals than in individuals with anxiety or mood disorders, may produce a more intense cascading of events. On the other hand, given the literature suggesting the confluence of several factors, stress reactivity may be just one factor (one that overlaps with internalizing disorders) in producing psychotic disorders; other factors may be necessary.

In earlier chapters, I have discussed how early difficulties may initiate a negative trajectory that becomes harder and harder to reverse as it progresses. Because we know that many individuals who develop schizophrenia or other psychotic disorders have experienced early adversity, this early stress may increase their vulnerability. However, it is also possible to imagine that highly sensitive children may experience their world as stressful and need to withdraw in order to manage that sense of stressfulness. Parents are likely to find the behavior of such children hard to understand and difficult to manage; parent–child conflict may well ensue. Such conflict will increase stress and produce behavioral difficulties (more likely conduct problems in boys and internalizing difficulties in girls). These strategies for regulating affects and behaviors may gradually become fixed patterns and lead to ongoing conflict within the family. Peer relations will be compromised by these patterns of affect and behavior regulation, and so will self-esteem. Whether individuals who eventually develop psychotic disorders have inherent difficulties that interfere with development and implementation of coping strategies is not clear, but it is likely. If so, maladaptive coping will disrupt their already compromised socioemotional development still further. If language disorders are present (as would be presumed in disorders affecting the left superior temporal gyrus), these will make use of language-based coping strategies more difficult. If there are other abnormalities that affect the processing of information, as has been suggested above, these stress-reactive individuals will be even more hampered in making sense of experiences and coping with normal demands.

Clearly, individuals who develop schizophrenia or other psychotic disorders appear to have deficits affecting many different systems. It is possible to view some if not all of these deficits as existing prior to the onset of symptoms. It is also possible to view many of these abnormalities as developing in the context of stress that cannot be modulated; this may lead to impairment in hippocampal function, and then to a cascading of dysfunctions in related circuits. Those individuals who have a genetic liability to develop psychotic disorders but who do not develop symptoms may have been supported from an early age in developing strategies that allow them to control their level of arousal and thus to avoid sustained stress exposure, which in itself may initiate this negative trajectory.

PART IV

Final Remarks

Chapter 12

Future Directions

$\mathbf{T}$he model I have presented in this book proposes that individuals vary in their likelihood of developing psychopathology. I have argued that those individuals who are stress-reactive—whether this arises from a genetic liability, from exposure to prenatal or perinatal circumstances that increase stress reactivity, or from sensitization by environmental stressors—possess a vulnerability that, in interaction with adverse developmental experience, creates difficulties with affect regulation. When such an individual is exposed to stressors that generate negative affect, psychopathology may readily develop as a coping compromise or solution. Interventions that improve the individual's capacity to deal constructively with affect should ameliorate the psychopathology.

Although I have necessarily had to engage in a certain amount of speculation based largely on my clinical experience, I have not been able to find studies contradicting the arguments I have presented in the preceding chapters. The absence of disproof does not prove the argument, of course. However, because the various literatures (which have developed in a largely independent fashion) all point in a similar direction, they provide support for the main thesis that affect regulation is a critical general factor in all major mental disorders. I hope that others will be as intrigued as I have been by these ideas, and that they will explore not only the main argument but many of the subarguments that are even less well developed.

If my speculations are correct, we can hypothesize that once the capacity to measure levels of arousal in the limbic circuits is refined, we should find the following:

1. Arousal, as measured in limbic circuits (particularly circuits that connect through the amygdala and hippocampus), will be high in the acute phases of all disorders and will not differentiate one disorder from another.

2. Arousal in limbic circuits should diminish as symptoms are alleviated, although in this regard it will be necessary to distinguish those symptoms that are related to arousal from those that may reflect deficit states or traits predisposing individuals to specific disorders.

3. Arousal will diminish with different forms of intervention, including removal from the source of stress. Interventions may, however, produce different effects on brain circuits as the arousal is diminishing. For example, psychotherapy may bring about more changes in the prefrontal cortex, hippocampus, and amygdala, whereas medication may have a greater influence on overall modulating systems, such as dopaminergic or serotonergic systems.

We can also expect that with improved neuroimaging, differences in prefrontal–limbic activity between disorders will emerge more clearly. There should be reduced left prefrontal activity in depression and deficit psychotic states (both of which involve withdrawal from activity), as opposed to anxiety states that do not include withdrawal. Using magnetic resonance imaging, Mayberg et al. (1999) recently demonstrated increased activity in limbic structures, accompanied by decreased activity in prefrontal areas (which they argued might reflect attentional difficulties), during sadness induction. This same pattern, which had been found in depressed subjects, was reversed with successful treatment. This type of study clearly supports the interaction between frontal and limbic circuits that I we have argued is a part of arousal and coping.

We should expect to find increased left prefrontal activity in states involving disinhibition or aggression, as compared to other disorders not involving aggression. Increased dopaminergic activity in left prefrontal–limbic circuits, and reduced serotonergic activity in these circuits, should also be expected in states involving aggression versus those predominantly involving withdrawal.

Lastly, familial and genetic studies should begin to show what factors or combination of factors are necessary and/or sufficient to produce psychopathology. An example of this type of study is the recent finding that whereas eye-tracking dysfunction occurs in both individuals with schizophrenia and their relatives at a higher rate than that in controls, the rate of obstetrical complications, which is high in schizo-phrenic subjects, is lower in their nonschizophrenic relatives than in the controls (Kinney, Levy, Yurgelun-Todd, Tramer, & Holzman, 1998). This type of study will necessarily require improvements in our capacity to measure both the biological and psychosocial factors dis-cussed in this book.

I began writing this treatise with a desire to make psychopatholo-gy more understandable. I end it now with the hope that these ideas may lead to more humane treatment of patients.

References

Abelson, J. L., & Curtis, G. C. (1996). Hypothalamic–pituitary–adrenal axis activity in panic disorder: Prediction of long-term outcome by pretreatment cortisol levels. *American Journal of Psychiatry, 153,* 69–73.

Achenbach, T. M., Edelbrock, C., & Howell, C. T. (1987). Empirically based assessment of the behavioral/emotional problems of 2- and 3-year-old children. *Journal of Abnormal Child Psychology, 15,* 629–650.

Adamec, R. E., & Stark-Adamec, C. (1989). Behavioral inhibition and anxiety: Dispositional, developmental, and neural aspects of the anxious personality of the domestic cat. In J. S. Reznick (Ed.), *Perspectives on behavioral inhibition* (pp. 93–124). Chicago: University of Chicago Press.

Adler, L. E., Olincy, A., Waldo, M., Harris, J. G., Griffith, J., Stevens, K., Flach, K., Nagamoto, H., Bickford, P., Leonard, S., & Freedman, R. (1998). Schizophrenia, sensory gating, and nicotine receptors. *Schizophrenia Bulletin, 24*(2), 189–202.

Adler, R., Hayes, M., Nolan, M., Lewin, T., & Raphael, B. (1991). Antenatal prediction of mother–infant difficulties. *Child Abuse and Neglect, 15,* 351–361.

Ainsworth, M. D. S., Bell, S. M., & Stayton, D. J. (1971). Individual differences in Strange Situation behavior of one-year-olds. In H. R. Schaffer (Ed.), *The origins of human social relations* (pp. 17–57). London: Academic Press.

Aitken, K. J., & Trevarthen, C. (1997). Self/other organization in human psychological development. *Development and Psychopathology, 9,* 653–677.

Akbarian, S., Kim, J. J., Potkin, S. G., Hagman, J. O., Tafazzoli, A., Bunney, W. E., & Jones, E. G. (1995). Gene expression for glutamic acid decarboxylase is reduced without loss of neurons in prefrontal cortex of schizophrenics. *Archives of General Psychiatry, 52,* 258–266.

Akiskal, H. S. (1991). An integrative perspective on recurrent mood disorders:

The mediating role of personality. In J. Becker & A. Kleinman (Eds.), *Psychosocial aspects of depression* (pp. 215–235). Hillsdale, NJ: Erlbaum.

Allen, A. J., Leonard, H. L., & Swedo, S. E. (1995). Case study: A new infection-triggered autoimmune subtype of pediatric OCD and Tourette's syndrome. *Journal of the American Academy of Child and Adolescent Psychiatry, 34,* 307–311.

Allen, J. P., Hauser, S. T., O'Connor, T. G., Bell, K. L., & Eickholt, C. (1996). The connection of observed hostile family conflict to adolescents' developing autonomy and relatedness with parents. *Development and Psychopathology, 8,* 425–442.

Allen, N. B., Lewinsohn, P. M., & Seeley, J. R. (1998). Prenatal and perinatal influences on risk for psychopathology in childhood and adolescence. *Development and Psychopathology, 10,* 513–529.

Allport, G. W. (1961). *Pattern and growth in personality.* New York: Holt, Rinehart & Winston.

Altemus, M., Smith, M. A., Aulakh, C. S., & Murphy, D. L. (1994/1995). Increased mRNA for corticotrophin releasing hormone in the amygdala of fawn-hooded rats: A potential animal model of anxiety. *Anxiety, 1,* 251–257.

Altorfer, A., Goldstein, M. J., Miklowitz, D. J., & Nuechterlein, K. H. (1992). Stress-indicative patterns of non-verbal behaviour: Their role in family interaction. *British Journal of Psychiatry, 161,* 103–113.

American Psychiatric Association. (1994). *Diagnostic and statistical manual of mental disorders* (4th ed.). Washington, DC: Author.

Andreasen, N. C. (1997). The role of the thalamus in schizophrenia. *Canadian Journal of Psychiatry, 42,* 27–33.

Andreasen, N. C., Arndt, S., Alliger, R., Miller, D., & Flaum, M. (1995). Symptoms of schizophrenia: Methods, meanings and mechanisms. *Archives of General Psychiatry, 52,* 341–351.

Andreasen, N. C., O'Leary, D. S., Flaum, M., Nopoulos, P., Watkins, G. L., Boles Ponto, L. L., & Hichwa, R. D. (1997). Hypofrontality in schizophrenia: Distributed dysfunctional circuits in neuroleptic-naive patients. *Lancet, 349,* 1730–1734.

Andreasen, N. C., Paradiso, S., & O'Leary D. S. (1998). "Cognitive dysmetria" as an integrative theory of schizophrenia: A dysfunction in cortical–subcortical–cerebellar circuitry? *Schizophrenia Bulletin, 24*(2), 203–218.

Arndt, S., Andreasen, N. C., Flaum, M., Miller, D., & Nopoulos, P. (1995). A longitudinal study of symptom dimensions in schizophrenia: Prediction and patterns of change. *Archives of General Psychiatry, 52,* 352–360.

Arnold, S. E. (1999). Neurodevelopmental abnormalities in schizophrenia: Insights from neuropathology. *Development and Psychopathology, 61,* 439–456.

Arnsten, A. F. T., & Goldman-Rakic, P. S. (1998). Noise stress impairs prefrontal cortical cognitive function in monkeys: Evidence for a hyperdopaminergic mechanism. *Archives of General Psychiatry, 55,* 362–368.

Asarnow, J. R., Goldstein, M., Tompson, M., & Guthrie, D. (1993). One-year outcomes of depressive disorders in child psychiatric in-patients: Evaluation of the prognostic power of a brief measure of expressed emotion. *Journal of Child Psychology and Psychiatry, 34,* 129–137.

Asendorpf, J. B. (1991). Development of inhibited children's coping with unfamiliarity. *Child Development, 62,* 1460–1474.

Atkinson, L., & Zucker, K. J. (Eds.). (1997). *Attachment and psychopathology.* New York: Guilford Press.

Avissar, S., Nechamkin, Y., Roitman, G., & Schreiber, G. (1998). Dynamics of ECT normalization of low G protein function and immunoreactivity in mononuclear leukocytes of patients with major depression. *American Journal of Psychiatry, 155,* 666–671.

Ballard, M. E., Cummings, E. M., & Larkin, K. (1993). Emotional and cardiovascular responses to adults' angry behavior and to challenging tasks in children of hypertensive and normotensive parents. *Child Development, 64,* 500–515.

Ballenger, J. C. (Speaker). (1998). Panic disorder [Cassette recording]. *Audio-Digest Psychiatry, 27*(18).

Bandura, A. (1991). Self-efficacy mechanism in physiological activation and health-promoting behavior. In J. Madden IV (Ed.), *Neurobiology of learning and affect* (pp. 229–269). New York: Raven Press.

Baron, M., & Gruen, R. S. (1991). Schizophrenia and affective disorder: Are they genetically linked? *British Journal of Psychiatry, 159,* 267–270.

Bates, J. E. (1994). Introduction. In J. E. Bates & T. D. Wachs (Eds.), *Temperament: Individual differences at the interface of biology and behavior* (pp. 1–16). Washington, DC: American Psychological Association.

Bates, J. E., & Bayles, K. (1984). Objective and subjective components in mothers' perceptions of their children from age 6 months to 3 years. *Merrill–Palmer Quarterly, 30,* 111–130.

Bates, J. E., Bayles, K., Bennett, D. S., Ridge, B., & Brown, M. M. (1991). Origins of externalizing behavior problems at eight years of age. In D. Pepler & K. Rubin (Eds.), *Development and treatment of childhood aggression* (pp. 93–120). Hillsdale, NJ: Erlbaum.

Bates, J. E., Freeland, C. A. B., & Lounsbury, M. L. (1979). Measurement of infant difficultness. *Child Development, 50,* 794–803.

Bates, J. E., Maslin, C. A., & Frankel, K. A. (1985). Attachment security, mother–child interaction, and temperament as predictors of behavior-problem ratings at age three years. In I. Bretherton & E. Waters (Eds.), Growing points of attachment theory and research. *Monographs of the Society for Research in Child Development, 50*(1–2, Serial No, 209), 167–193.

Baumrind, D. (1989). Rearing competent children. In W. Damon (Ed.), *Child development today and tomorrow* (pp. 349–378). San Francisco: Jossey-Bass.

Baxter, L. R., Schwartz, J. M., Bergman, K. S., Szuba, M. P., Guze, B. H., & Mazziotta, J. C. (1992). Caudate glucose metabolic rate changes with both drug and behavior therapy for obsessive–compulsive disorder. *Archives of General Psychiatry, 49,* 681–689.

Beardslee, W. R., Versage, E. M., & Gladstone, T. R. G. (1998). Children of affectively ill parents: A review of the past 10 years. *Journal of the American Academy of Child and Adolescent Psychiatry, 37,* 1134–1141.

Bebbington, P., & Kuipers, L. (1994). The predictive utility of expressed emotion in schizophrenia: An aggregate analysis. *Psychological Medicine, 24,* 707–718.

Bechara, A., Tranel, D., Damasio, H., Adolphs, R., Rockland, C., & Damasio, A. R. (1995). Double dissociation of conditioning and declarative knowledge relative to the amygdala and hippocampus in humans. *Science, 269,* 1115–1118.

Bechara, A., Tranel, D., Damasio, H., & Damasio, A. R. (1996). Failure to respond autonomically to anticipated future outcomes following damage to prefrontal cortex. *Cerebral Cortex, 6,* 215–225.

Beck, A. T. (1971). Cognition, affect, and psychopathology. *Archives of General Psychiatry, 24,* 495–500.

Beebe, B. (1993, October). *A dyadic systems view of communcation: Contributions from infant research to adult treatment.* Paper presented at the Self Psychology Conference, Toronto.

Beeghly, M., & Cicchetti, D. (1994). Child maltreatment, attachment, and the self system: Emergence of an internal state lexicon in toddlers at high social risk. *Development and Psychopathology, 6,* 5–30.

Beidel, D. C., & Turner, S. M. (1997). At risk for anxiety: 1. Psychopathology in the offspring of anxious parents. *Journal of the American Academy of Child and Adolescent Psychiatry, 36,* 918–924.

Beiser, M., & Iacono, W. G. (1990). An update on the epidemiology of schizophrenia. *Canadian Journal of Psychiatry, 35,* 657–668.

Beitchman, J. H., Brownlie, E. B., & Wilson, B. (1996). Linguistic impairment and psychiatric disorder: Pathways to outcome. In J. H. Beitchman, N. J. Cohen, M. M. Konstantareas, & R. Tannock (Eds.), *Language, learning, and behavior disorders* (pp. 493–514). New York: Cambridge University Press.

Beitman, B. D. (1992). Integration through fundamental similarities and useful differences among the schools. In J. C. Norcross & M. R. Goldfried (Eds.), *Handbook of psychotherapy integration* (pp. 202–230). New York: Basic Books.

Belsky, J., Rosenberger, K., & Crnic, K. (1995). The origins of attachment security: "Classical" and contextual determinants. In S. Goldberg, R. Muir, & J. Kerr (Eds.), *Attachment theory: Social, developmental, and clinical perspectives* (pp. 153–183). Hillsdale, NJ: Analytic Press.

Belsky, J., & Rovine, M. (1987). Temperament and attachment security in the strange situation: An empirical rapprochement. *Child Development, 58,* 787–795.

Bench, C. J., Friston, K. J., Brown, R. G., Frackowiak, R. S. J., & Dolan, R. J. (1993). Regional cerebral blood flow in depression measured by positron emission tomography: The relationship with clinical dimensions. *Psychological Medicine, 23,* 579–590.

Bender, L. (1947). Childhood schizophrenia: Clinical study of 100 schizophrenic children. *American Journal of Orthopsychiatry, 17,* 40–56.

Benes, F. M. (1998). Model generation and testing to probe neural circuitry in the cingulate cortex of postmortem schizophrenic brain. *Schizophrenia Bulletin, 24*(2), 219–230.

Benjamin, J., Li, L., Patterson, C., Greenberg, B. D., Murphy, D. L., & Hamer, D. (1996). Population and familial association between the D4 dopamine receptor gene and measures of novelty seeking. *Nature Genetics, 12,* 81–84.

Benoit, D., & Parker, K. C. H. (1994). Stability and transmission of attachment across three generations. *Child Development, 65*, 1444–1456.

Bergman, A. J., Harvey, P. D., Mitropoulou, V., Aronson, A., Marder, D., Silverman, J., Trestman, R., & Siever, L. J. (1996). The factor structure of schizotypal symptoms in a clinical population. *Schizophrenia Bulletin, 22*(3), 501–510.

Bernstein, V. J., & Hans, S. L. (1994). Predicting the developmental outcome of two-year-old children born exposed to methadone: Impact of social-environmental risk factors. *Journal of Clinical Child Psychology, 23*, 349–359.

Berntson, G. G., Cacioppo, J. T., & Quigley, K. S. (1991). Autonomic determinism: The modes of autonomic control, the doctrine of autonomic space, and the laws of autonomic constraint. *Psychological Review, 98*, 459–487.

Berridge, C. W., Arnsten, A. F. T., & Foote, S. L. (1993). Noradrenergic modulation of cognitive function: Clinical implications of anatomical, electrophysiological and behavioural studies in animal models. *Psychological Medicine, 23*, 557–564.

Biederman, J., Rosenbaum, J. F., Bolduc-Murphy, E. A., Faraone, S. V., Chaloff, J., & Hirshfeld, D. R. (1993). A 3-year follow-up of children with and without behavioral inhibition. *Journal of the American Academy of Child and Adolescent Psychiatry, 32*, 814–821.

Biederman, J., Rosenbaum, J. F., Hirshfeld, D. R., Faraone, S. V., Bolduc, E. A., Gersten, M., Meminger, S. R., Kagan, J., Snidman, N., & Reznick, J. S. (1990). Psychiatric correlates of behavioral inhibition in young children of parents with and without psychiatric disorders. *Archives of General Psychiatry, 47*, 21–26.

Bierman, K. L., & Wargo, J. B. (1995). Predicting the longitudinal course associated with aggressive–rejected, aggressive (nonrejected), and rejected (nonagressive) status. *Development and Psychopathology, 7*, 669–713.

Bion, W. (1978). *Second thoughts*. London: Heinemann.

Black, J. E., Jones, T. A., Nelson, C. A., & Greenough, W. T. (1998). Neuronal plasticity and the developing brain. In N. E. Alessi, J. T. Coyle, S. I. Harrison, & S. Eth (Series Eds.) & J. D. Noshpitz (Vol. Ed.), *Handbook of child and adolescent psychiatry: Vol. 6. Basic psychiatric science* (pp. 31–53). New York: Wiley.

Blanchard, J. J., Mueser, K. T., & Bellack, A. S. (1998). Anhedonia, positive and negative affect, and social functioning in schizophrenia. *Schizophrenia Bulletin, 24*(4), 413–424.

Bogerts, B. (1997). The temporolimbic system theory of positive schizophrenic symptoms. *Schizophrenia Bulletin, 23*(3), 423–435.

Bohman, M. (1995). Predisposition to criminality: Swedish adoption studies in retrospect. In G. R. Bock & J. A. Goode (Eds.), *Genetics of criminal and antisocial behaviour* (Ciba Foundation Symposium No. 194, pp. 99–114). Chichester, England: Wiley.

Bolig, R., Price, C. S., O'Neill, P. L., & Suomi, S. J. (1992). Subjective assessment of reactivity level and personality traits of rhesus monkeys. *International Journal of Primatology, 13*, 287–306.

Borod, J. C. (1992). Interhemispheric and intrahemispheric control of emotion: A focus on unilateral brain damage. *Journal of Consulting and Clinical Psychology*, *60*(3), 339–348.

Bowlby, J. (1969). *Attachment and loss: Vol. 1. Attachment.* New York: Basic Books.

Bowlby, J. (1973). *Attachment and loss: Vol. 2. Separation: Anxiety and anger.* New York: Basic Books.

Bowlby, J. (1980). *Attachment and loss: Vol. 3. Sadness and depression.* Harmondsworth, England: Penguin.

Bracha, H. S., Torrey, E. F., Gottesman, I. I., Bigelow, L. B., & Cunniff, C. (1992). Second-trimester markers of fetal size in schizophrenia: A study of monozygotic twins. *American Journal of Psychiatry*, *149*, 1355–1361.

Bradley, R. H., & Casey, P. H. (1992). Family environment and behavioral development of low-birthweight children. *Developmental Medicine and Child Neurology*, *32*, 822–832.

Bradley, S. J. (1985). Gender disorders in childhood: A formulation. In B. W. Steiner (Ed.), *Gender dysphoria: Development, research, management* (pp. 175–188). New York: Plenum Press.

Bradley, S. J. (1990). Affect regulation and psychopathology: Bridging the mind–body gap. *Canadian Journal of Psychiatry*, *35*, 540–547.

Braff, D. L., Grillon, C., & Geyer, M. A. (1992). Gating and habituation of the startle reflex in schizophrenic patients. *Archives of General Psychiatry*, *49*, 206–215.

Braff, D. L., Heaton, R., Kuck, J., Cullum, M., Moranville, J., Grant, I., & Zisook, S. (1991). The generalized pattern of neuropsychological deficits in outpatients with chronic schizophrenia with heterogeneous Wisconsin Card Sorting Test results. *Archives of General Psychiatry*, *48*, 891–898.

Braungart-Rieker, J., Rende, R. D., Plomin, R., DeFries, J. C., & Fulker, D. W. (1995). Genetic mediation of longitudinal associations between family environment and childhood behavior problems. *Development and Psychopathology*, *7*, 233–245.

Breier, A., Buchanan, R. W., Elkashef, A., Munson, R. C., Kirkpatrick, B., & Gellad, F. (1992). Brain morphology and schizophrenia: A magnetic resonance imaging study of limbic, prefrontal cortex, and caudate structures. *Archives of General Psychiatry*, *49*, 921–926.

Breier, A., Schreiber, J. L., Dyer, J., & Pickar, D. (1991). National Institute of Mental Health longitudinal study of chronic schizophrenia: Prognosis and predictors of outcome. *Archives of General Psychiatry*, *48*, 239–246.

Brennan, P. A., Raine, A., Schulsinger, F., Kirkegaard-Sorensen, L., Knop, J., Hutchings, B., Rosenberg, R., & Mednick, S. A. (1997). Psychophysiological protective factors for male subjects at high risk for criminal behavior. *American Journal of Psychiatry*, *154*, 853–855.

Breslau, N. (1990). Does brain dysfunction increase children's vulnerability to environmental stress? *Archives of General Psychiatry*, *47*, 15–20.

Breslau, N. (1995). Psychiatric sequelae of low birth weight. *Epidemiologic Reviews*, *17*, 96–106.

Breslau, N., Chilcoat, H. D., Kessler, R. C., & Davis, G. C. (1999). Previous exposure to trauma and PTSD effects of subsequent trauma: Results from the Detroit Area Survey of Trauma. *American Journal of Psychiatry*, *156*, 902–907.

Breslau, N., & Davis, G. C. (1992). Posttraumatic stress disorder in an urban population of young adults: Risk factors for chronicity. *American Journal of Psychiatry, 149,* 671–675.

Bretherton, I. (1995). The origins of attachment theory: John Bowlby and Mary Ainsworth. In S. Goldberg, R. Muir, & J. Kerr (Eds.), *Attachment theory: Social, developmental, and clinical perspectives* (pp. 45–84). Hillsdale, NJ: Analytic Press.

Broberg, A., Lamb, M. E., & Hwang, P. (1990). Inhibition: Its stability and correlates in sixteen- to forty-month-old children. *Child Development, 61,* 1153–1163.

Brown, A. S., Susser, E. S., Lin, S. P., Neugebauer, R., & Gorman, J. M. (1995). Increased risk of affective disorders in males after second trimester prenatal exposure to the Dutch hunger winter of 1944–45. *British Journal of Psychiatry, 166,* 601–606.

Brown, G. W., Birley, J. L. T., & Wing, J. K. (1972). Influence of family life on the course of schizophrenic disorders: A replication. *British Journal of Psychiatry, 121,* 241–258.

Brown, G. W., Bifulco, A., & Andrews, B. (1990). Self-esteem and depression: III. Aetiological issues. *Social Psychiatry and Psychiatric Epidemiology, 25,* 235–243.

Brown, G. W., & Harris, T. (1978). *Social origins of depression.* London: Tavistock.

Brown, G. W., & Harris, T. O. (1993). Aetiology of anxiety and depressive disorders in an inner-city population: 1. Early adversity. *Psychological Medicine, 23,* 143–154.

Brown, G. W., Harris, T. O., & Eales, M. J. (1993). Aetiology of anxiety and depressive disorders in an inner-city population: 2. Comorbidity and adversity. *Psychological Medicine, 23,* 155–165.

Brown, G. W., Harris, T. O., Hepworth, C., & Robinson, R. (1994). Clinical and psychosocial origins of chronic depressive episodes: II. A patient enquiry. *British Journal of Psychiatry, 165,* 457–465.

Brown, G. W., & Moran, P. (1994). Clinical and psychosocial origins of chronic depressive episodes: I. A community survey. *British Journal of Psychiatry, 165,* 447–456.

Brown, G. W., & Moran, P. (1998). Emotion and the etiology of depressive disorders. In W. F. Flack & J. D. Laird (Eds.), *Emotions in psychopathology: Theory and research* (pp. 171–184). New York: Oxford University Press.

Brown, T. A. (1997). The nature of generalized anxiety disorder and pathological worry: Current evidence and conceptual models. *Canadian Journal of Psychiatry, 42,* 817–825.

Brown, T. A., Chorpita, B. F., & Barlow, D. H. (1998). Structural relationships among dimensions of the DSM-IV anxiety and mood disorders and dimensions of negative affect, positive affect, and autonomic arousal. *Journal of Abnormal Psychology, 107,* 179–192.

Buchanan, R. W., & Carpenter, W. T., Jr. (1997). The neuroanatomies of schizophrenia. *Schizophrenia Bulletin, 23*(3), 367–372.

Buchanan, R. W., Strauss, M. E., Breier, A., Kirkpatrick, B., & Carpenter, W. T. (1997). Attentional impairments in deficit and nondeficit forms of schizophrenia. *American Journal of Psychiatry, 154,* 363–370.

Buchsbaum, M. S., & Hazlett, E. A. (1998). Positron emission tomography studies of abnormal glucose metabolism in schizophrenia. *Schizophrenia Bulletin, 24*(3), 343–364.

Bugental, D. B. (1992). Affective and cognitive processes within threat-oriented family systems. In I. E. Sigel, A. McGillicuddy-de Lisi, & J. J. Goodnow (Eds.), *Parental belief systems: The psychological consequences for children* (2nd ed., pp. 219–248). Hillsdale, NJ: Erlbaum.

Bugental, D. B., Mantyla, S. M., & Lewis, J. (1989). Parental attributions as moderators of affective communication to children at risk for physical abuse. In D. Cicchetti & V. Carlson (Eds.), *Child maltreatment: Theory and research on the causes and consequences of child abuse and neglect* (pp. 254–279). New York: Cambridge University Press.

Buss, A. H., & Plomin, R. (1984). *Temperament: Early developing personality traits.* Hillsdale, NJ: Erlbaum.

Cadoret, R. J., Yates, W. R., Troughton, E., Woodworth, G., & Stewart, M. A. (1995a). Adoption study demonstrating two genetic pathways to drug abuse. *Archives of General Psychiatry, 52,* 42–52.

Cadoret, R. J., Yates, W. R., Troughton, E., Woodworth, G., & Stewart, M. A. (1995b). Genetic–environmental interaction in the genesis of aggressivity and conduct disorders. *Archives of General Psychiatry, 52,* 916–936.

Calkins, S. D., & Fox, N. A. (1992). The relations among infant temperament, security of attachment, and behavioral inhibition at twenty-four months. *Child Development, 63,* 1456–1472.

Campbell, S. B., Pierce, E. W., Moore, G., Marakovitz, S., & Newby, K. (1996). Boys' externalizing problems at elementary school age: Pathways from early behavior problems, maternal control, and family stress. *Development and Psychopathology, 8,* 701–719.

Campos, J. J., Barrett, K. C., Lamb, M. E., Goldsmith, H. H., & Stenberg, C. (1983). Socioemotional development. In P. H. Mussen (Series Ed.) & M. M. Haith (Vol. Ed.), *Handbook of child psychology: Vol. 2. Infancy and developmental psychobiology* (4th ed., pp. 783–917). New York: Wiley.

Campos, J. J., Campos, R. G., & Barrett, K. C. (1989). Emergent themes in the study of emotional development and emotion regulation. *Developmental Psychology, 25,* 394–402.

Cannon, T. D., Mednick, S. A., Parnas, J., Schulsinger, F., Praestholm, J., & Vestergaard, A. (1993). Developmental brain abnormalities in the offspring of schizophrenic mothers: I. Contributions of genetic and perinatal factors. *Archives of General Psychiatry, 50,* 551–564.

Cannon, T. D., Rosso, I. M., Bearden, C. E., Sanchez, L. E., & Hadley, T. (1999). A prospective cohort study of neurodevelopmental processes in the genesis and epigenesis of schizophrenia. *Development and Psychopathology, 11,* 467–485.

Caplan, R. (1996). Discourse deficits in schizophrenia. In J. H. Beitchman, N. J. Cohen, M. M. Konstantareas, & R. Tannock (Eds.), *Language, learning, and behavior disorders* (pp. 157–177). New York: Cambridge University Press.

Carek, D. J. (1990). Affect in psychodynamic psychotherapy. *American Journal of Psychotherapy, 44,* 274–282.

Carey, W. B., & McDevitt, S. C. (1978). Revision of the Infant Temperament Questionnaire. *Pediatrics, 61,* 735–739.

Carlson, E. A., Jacobvitz, D., & Sroufe, L. A. (1995). A developmental investigation of inattentiveness and hyperactivity. *Child Development, 66,* 37–54.

Carlsson, M., & Carlsson, A. (1990). Interactions between glutamatergic and monoaminergic systems within the basal ganglia: Implications for schizophrenia and Parkinson's disease. *Trends in Neuroscience, 13,* 272–276.

Carpenter, W. T., Heinrichs, D. W., & Wagman, A. M. I. (1988). Deficit and nondeficit forms of schizophrenia: The concept. *American Journal of Psychiatry, 145,* 578–583.

Carter, C. S., Perlstein, W., Ganguli, R., Brar, J., Mintun, M., & Cohen, J. D. (1998). Functional hyperfrontality and working memory dysfunction in schizophrenia. *American Journal of Psychiatry, 155,* 1285–1287.

Caspi, A., Henry, B., McGee, R. O., Moffitt, T. E., & Silva, P. A. (1995). Temperamental origins of child and adolescent behavior problems: From age three to age fifteen. *Child Development, 66,* 55–68.

Cassidy, J. (1992). *Generalized anxiety disorder and attachment.* Unpublished manuscript.

Cassidy, J. (1994). Emotion regulation: Influences of attachment relationships. In N. A. Fox (Ed.), The development of emotion regulation: Biological and behavioral considerations. *Monographs of the Society for Research in Child Development, 59*(2–3), 228–249.

Cassidy, J., & Kobak, R. R. (1988). Avoidance and its relation to other defensive processes. In J. Belsky & T. Nezworski (Eds.), *Clinical implications of attachment* (pp. 300–323). Hillsdale, NJ: Erlbaum.

Cassidy, J., & Marvin, R. S., with the Attachment Working Group of the MacArthur Network on the Transition from Infancy to Early Childhood. (1992). *Attachment organization in three- and four-year-olds: Coding guidelines* (rev. ed.). Unpublished manuscript, University of Virginia.

Changeux, J. P., & Dehaene, S. (1989). Neuronal models of cognitive functions. *Cognition, 33,* 63–109.

Chapman, J. P., & Chapman, L. J. (1996). The psychometric assessment of schizophrenia proneness. In S. Matthysse, D. L. Levy, J. Kagan, & F. M. Benes (Eds.), *Psychopathology: The evolving science of mental disorder* (pp. 313–333). New York: Cambridge University Press.

Charney, D. S., Deutch, A. Y., Krystal, J. H., Southwick, S. M., & Davis, M. (1993). Psychobiologic mechanisms of posttraumatic stress disorder. *Archives of General Psychiatry, 50,* 294–305.

Chess, S., & Thomas, A. (1984). *Origins and evolution of behavior disorders from infancy to early adult life.* New York: Brunner/Mazel.

Chua, S. E., & McKenna, P. J. (1995). Schizophrenia—a brain disease?: A critical review of structural and functional cerebral abnormality in the disorder. *British Journal of Psychiatry, 166,* 563–582.

Chugani, H. T. (1994). Development of regional brain glucose metabolism in relation to behavior and plasticity. In G. Dawson & K. W. Fischer (Eds.), *Human behavior and the developing brain* (pp. 153–175). New York: Guilford Press.

Ciaranello, R. D., Aimi, J., Dean, R. R., Morilak, D. A., Porteus, M. H., & Cicchetti, D. (1995). Fundamentals of molecular neurobiology. In D. Cicchetti & D. J. Cohen (Eds.), *Developmental psychopathology: Vol. 1. Theory and methods* (pp. 109–160). New York: Wiley.

Cicchetti, D. (1989). How research on child maltreatment has informed the study of child development: Perspectives from developmental psychology. In D. Cicchetti & V. Carlson (Eds.), *Child maltreatment: Theory and research on the causes and consequences of child abuse and neglect* (pp. 377–431). New York: Cambridge University Press.

Cicchetti, D., & Aber, J. L. (1986). Early precursors of later depression: An organizational perspective. In L. Lipsitt & C. Rovee-Collier (Eds.), *Advances in infancy* (Vol. 4, pp. 87–137). Norwood, NJ: Ablex.

Cicchetti, D., & Beeghly, M. (1987). Symbolic development in maltreated youngsters: An organizational perspective. *New Directions for Child Development, 36,* 5–29.

Cicchetti, D., & Rogosch, F. A. (1996). Equifinality and multifinality in developmental psychopathology. *Development and Psychopathology, 8,* 597–600.

Cicchetti, D., & Toth, S. (1995). Child maltreatment and attachment organization. In S. Goldberg, R. Muir, & J. Kerr (Eds.), *Attachment theory: Social, developmental, and clinical perspectives* (pp. 279–308). Hillsdale, NJ: Analytic Press.

Cicchetti, D., & Tucker, D. (1994). Development and self-regulatory structures of the mind. *Development and Psychopathology, 6,* 533–549.

Clark, C. R., Geffen, G. M., & Geffen, L. B. (1987a). Catecholamines and attention: I. Animal and clinical studies. *Neuroscience & Biobehavioral Reviews, 11,* 341–352.

Clark, C. R., Geffen, G. M., & Geffen, L. B. (1987b). Catecholamines and attention: II. Pharmacological studies in normal humans. *Neuroscience and Biobehavioral Reviews, 11,* 353–364.

Clark, D. A., & Steer, R. A. (1996). Empirical status of the cognitive model of anxiety and depression. In P. M. Salkovskis (Ed.), *Frontiers of cognitive therapy* (pp. 75–96). New York: Guilford Press.

Clark, L. A., & Watson, D. (1991a). Theoretical and empirical issues in differentiating depression from anxiety. In J. Becker & A. Kleinman (Eds.), *Psychosocial aspects of depression* (pp. 39–65). Hillsdale, NJ: Erlbaum.

Clark, L. A., & Watson, D. (1991b). A tripartite model of anxiety and depression: Psychometric evidence and taxonomic implications. *Journal of Abnormal Psychology, 100,* 316–336.

Clarke, A. S., Kammerer, C. M., George, K. P., Kupfer, D. J., McKinney, W. T., Spence, M. A., & Kraemer, G. W. (1995). Evidence for heritability of biogenic amine levels in the cerebrospinal fluid of rhesus monkeys. *Biological Psychiatry, 38,* 572–577.

Clarke, A. S., & Schneider, M. L. (1993). Prenatal stress has long-term effects on behavioral responses to stress in juvenile rhesus monkeys. *Developmental Psychobiology, 26,* 293–304.

Clarke, A. S., Soto, A., Bergholz, T., & Schneider, M. L. (1996). Maternal gestational stress alters adaptive and social behavior in adolescent Rhesus monkey offspring. *Infant Behavior and Development, 19,* 451–461.

Cloninger, C. R. (1987). A systematic method for clinical description and classification of personality variants: A proposal. *Archives of General Psychiatry, 44,* 573–588.

Cloninger, C. R., Adolfsson, R., & Svrakic, N. M. (1996). Mapping genes for human personality. *Nature Genetics, 12,* 3–4.

Clyman, R. B. (1992). The procedural organization of emotions: A contribution from cognitive science to the psychoanalytic theory of therapeutic action. In T. Shapiro & R. N. Emde (Eds.), *Affect: Psychoanalytic perspectives* (pp. 349–382). Madison, CT: International Universities Press.

Cohen, N. J. (1996). Unsuspected language impairments in psychiatrically disturbed children: Developmental issues and associated conditions. In J. H. Beitchman, N. J. Cohen, M. M. Konstantareas, & R. Tannock (Eds.), *Language, learning, and behavior disorders* (pp. 105–127). New York: Cambridge University Press.

Coie, J., Terry, R., Lenox, K., Lochman, J., & Hyman, C. (1995). Childhood peer rejection and aggression as predictors of stable patterns of adolescent disorder. *Development and Psychopathology, 7,* 697–713.

Cole, P. M., Michel, M. K., & Teti, L. O. (1994). The development of emotion regulation and dysregulation: A clinical perspective. In N. A. Fox (Ed.), The development of emotion regulation: Biological and behavioral considerations. *Monographs of the Society for Research in Child Development, 59*(2–3, Serial No. 240), 73–100.

Cole, P. M., & Putnam, F. W. (1992). Effect of incest on self and social functioning: A developmental psychopathology perspective. *Journal of Consulting and Clinical Psychology, 60,* 174–184.

Cole, P. M., & Zahn-Waxler, C. (1992). Emotional dysregulation in disruptive behavior disorders. In D. Cicchetti & S. L. Toth (Eds.), *Developmental perspectives on depression* (pp. 173–209). Rochester, NY: University of Rochester Press.

Constantino, J. N., Morris, J. A., & Murphy, D. L. (1997). CSF 5-HIAA and family history of antisocial personality disorder in newborns. *American Journal of Psychiatry, 154,* 1771–1773.

Coplan, J. D., Rosenblum, L. A., & Gorman, J. M. (1995). Primate models of anxiety: Longitudinal perspectives. *Psychiatric Clinics of North America, 18,* 727–743.

Coplan, J. D., Trost, R. C., Owens, M. J., Cooper, T. B., Gorman, J. M., Nemeroff, C. B., & Rosenblum, L. A. (1998). Cerebrospinal fluid concentrations of somatostatin and biogenic amines in grown primates reared by mothers exposed to manipulated foraging conditions. *Archives of General Psychiatry, 55,* 473–477.

Cornblatt, B. A., Lenzenweger, M. F., Dworkin, R. H., & Erlenmeyer-Kimling, L. (1992). Childhood attentional dysfunctions predict social deficits in unaffected adults at risk for schizophrenia. *British Journal of Psychiatry, 161,* 59–64.

Cornblatt, B., Obuchowski, M., Roberts, S., Pollack, S., & Erlenmeyer-Kimling, L. (1999). Cognitive and behavioral precursors of schizophrenia. *Development and Psychopathology, 11,* 487–508.

Coryell, W., Keller, M., Lavori, P., & Endicott, J. (1990a). Affective syndromes, psychotic features and prognosis: I. Depression. *Archives of General Psychiatry, 47,* 651–657.

Coryell, W., Keller, M., Lavori, P., & Endicott, J. (1990b). Affective syndromes, psychotic features, and prognosis: II. Mania. *Archives of General Psychiatry, 47,* 658–662.

Crittenden, P. M. (1992). *Classification of quality of attachment for preschool-aged children.* Unpublished coding manual. (Available from P.M. Crittenden, 9481 S.W. 147 St., Miami, FL 33176.)

Crittenden, P. M. (1995). Attachment and psychopathology. In S. Goldberg, R. Muir, & J. Kerr (Eds.), *Attachment theory: Social, developmental, and clinical perspectives* (pp. 367–406). Hillsdale, NJ: Analytic Press.

Crittenden, P. M., & Ainsworth, M. D. S. (1989). Child maltreatment and attachment theory. In D. Cicchetti & V. Carlson (Eds.), *Child maltreatment: Theory and research on the causes and consequences of child abuse and neglect* (pp. 432–463). New York: Cambridge University Press.

Crockenberg, S. B. (1981). Infant irritability, mother responsiveness, and social support influences on the security of infant–mother attachment. *Child Development, 52,* 857–865.

Crow, T. J. (1980). Molecular pathology of schizophrenia: More than one disease process? *British Medical Journal, 280,* 1–9.

Crow, T. J. (1986). The continuum of psychosis and its implication for the structure of the gene. *British Journal of Psychiatry, 149,* 419–429.

Cummings, E. M., & Cummings, J. L. (1988). A process-oriented approach to children's coping with adults' angry behavior. *Developmental Review, 8,* 296–321.

Cummings, E. M., & Davies, P. T. (1994). Maternal depression and child development. *Journal of Child Psychology and Psychiatry, 35,* 73–112.

Cummings, E. M., Iannotti, R. J., & Zahn-Waxler, C. (1985). Influence of conflict between adults on the emotions and aggression of young children. *Developmental Psychology, 21,* 495–507.

Cummings, E. M., Simpson, K. S., & Wilson, A. (1993). Children's responses to interadult anger as a function of information about resolution. *Developmental Psychology, 29,* 978–985.

Cutler, J. L., & Siris, S. G. (1991). "Panic-like" symptomatology in schizophrenic and schizoaffective patients with postpsychotic depression: Observations and implications. *Comprehensive Psychiatry, 32,* 465–473.

Czobor, P., & Volavka, J. (1996). Positive and negative symptoms: Is their change related? *Schizophrenia Bulletin, 22*(4), 577–590.

Dadds, M. R., Rosenthal Gaffney, L., Kenardy, J., Oei, T. P. S., & Evans, L. (1993). An exploration of the relationship between expression of hostility and the anxiety disorders. *Journal of Psychiatric Research, 27,* 17–26.

Davidson, R. J. (1992). Cerebral asymmetry and affective disorders: A developmental perspective. In D. Cicchetti & S. L. Toth (Eds.), *Rochester Symposium on Developmental Psychopathology: Vol. 2. Internalizing and externalizing expressions of dysfunction* (pp. 123–154). Hillsdale, NJ: Erlbaum.

Davidson, R. J., & Fox, N. A. (1989). Frontal brain asymmetry predicts infants' response to maternal separation. *Journal of Abnormal Psychology, 98,* 127–131.

Davis, J. O., Phelps, J. A., & Bracha, H. S. (1995). Prenatal development of monozygotic twins and concordance for schizophrenia. *Schizophrenia Bulletin, 21,* 357–366.

Dawson, G. (1994). Frontal electroencephalographic correlates of individual differences in emotion expression in infants: A brain systems perspective on emotion. In N. A. Fox (Ed.), The development of emotion regulation: Biological and behavioral considerations. *Monographs of the Society for Research in Child Development, 59*(2–3, Serial No. 240), 135–151.

Dawson, G., Frey, K., Self, J., Panagiotides, H., Hessl, D., Yamada, G., & Rinaldi, J. (1991). Frontal brain electrical activity in infants of depressed and non-depressed mothers: Relation to variations in infant behavior. *Development and Psychopathology, 11,* 589–605.

Dawson, G., Klinger, L. G., Panagiotides, H., Spieker, S., & Frey, K. (1992). Infants of mothers with depressive symptoms: Electroencephalographic and behavioral findings related to attachment status. *Development and Psychopathology, 4,* 67–80.

Dawson, M. E. (1990). Psychophysiology at the interface of clinical science, cognitive science, and neuroscience (Presidential Address). *Psychophysiology, 27,* 243–255.

Deater-Deckard, K., Dodge, K. A., Bates, J. E., & Pettit, G. S. (1998). Multiple risk factors in the development of externalizing behavior problems: Group and individual differences. *Development and Psychopathology, 10,* 469–493.

De Kloet, E. R. (1991). Brain corticosteroid receptor balance and homeostatic control. *Frontiers in Neuroendocrinology, 12,* 95–164.

Derryberry, D., & Reed, M. (1996). Regulatory processes and the development of cognitive representations. *Development and Psychopathplogy, 8,* 215–234.

Derryberry, D., & Rothbart, M. K. (1997). Reactive and effortful processes in the organization of temperament. *Development and Psychopathplogy, 9,* 633–652.

Diamond, S. (1957). *Personality and temperament.* New York: Harper.

DiLalla, D. L., & Gottesman, I. I. (1995). Normal personality characteristics in identical twins discordant for schizophrenia. *Journal of Abnormal Psychology, 104,* 490–499.

Dinan, T. (1994). Glucocortoids and the genesis of depressive illness: A psychobiological model. *British Journal of Psychiatry, 164,* 365–371.

Dishion, T. J., Andrews, D. W., & Crosby, L. (1995). Antisocial boys and their friends in early adolescence: Relationship characteristics, quality, and interactional process. *Child Development, 66,* 139–151.

Dishion, T. J., French, D. C., & Patterson, G. R. (1995). The development and ecology of antisocial behavior. In D. Cicchetti & D. Cohen (Eds.), *Developmental psychopathology: Vol. 2. Risk disorder and adaptation* (pp. 421–471). New York: Wiley.

Dishion, T. J., Loeber, R., Stouthamer-Loeber, M., & Patterson, G. R. (1984). Skill deficits and male adolescent delinquency. *Journal of Abnormal Child Psychology, 12,* 37–54.

Doane, J. A., West, K. L., Goldstein, M. J., Rodnick, E. H., & Jones, J. E. (1981). Parental communication deviance and affective style: Predictors of subsequent schizophrenia spectrum disorders in vulnerable adolescents. *Archives of General Psychiatry, 38,* 679–685.

Dodge, K. A. (1993). Social-cognitive mechanisms in the development of conduct disorder and depression. *Annual Review of Psychology, 44,* 559–584.

Doering, S., Muller, E., Kopcke, W., Pietzcker, A., Gaebel, W., Linden, M., Muller, P., Muller-Spahn, F., Tegeler, J., & Schussler, G. (1998). Predictors of relapse and rehospitalization in schizophrenia and schizoaffective disorder. *Schizophrenia Bulletin, 24*(1), 87–98.

Dolan, R. J., Bench, C. J., Liddle, P. F., Friston, K. J., Frith, C. D., Grasby, P. M., & Frackowiak, R. S. J. (1993). Dorsolateral prefrontal cortex dysfunction in the major psychoses: Symptom or disease specificity? *Journal of Neurology, Neurosurgery and Psychiatry, 56,* 1290–1294.

Done, D. J., Crow, T. J., Johnstone, E. C., & Sacker, A. (1994). Childhood antecedents of schizophrenia and affective illness: Social adjustment at ages 7 and 11. *British Medical Journal, 309,* 699–703.

Donovan, W. L., & Leavitt, L. A. (1989). Maternal self-efficiency and infant attachment: Integrating physiology, perceptions and behavior. *Child Development, 60,* 460–472.

Downey, G., & Coyne, J. C. (1990). Children of depressed parents: An integrative review. *Psychological Bulletin, 108,* 50–76.

Dozier, M., & Kobak, R. R. (1992). Psychophysiology in attachment interviews: Converging evidence for deactivating strategies. *Child Development, 63,* 1473–1480.

Dwork, A. J. (1997). Postmortem studies of the hippocampal formation in schizophrenia. *Schizophrenia Bulletin, 23*(3), 385–402.

Dworkin, R. H., Green, S. R., Small, N. E., Warner, M. L., Cornblatt, B. A., & Erlenmeyer-Kimling, L. (1990). Positive and negative symptoms and social competence in adolescents at risk for schizophrenia and affective disorder. *American Journal of Psychiatry, 147,* 1234–1236.

Eagle, M. (1995). The developmental perspectives of attachment and psychoanalytic theory. In S. Goldberg, R. Muir, & J. Kerr (Eds.), *Attachment theory: Social, developmental, and clinical perspectives* (pp. 123–150). Hillsdale, NJ: Analytic Press.

Eaves, L. J., Silberg, J. L., Meyer, J. M., & Maes, H. H. (1997). Genetics and developmental psychopathology: 2. The main effects of genes and environment on behavioral problems in the Virginia Twin Study of Adolescent Behavioral Development. *Journal of Child Psychology and Psychiatry, 38,* 965–980.

Ebstein, R., Novick, O., Umansky, R., Priel, B., Osher, Y., Blaine, D., Bennett, E. R., Nemanov, L., Katz, M., & Belmaker, R. H. (1996). Dopamine D4 receptor (D4DR) exon III polymorphism associated with the human personality trait of novelty seeking. *Nature Genetics, 12,* 78–80.

Edelman, G. M. (1987). *Neural Darwinism: The theory of neuronal group selection.* New York: Basic Books.

Eggers, C., & Bunk, D. (1997). The long-term course of childhood-onset schizophrenia: A 42-year followup. *Schizophrenia Bulletin, 23*(1), 105–117.

Eisenberg, N., Fabes, R. A., Guthrie, I. K., Murphy, B. C., Maszk, P., Holmgren, R., & Suh, K. (1996). The relations of regulation and emotionality to problem behavior in elementary school children. *Development and Psychopathology, 8,* 141–162.

Eisenberg, N., Fabes, R. A., Nyman, M., Bernzweig, J., & Pinuelas, A. (1994). The relations of emotionality and regulation to children's anger-related reactions. *Child Development, 65,* 109–128.

Ekelund, J., Lichtermann, D., Jarvelin, M.-R., & Peltonen, L. (1999). Association between novelty seeking and the type 4 dopamine receptor gene in a large Finnish cohort sample. *American Journal of Psychiatry, 156,* 1453–1455.

Ekman, P., & Davidson, R. J. (Eds.). (1994). *The nature of emotion: Fundamental questions.* New York: Oxford University Press.

Eley, T. C., Deater-Deckard, K., Fombonne, E., Fulker, D. W., & Plomin, R. (1998). An adoption study of depressive symptoms in middle childhood. *Journal of Child Psychology and Psychiatry, 39,* 337–345.

Elkin, I., Shea, T., Watkins, J. T., Imber, S. D., Sotsky, S. M., & Collins, J. F. (1989). National Institute of Mental Health Treatment of Depression Collaborative Research Program: General effectiveness of treatments. *Archives of General Psychiatry, 46,* 971–982.

El-Sheikh, M., Cummings, E. M., & Goetsch, V. L. (1989). Coping with adults' angry behavior: Behavioral, physiological, and verbal responses in preschoolers. *Developmental Psychology, 25,* 490–498.

Emde, R. N. (1989). The infant's relationship experience: Developmental and affective aspects. In A. J. Sameroff & R. N. Emde (Eds.), *Relationship disturbances in early childhood: A developmental approach* (pp. 35–51). New York: Basic Books.

Erikson, D. H., Beiser, M., Iacono, W. G., Fleming, J. A. E., & Lin, T.-L. (1989). The role of social relationships in the course of first-episode schizophrenia and affective psychosis. *American Journal of Psychiatry, 146,* 1456–1461.

Erickson, M. F., Egeland, B., & Pianta, R. (1989). The effects of maltreatment on the development of young children. In D. Cicchetti & V. Carlson (Eds.), *Child maltreatment: Theory and research on the causes and consequences of child abuse and neglect* (pp. 647–684). New York: Cambridge University Press.

Erickson, M. F., Sroufe, L. A., & Egeland, B. (1985). The relationship between quality of attachment and behavior problems in a preschool high-risk sample. In I. Bretherton & E. Waters (Eds.), Growing points of attachment theory and research. *Monographs of the Society for Research in Child Development, 50*(1–2, Serial No. 209), 147–166.

Erlenmeyer-Kimling, L., & Cornblatt, B. (1987). High-risk research in schizophrenia: A summary of what has been learned. *Journal of Psychiatric Research, 21,* 404–411.

Erlenmeyer-Kimling, L., Cornblatt, B. A., Rock, D., Roberts, S., Bell, M., & West, A. (1993). The New York High-Risk Project: Anhedonia, attentional deviance, and psychopathology. *Schizophrenia Bulletin, 19,* 141–153.

Erlenmeyer-Kimling, L., Squires-Wheeler, E., Adamo, U. H., Bassett, A. S., Cornblatt, B. A., Kestenbaum, C. J., Rock, D., Roberts, S. A., & Gottesman, I. I. (1995). The New York High-Risk Project: Psychoses and cluster A personality disorders in offspring of schizophrenic parents at 23 years of follow-up. *Archives of General Psychiatry, 52,* 857–865.

Estrada, P., Arsenio, W. F., Hess, R. D., & Holloway, S. D. (1987). Affective quality of the mother–child relationship: Longitudinal consequences for children's school-relevant cognitive functioning. *Developmental Psychology, 23,* 210–215.

Eysenck, H. J. (1967). *The biological basis of personality.* Springfield, IL: Thomas.

Fabes, R. A., & Eisenberg, N. (1992). Young children's emotional arousal and anger/aggressive behaviors. In A. Fraczek & H. Zumkley (Eds.), *Socialization and aggression: Recent research in psychology* (pp. 85–101). New York: Springer-Verlag.

Fagot, B. I., & Leve, L. D. (1998). Teacher ratings of externalizing behavior at school entry for boys and girls: Similar early predictors and different correlates. *Journal of Child Psychology and Psychiatry, 39,* 555–566.

Fagot, B. I., & Pears, K. C. (1996). Changes in attachment during the third year: Consequences and predictions. *Development and Psychopathology, 8,* 325–344.

Fairbanks, L. A., & McGuire, M. T. (1993). Maternal protectiveness and response to the unfamiliar in vervet monkeys. *American Journal of Primatology, 30,* 119–129.

Fergusson, D. M., & Lynskey, M. T. (1997). Early reading difficulties and later conduct problems. *Journal of Child Psychology and Psychiatry, 38,* 899–907.

Fergusson, D. M., Lynskey, M. T., & Horwood, L. J. (1996). Origins of comorbidity between conduct and affective disorders. *Journal of the American Academy of Child and Adolescent Psychiatry, 35,* 451–460.

Feshbach, N. D. (1989). The construct of empathy and the phenomenon of physical maltreatment of children. In D. Cicchetti & V. Carlson (Eds.), *Child maltreatment: Theory and research on the causes and consequences of child abuse and neglect* (pp. 349–373). New York: Cambridge University Press.

Field, T. (1989). Maternal depression effects on infant interaction and attachment behavior. In D. Cicchetti (Ed.), *Rochester Symposium on Developmental Psychopathology: Vol. 1. The emergence of a discipline* (pp. 139–163). Hillsdale, NJ: Erlbaum.

Field, T. (1994). The effects of mother's physical and emotional unavailability on emotion regulation. In N. A. Fox (Ed.), The development of emotion regulation: Biological and behavioral considerations. *Monographs of the Society for Research in Child Development, 59*(2–3, Serial No. 240), 208–227.

Field, T. (1995). Infants of depressed mothers. *Infant Behavior and Development, 18,* 1–13.

Fish, B., Marcus, J., Hans, S. L., Auerbach, J. G., & Perdue, S. (1992). Infants at risk for schizophrenia: Sequelae of a genetic neurointegrative defect. A review and replication analysis of pandysmaturation in the Jerusalem Infant Development Study. *Archives of General Psychiatry, 49,* 221–235.

Foa, E. B., Riggs, D. S., & Gershuny, B. S. (1995). Arousal, numbing and intrusion: Symptom structure of PTSD following assault. *American Journal of Psychiatry, 152,* 116–120.

Fonagy, P., Steele, M., Steele, H., Leigh, T., Kennedy, R., Mattoon, G., & Target, M. (1995). Attachment, the reflective self, and borderline states: The predictive specificity of the Adult Attachment Interview and pathological emotional development. In S. Goldberg, R. Muir, & J. Kerr (Eds.), *Attachment theory: Social, developmental, and clinical perspectives* (pp. 233–278). Hillsdale, NJ: Analytic Press.

Fonagy, P., Target, M., Steele, M., Steele, H., Leigh, T., Levinson, A., & Kennedy, R. (1997). Morality, disruptive behavior, borderline personality disorder, crime, and their relationships to security of attachment. In L. Atkinson & K. J. Zucker (Eds.), *Attachment and psychopathology* (pp. 223–274). New York: Guilford Press.

Fox, N. A. (1994). Dynamic cerebral processes underlying emotion regulation. In N. A. Fox (Ed.), The development of emotion regulation: Biological and behavioral considerations. *Monographs of the Society for Research in Child Development, 59*(2–3, Serial No. 240), 152–166.

Fox, N. A., & Davidson, R. J. (1987). Electroencephalogram asymmetry in response to the approach of a stranger and maternal separation in 10-month-old infants. *Developmental Psychology, 23*, 233–240.

Fox, N. A., Schmidt, L. A., Calkins, S. D., Rubin, K. H., & Coplan, R. J. (1996). The role of frontal activation in the regulation and dysregulation of social behavior during the preschool years. *Development and Psychopathology, 8*, 89–102.

Frank, J. (1973). *Persuasion and healing* (rev. ed.). Baltimore: Johns Hopkins University Press.

Fremmer-Bombik, E., & Grossmann, K. E. (1993). Über die lebenslange Bedeutung früher Bindungserfahrungen [About the life-long meaning of early attachment experiences]. In H. G. Petzold (Ed.), *Frühe scheidigungen-späte Folgen?: Psychotherapie und babyforschung* (pp. 83–150). Band 1. Paderborn: Funfermann Verlag.

Frenkel, E., Kugelmass, S., Nathan, M., & Ingraham, L. J. (1995). Locus of control and mental health in adolescence and adulthood. *Schizophrenia Bulletin, 21*, 219–226.

Frijda, N. H. (1993). Moods, emotion episodes, and emotions. In M. Lewis & J. M. Haviland (Eds.), *Handbook of emotions* (pp. 381–403). New York: Guilford Press.

Frith, C. D. (1979). Consciousness, information processing and schizophrenia. *British Journal of Psychiatry, 134*, 225–235.

Frith, C. D., & Done, D. J. (1988). Towards a neuropsychology of schizophrenia. *British Journal of Psychiatry, 153*, 437–443.

Frodi, A., Bridges, L., & Shonk, S. (1989). Maternal correlates of infant temperament ratings and of infant–mother attachment: A longitudinal study. *Infant Mental Health Journal, 10*, 273–289.

Fullard, W., McDevitt, S. C., & Carey, W. B. (1978). *Toddler Temperament Scale*. Unpublished manuscript, Temple University.

Fuller, J. L., & Thompson, W. R. (1960). *Behavior genetics*. New York: Wiley.

Gable, S., & Isabella, R. A. (1992). Maternal contributions to infant regulation of arousal. *Infant Behavior and Development, 15*, 95–107.

Gannon, L., Banks, J., Shelton, D., & Luchetta, T. (1989). The mediating effects of psychophysiological reactivity and recovery on the relationship between environmental stress and illness. *Journal of Psychosomatic Research, 33*, 167–175.

Garcia-Coll, C., Kagan, J., & Reznick, J. S. (1984). Behavioral inhibition in young children. *Child Development, 55,* 1005–1019.

Garfield, S. L. (1992). Eclectic psychotherapy: A common factors approach. In J. C. Norcross & M. R. Goldfried (Eds.), *Handbook of psychotherapy integration* (pp. 169–201). New York: Basic Books.

Garvey, M., Noyes, R., Jr., Anderson, D., & Cook, B. (1991). Examination of comorbid anxiety in psychiatric inpatients. *Comprehensive Psychiatry, 32,* 277–282.

Ge, X., Best, K. M., Conger, R. D., & Simons, R. L. (1996). Parenting behaviors and the occurrence and co-occurrence of adolescent depressive symptoms and conduct problems. *Developmental Psychology, 32,* 717–731.

George, M. S., Ketter, T. A., Parekh, P. I., Horwitz, B., Herscovitch, P., & Post, R. M. (1995). Brain activity during transient sadness and happiness in healthy women. *American Journal of Psychiatry, 152,* 341–351.

Geracioti, T. D., Loosen, P. T., Ekhator, N. N., Schmidt, D., Chambliss, B., Baker, D. G., Kasckow, J. W., Richtand, N. M., Keck, P. E., & Ebert, M. H. (1997). Uncoupling of serotonergic and noradrenergic systems in depression: Preliminary evidence from continuous cerebrospinal fluid sampling. *Depression and Anxiety, 6,* 89–94.

Gersten, M. (1989). Behavioral inhibition in the classroom. In J. S. Reznick (Ed.), *Perspectives on behavioral inhibition* (pp. 71–91). Chicago: University of Chicago Press.

Gillberg, I. C., Gillberg, C., & Groth, J. (1989). Children with minor neurodevelopmental disorders: V. Neurodevelopmental profiles at age 13. *Developmental Medicine and Child Neurology, 31,* 14–24.

Giron, M., & Gomez-Beneyto, M. (1998). Relationship between empathic family attitude and relapse in schizophrenia: A 2-year followup prospective study. *Schizophrenia Bulletin, 24*(4), 619–627.

Gjone, H., & Stevenson, J. (1997). A longitudinal study of temperament and behavior problems: Common genetic or environmental influences? *Journal of the American Academy of Child and Adolescent Psychiatry, 36,* 1448–1456.

Gloor, P. (1986). Role of the human limbic system in perception, memory and affect: Lessons from temporal lobe epilepsy. In B. K. Doane & K. E. Livingston (Eds.), *The limbic system: Functional organization and clinical disorders* (pp. 159–169). New York: Raven Press.

Goldberg, S. (1996, February). *A tale of two stories: Temperament, attachment and affect regulation.* Paper presented at the GRIP Symposium on Emotion Regulation, Temperament and Attachment, University of Montréal.

Goldberg, S. (1997). Attachment and childhood behavior problems in normal, at-risk, and clinical samples. In L. Atkinson & K. J. Zucker (Eds.), *Attachment and psychopathology* (pp. 171–195). New York: Guilford Press.

Goldberg, S., MacKay-Soroka, S., & Rochester, M. (1994). Affect, attachment and maternal responsiveness. *Infant Behavior and Development, 17,* 335–339.

Goldberg, S., Muir, R., & Kerr, J. (Eds.). (1995). *Attachment theory: Social, developmental, and clinical perspectives.* Hillsdale, NJ: Analytic Press.

Goldman-Rakic, P. S., & Selemon, L. D. (1997). Functional and anatomical aspects of prefrontal pathology in schizophrenia. *Schizophrenia Bulletin, 23*(3), 437–458.

Goldsmith, H. H. (1994). Parsing the emotional domain from a developmental perspective. In P. Ekman & R. J. Davidson (Eds.), *The nature of emotion* (pp. 60–73). New York: Oxford University Press.

Goodyer, I. M., Ashby, L., Altham, P. M. E., Vize, C., & Cooper, P. J. (1993). Temperament and major depression in 11 to 16 year olds. *Journal of Child Psychology and Psychiatry, 34,* 1409–1423.

Goodyer, J. M., Herbert, J., Secher, S. M., & Pearson, J. (1997). Short-term outcome of major depression: I. Comorbidity and severity at presentation as predictors of persistent disorder. *Journal of the American Academy of Child and Adolescent Psychiatry, 36,* 179–187.

Gorman, J. M., Liebowitz, M. R., Fyer, A. J., & Stein, J. (1989). A neuroanatomical hypothesis for panic disorder. *American Journal of Psychiatry, 146,* 148–161.

Gorman-Smith, D., & Tolan, P. (1998). The role of exposure to community violence and developmental problems among inner city youth. *Development and Psychopathology, 10,* 101–116.

Gould, R. A., Buckminster, S., Pollack, M. H., Otto, M. W., & Yap, L. (1997). Cognitive-behavioral and pharmacological treatment for social phobia: A meta-analysis. *Clinical Psychology: Science and Practice, 4,* 291–306.

Graham, Y. P., Heim, C., Goodman, S. H., Miller, A. H., & Nemeroff, C. B. (1999). The effects of neonatal stress on brain development: Implications for psychopathology. *Development and Psychopathology, 11,* 545–565.

Gray, J. A. (1987). *The psychology of fear and stress* (2nd ed.). Cambridge, England: Cambridge University Press.

Gray, J. A. (1991). Neural systems, emotion and personality. In J. Madden IV (Ed.), *Neurobiology of learning and affect* (pp. 273–306). New York: Raven Press.

Graybiel, A. M. (1997). The basal ganglia and cognitive pattern generators. *Schizophrenia Bulletin, 23,* 459–469.

Greenberg, L. S., Rice, L. N., & Elliott, R. (1993). *Facilitating emotional change: The moment-by-moment process.* New York: Guilford Press.

Greenberg, M. T., DeKlyen, M., Speltz, M. L., & Endriga, M. C. (1997). The role of attachment processes in externalizing psychopathology in young children. In L. Atkinson & K. J. Zucker (Eds.), *Attachment and psychopathology* (pp. 196–222). New York: Guilford Press.

Greenberg, M. T., Kusche, C. A., & Speltz, M. (1992). Emotional regulation, self-control, and psychopathology: The role of relationships in early childhood. In D. Cicchetti & S. L. Toth (Eds.), *Rochester Symposium on Developmental Psychopathology: Vol. 2. Internalizing and externalizing expressions of dysfunction* (pp. 21–55). Hillsdale, NJ: Erlbaum.

Greenough, W. T., Black, J. E., & Wallace, C. S. (1987). Experience and brain development. *Child Development, 58,* 539–559.

Grillon, C., Courchesne, E., Ameli, R., Geyer, M. A., & Braff, D. L. (1990). Increased distractibility in schizophrenic patients: Electrophysiologic and behavioral evidence. *Archives of General Psychiatry, 47,* 171–179.

Grossmann, K. (1995). The evolution and history of attachment research and theory. In S. Goldberg, R. Muir, & J. Kerr (Eds.), *Attachment theory: Social, developmental, and clinical perspectives* (pp. 85–121). Hillsdale, NJ: Analytic Press.

Grossmann, K. E., Grossmann, K., & Schwann, A. (1986). Capturing the wider view of attachment: A reanalysis of Ainsworth's Strange Situation. In C. E. Izard & P. B. Read (Eds.), *Measuring emotions in infants and children* (pp. 124–171). New York: Cambridge University Press.

Gunnar, M. R. (1992). Reactivity of the hypothalamic–pituitary–adrenocortical system to stressors in normal infants and children. *Pediatrics, 90,* 491–497.

Gunnar, M. R., & Barr, R. G. (1998). Stress, early brain development, and behavior. *Infants and Young Children, 11,* 1–14.

Gunnar, M. R., Brodersen, L., Krueger, K., & Rigatuso, J. (1996). Dampening of adrenocortical responses during infancy: Normative changes and individual differences. *Child Development, 67,* 877–889.

Gunnar, M. R., Brodersen, L., Nachmias, M., Buss, K., & Rigatuso, J. (1996). Stress reactivity and attachment security. *Developmental Psychobiology, 29,* 191–204.

Gunnar, M., Mangelsdorf, S., Kestenbaum, R., Lang, S., Larson, M., & Andreas, D. (1989). Stress and coping in early development. In D. Cicchetti (Ed.), *Rochester Symposium on Developmental Psychopathology: Vol. 1. The emergence of a discipline* (pp. 119–138). Hillsdale, NJ: Erlbaum.

Haber, S. N., & Fudge, J. L. (1997). The interface between dopamine neurons and the amygdala: Implications for schizophrenia. *Schizophrenia Bulletin, 23,* 471–482.

Hammen, C. L. (1992). The family-environmental context of depression: A perspective on children's risk. In D. Cicchetti & S. L. Toth (Eds.), *Developmental perspectives on depression* (pp. 251–281). Rochester: University of Rochester Press.

Hammen, C. L., Burge, D., Daley, S. E., Davila, J., Paley, B., & Rudolph, K. D. (1995). Interpersonal attachment cognitions and prediction of symptomatic responses to interpersonal stress. *Journal of Abnormal Psychology, 104,* 436–443.

Hammen, C. L., Burge, D., & Stansbury, K. (1990). Relationship of mother and child variables to child outcomes in a high-risk sample: A causal modeling analysis. *Developmental Psychology, 26,* 24–30.

Hammen, C. L., & Goodman-Brown, T. (1990). Self-schemas and vulnerability to specific life stress in children at risk for depression. *Cognitive Research and Therapy, 14,* 215–227.

Hare, R. D. (1975). Electrodermal and cardiovascular correlates of psychopathy. In R. D. Hare & D. Schalling (Eds.), *Psychopathic behavior: Approaches to research* (pp. 107–144). New York: Wiley.

Harrington, R., Rutter, M., Weissman, M., Fudge, H., Groothues, C., Bredenkamp, D., Pickles, A., Rende, R., & Wickramaratne, P. (1997). Psychiatric disorders in the relatives of depressed probands: I. Comparison of prepubertal, adolescent and early adult onset cases. *Journal of Affective Disorders, 42,* 9–22.

Harris, J. C. (1995). *Developmental neuropsychiatry: Vol. 1. Fundamentals.* New York: Oxford University Press.

Harris, T., Brown, G. W., & Bifulco, A. (1987). Loss of parent in childhood and adult psychiatric disorder: The role of social class position and premarital pregnancy. *Psychological Medicine, 17,* 163–183.

Harter, S., & Whitesell, N. R. (1996). Multiple pathways to self-reported depression and psychological adjustment among adolescents. *Development and Psychopathology, 8,* 761–777.

Heard, H. L., & Linehan, M. M. (1993). Problems of self and borderline personality disorder: A dialectical behavioral analysis. In Z. V. Segal & S. J. Blatt (Eds.), *The self in emotional distress: Cognitive and psychodynamic perspectives* (pp. 301–325). New York: Guilford Press.

Heath, A. C., Cloninger, C. R., & Martin, N. G. (1994). Testing a model for the genetic structure of personality: A comparison of the personality systems of Cloninger and Eysenck. *Journal of Personality and Social Psychology, 66,* 762–775.

Heckers, S. (1997). Neuropathology of schizophrenia: Cortex, thalamus, basal ganglia, and neurotransmitter-specific projection systems. *Schizophrenia Bulletin, 23*(3), 403–421.

Henn, F. (1994, January). *Discussion.* Paper presented at the Seventh Biennial European Workshop on Schizophrenia. Les Diablerets, Switzerland.

Henning, K., Leitenberg, H., Coffey, P., Bennett, T., & Jankowski, M. K. (1997). Long-term psychological adjustment to witnessing interparental physical conflict during childhood. *Child Abuse and Neglect, 21,* 501–515.

Henriques, J. B., & Davidson, R. J. (1990). Regional brain electrical asymmetries discriminate between previously depressed and healthy control subjects. *Journal of Abnormal Psychology, 99,* 22–31.

Heuser, I., Bissette, G., Dettling, M., Schweiger, U., Gotthardt, U., Schmider, J., Lammers, C.-H., Nemeroff, C. B., & Holsboer, F. (1998). Cerebrospinal fluid concentrations of corticotrophin releasing hormone, vasopressin, and somatostatin in depressed patients and healthy controls: Response to amitriptyline treatment. *Depression and Anxiety, 8,* 71–79.

Hewitt, J. K., Silberg, J. L., Rutter, M., Simonoff, E., Meyer, J. M., Maes, H., Pickles, A., Neale, M. C., Loeber, R., Erickson, M. T., Kendler, K. S., Truett, K. R., & Eaves, L. J. (1997). Genetics and developmental psychopathology: 1. Phenotypic assessment in the Virginia Twin Study of Adolescent Behavioral Development. *Journal of Child Psychology and Psychiatry, 38,* 943–963.

Hibbs, E. D., Hamburger, S. D., Lenane, M., Rapoport, J. L., Kruesi, M. J. P., Keysor, C. S., & Goldstein, M. J. (1991). Determinants of expressed emotion in families of disturbed and normal children. *Journal of Child Psychology and Psychiatry, 32,* 757–770.

Hibbs, E. D., Zahn, T. P., Hamburger, S. D., Kruesi, M. J. P., & Rapoport, J. L. (1992). Parental expressed emotion and psychophysiological reactivity in disturbed and normal children. *British Journal of Psychiatry, 160,* 504–510.

Higley, J. D., & Suomi, J. S. (1989). Temperamental reactivity in non-human primates. In G. A. Kohnstamm, J. E. Bates, & M. K. Rothbart (Eds.), *Temperament in childhood* (pp. 153–167). Chichester, England: Wiley.

Hinshaw, S. P., & Melnick, S. A. (1995). Peer relationships in boys with attention-deficit hyperactivity disorder with and without comorbid aggression. *Development and Psychopathology, 7,* 627–647.

Hirshfeld, D. R., Biederman, J., Brody, L., Faraone, S. V., & Rosenbaum, J. F. (1997). Expressed emotion toward childen with behavioral inhibition: Associations with maternal anxiety disorder. *Journal of the American Academy of Child and Adolescent Psychiatry, 36,* 910–917.

Hirshfeld, D. R., Rosenbaum, J. F., Biederman, J., Bolduc, E. A., Faraone, S. V., & Snidman, N. (1992). Stable behavioral inhibition and its association with anxiety disorder. *Journal of the American Academy of Child and Adolescent Psychiatry, 31,* 103–111.

Hirschfeld, R. M. A., Klerman, G. L., Lavori, P., Keller, M. B., Griffith, P., & Coryell, W. (1989). Premorbid personality assessments of first onset of major depression. *Archives of General Psychiatry, 46,* 345–350.

Hoehn-Saric, R., & McLeod, D. R. (1993). Somatic manifestations of normal and pathological anxiety. In R. Hoehn-Saric & D. R. McLeod (Eds.), *Biology of anxiety disorders* (pp. 177–222). Washington, DC: American Psychiatric Press.

Hoehn-Saric, R., McLeod, D. R., & Hipsley, P. (1995). Is hyperarousal essential to obsessive–compulsive disorder?: Diminished physiologic flexibility, but not hyperarousal, characterizes patients with obsessive–compulsive disorder. *Archives of General Psychiatry, 52,* 688–693.

Hofer, M. A. (1987). Early social relationships: A psychobiologist's view. *Child Development, 58,* 633–647.

Hofer, M. (1995). Hidden regulators: Implications for a new understanding of attachment, separation, and loss. In S. Goldberg, R. Muir, & J. Kerr (Eds.), *Attachment theory: Social, developmental, and clinical perspectives* (pp. 203–231). Hillsdale, NJ: Analytic Press.

Hollis, C. (1995). Child and adolescent (juvenile onset) schizophrenia: A case study of premorbid developmental impairments. *British Journal of Psychiatry, 166,* 489–495.

Holmes, J. (1993). Attachment theory: A biological basis for psychotherapy? *British Journal of Psychiatry, 163,* 430–438.

Hooley, J. M., & Teasdale, J. D. (1989). Predictors of relapse in unipolar depressives: Expressed emotion, marital distress, and perceived criticism. *Journal of Abnormal Psychology, 98,* 229–235.

Horowitz, M., Fridhandler, B., & Stinson, C. (1992). Person schemas and emotions. In T. Shapiro & R. N. Emde (Eds.), *Affect: Psychoanalytic perspectives* (pp. 173–208). Madison, CT: International Universities Press.

Hudson, J. I., & Pope, H. G. (1990). Affective spectrum disorder: Does antidepressant response identify a family of disorders with a common pathophysiology? *American Journal of Psychiatry, 147,* 552–564.

Hultman, C. M., Öhman, A., Cnattingius, S., Wieselgren, I., & Lindstrom, L. H. (1997). Prenatal and neonatal risk factors for schizophrenia. *British Journal of Psychiatry, 170,* 128–133.

Huttenlocher, P. R. (1994). Synaptogenesis in human cerebral cortex. In G. Dawson & K. W. Fischer (Eds.), *Human behavior and the developing brain* (pp. 137–152). New York: Guilford Press.

Hyde, L. (1983) *The gift: Imagination and the erotic life of property.* New York: Random House

Hyman, S. E., & Nestler, E. J. (1996). Initiation and adaptation: A paradigm for understanding psychotropic drug action. *American Journal of Psychiatry, 153,* 151–162.

Ingram, R. E., Miranda, J., & Segal, Z. V. (1998). *Cognitive vulnerability to depression.* New York: Guilford Press.

Insel, T. R. (1997). A neurobiological basis of social attachment. *American Journal of Psychiatry, 154,* 726–735.

Izard, C. E. (1971). *The face of emotion.* New York: Appleton- Century-Crofts.

Izard, C. E., Haynes, O. M., Chisholm, G., & Baak, K. (1991). Emotional determinants of infant–mother attachment. *Child Development, 62,* 906–917.

Izard, C. E., Libero, D. Z., Putnam, P., & Haynes, O. M. (1993). Stability of emotion experiences and their relations to traits of personality. *Journal of Personality and Social Psychology, 64,* 847–860.

Jacobsen, L. K., & Rapoport, J. L. (1998). Research update. Childhood-onset schizophrenia: Implications of clinical and neurobiological research. *Journal of Child Psychology and Psychiatry, 39,* 101–113.

Jacobson, N. S., Dobson, K. S., Truax, P. A., Addis, M. E., Koerner, K., Gollan, J. K., Gortner, E., & Prince, S. E. (1996). A component analysis of cognitive-behavioral treatment for depression. *Journal of Consulting and Clinical Psychology, 64,* 295–304.

Jacobvitz, D., & Sroufe, L. A. (1987). The early caregiver–child relationship and attention-deficit disorder with hyperactivity in kindergarten: A prospective study. *Child Development, 58,* 1496–1504.

Javitt, D. C., Doneshka, P., Grochowski, S., & Ritter, W. (1995). Impaired mismatch negativity generation reflects widespread dysfunction of working memory in schizophrenia. *Archives of General Psychiatry, 52,* 550–558.

Johnson, E. O., Kamilaris, T. C., Chrousos, G. P., & Gold, P. W. (1992). Mechanisms of stress: A dynamic overview of hormonal and behavioral homeostasis. *Neuroscience and Biobehavioral Reviews, 16,* 115–130.

Johnston, M. V., & Singer, H. S. (1982). Brain neurotransmitters and neuromodulators in pediatrics. *Pediatrics, 70,* 57–68.

Johnstone, E. C., MacMillan, J. F., Frith, C. D., Benn, D. K., & Crow, T. J. (1990). Further investigation of the predictors of outcome following first schizophrenic episodes. *British Journal of Psychiatry, 157,* 182–189.

Jones, E. G. (1997). Cortical development and thalamic pathology in schizophrenia. *Schizophrenia Bulletin, 23,* 483–501.

Jones, N. A., Field, T., Fox, N., Lindy, B., & Davalos, M. (1997). EEG activation in 1-month-old infants of depressed mothers. *Development and Psychopathology, 9,* 491–505.

Kafka, P. M. (1997). A monoamine hypothesis for the pathophysiology of paraphilic disorders. *Archives of Sexual Behavior, 26,* 343–358.

Kagan, J. (1989). The concept of behavioral inhibition to the unfamiliar. In J. S.

Reznick (Ed.), *Perspectives on behavioral inhibition* (pp. 1–23). Chicago: University of Chicago Press.

Kagan, J. (1994). Of the nature of emotion. In N. A. Fox (Ed.), The development of emotion regulation: Biological and behavioral considerations. *Monographs of the Society for Research in Child Development, 59*(2–3, Serial No. 240), 7–24.

Kagan, J., Kearsley, R., & Zelazo, P. (1978). *Infancy: Its place in human development.* Cambridge, MA: Harvard University Press.

Kagan, J., & Moss, H. A. (1962). *Birth to maturity.* New York: Wiley.

Kagan, J., Reznick, J. S., Clarke, C., Snidman, N., & Garcia-Coll, C. (1984). Behavioral inhibition to the unfamiliar. *Child Development, 55,* 2212–2225.

Kagan, J., Reznick, J. S., & Gibbons, J. (1989). Inhibited and uninhibited types of children. *Child Development, 60,* 838–845.

Kagan, J., Reznick, J. S., & Snidman, N. (1987). The physiology and psychology of behavioral inhibition in children. *Child Development, 58,* 1459–1473.

Kagan, J., Reznick, J. S., Snidman, N., Gibbons, J., & Johnson, M. O. (1988). Childhood derivatives of inhibition and lack of inhibition to the unfamiliar. *Child Development, 59,* 1580–1589.

Kagan, J., Snidman, N., & Arcus, D. M. (1992). Initial reactions to unfamiliarity. *Current Directions in Psychological Science, 1*(6), 171–174.

Kagan, J., Snidman, N., Zentner, M., & Peterson, E. (1999). Infant temperament and anxious symptoms in schoolage children. *Development and Psychopathology, 11,* 209–224.

Kaneko, W. M., Riley, E. P., & Ehlers, C. L. (1993). Electrophysiological and behavioral findings in rats prenatally exposed to alcohol. *Alcohol, 10,* 169–178.

Kaneko, W. M., Riley, E. P., & Ehlers, C. L. (1994). Behavioral and electrophysiological effects of early repeated maternal separation. *Depression, 2,* 43–53.

Kaneko, W. M., Riley, E. P., & Ehlers, C. L. (1996–1997). Effects of artificial rearing on electrophysiology and behavior in adult rats. *Depression and Anxiety, 4,* 279–288.

Karen, R. (1990, February). Becoming attached. *Atlantic Monthly,* pp. 35–70.

Kaufman, J., & Zigler, E. (1989). The intergenerational transmission of child abuse. In D. Cicchetti & V. Carlson (Eds.), *Child maltreatment: Theory and research on the causes and consequences of child abuse and neglect* (pp. 129–150). New York: Cambridge University Press.

Kavanagh, D. J. (1992). Recent developments in expressed emotion and schizophrenia. *British Journal of Psychiatry, 160,* 601–620.

Kazdin, A. E. (1997). Practitioner review: Psychosocial treatments for conduct disorder in children. *Journal of Child Psychology and Psychiatry, 38,* 161–178.

Keenan, K., Loeber, R., Zhang, Q., Stouthamer-Loeber, M., & Van Kammen, W. B. (1995). The influence of deviant peers on the development of boys' disruptive and delinquent behavior: A temporal analysis. *Development and Psychopathology, 7,* 715–726.

Kelvin, R. G., Goodyer, I. M., & Altham, P. M. E. (1996). Temperament and psychopathology amongst siblings of probands with depressive and anxiety disorders. *Journal of Child Psychology and Psychiatry, 37,* 543–550.

Kendell, R. E., Juszczak, E., & Cole, S. K. (1996). Obstetric complications and schizophrenia: A case control study based on standardised obstetric records. *British Journal of Psychiatry, 168,* 556–561.

Kendler, K. S., Heath, A. C., Martin, N. G., & Eaves, L. J. (1987). Symptoms of anxiety and symptoms of depression: Same genes, different environments? *Archives of General Psychiatry, 44,* 451–457.

Kendler, K. S., Kessler, R. C., Heath, A. C., Neale, M. C., & Eaves, L. J. (1991). Coping: A genetic epidemiological investigation. *Psychological Medicine, 21,* 337–346.

Kendler, K. S., Kessler, R. C., Neale, M. C., Heath, A. C., & Eaves, L. J. (1993). The prediction of major depression in women: Toward an integrated etiologic model. *American Journal of Psychiatry, 150,* 1139–1148.

Kendler, K. S., Kessler, R. C., Walters, E. E., MacLean, C., Neale, M. C., Heath, A. C., & Eaves, L. (1995). Stressful life events, genetic liability, and onset of an episode of major depression in women. *American Journal of Psychiatry, 152,* 833–842.

Kendler, K. S., McGuire, M., Gruenberg, A. M., & Walsh, D. (1995). Schizotypal symptoms and signs in the Roscommon Family Study: Their factor structure and familial relationship with psychotic and affective disorders. *Archives of General Psychiatry, 52,* 296–303.

Kendler, K. S., Neale, M. C., Kessler, R. C., Heath, A. C., & Eaves, L. J. (1992a). Major depression and generalized anxiety disorder: Same genes, partly different environments? *Archives of General Psychiatry, 49,* 716–722.

Kendler, K. S., Neale, M. C., Kessler, R. C., Heath, A. C., & Eaves, L. J. (1992b). The genetic epidemiology of phobias in women: The interrelationship of agoraphobia, social phobia, situational phobia, and simple phobia. *Archives of General Psychiatry, 49,* 273–281.

Kendler, K. S., Neale, M. C., Kessler, R. C., Heath, A. C., & Eaves, L. J. (1992c). Childhood parental loss and adult psychopathology in women: A twin study perspective. *Archives of General Psychiatry, 49,* 109–116.

Kendler, K. S., Neale, M. C., Kessler, R. C., Heath, A. C., & Eaves, L. J. (1993). A longitudinal twin study of personality and major depression in women. *Archives of General Psychiatry, 50,* 853–862.

Kendler, K. S., Ochs, A. L., Gorman, A. M., Hewitt, J. K., Ross, D. E., & Mirsky, A. F. (1991). The structure of schizotypy: A pilot multitrait twin study. *Psychiatry Research, 36,* 19–36.

Kendler, K. S., Thacker, L., & Walsh, D. (1996). Self-report measures of schizotypy as indices of familial vulnerability to schizophrenia. *Schizophrenia Bulletin, 22*(3), 511–520.

Kendler, K. S., & Walsh, D. (1995). Schizophreniform disorder, delusional disorder and psychotic disorder not otherwise specified: Clinical features, outcome and familial psychopathology. *Acta Psychiatrica Scandinavica, 91,* 370–378.

Kendler, K. S., Walters, E. E., Neale, M. C., Kessler, R. C., Heath, A. C., & Eaves, L. J. (1995). The structure of the genetic and environmental risk factors for six major psychiatric disorders in women: Phobia, generalized anxiety disorder, panic disorder, bulimia, major depression, and alcoholism. *Archives of General Psychiatry, 52,* 374–383.

Kendziora, K. T., & O'Leary, S. G. (1993). Dysfunctional parenting as a focus for prevention and treatment of child behavior problems. In R. H. Ollendick & R. J. Prinz (Eds.), *Advances in clinical psychology* (Vol. 15, pp. 175–206). New York: Plenum Press.

Kennedy, S. H., Javanmard, M., & Vaccarino, F. J. (1997). A review of functional neuroimaging in mood disorders: Positron emission tomography and depression. *Canadian Journal of Psychiatry, 42,* 467–475.

Kerr, M., Tremblay, R. E., Pagani, L., & Vitaro, F. (1997). Boys' behavioral inhibition and the risk of later delinquency. *Archives of General Psychiatry, 54,* 809–816.

Kessler, R. C., Davis, C. G., & Kendler, K. S. (1997). Childhood adversity and adult psychiatric disorder in the U.S. National Comorbidity Survey. *Psychological Medicine, 27,* 1101–1119.

Kessler, R. C., & Walters, E. E. (1998). Epidemiology of DSM-III-R major depression and minor depression among adolescents and young adults in the National Comorbidity Survey. *Depression and Anxiety, 7,* 3–14.

Ketter, T. A., George, M. S., Kimbrell, T. A., Benson, E., & Post, R. M. (1996). Functional brain imaging, limbic function, and affective disorders. *The Neuroscientist, 2,* 55–65.

Kingston, L., & Prior, M. (1995). The development of patterns of stable, transient, and school-age onset aggressive behavior in young children. *Journal of the American Academy of Child and Adolescent Psychiatry, 34,* 348–358.

Kinney, D. K., Levy, D. L., Yurgelun-Todd, D. A., Tramer, S. J., & Holzman, P. S. (1998). Inverse relationship of perinatal complications and eye tracking dysfunction in relatives of patients with schizophrenia: Evidence for a two-factor model. *American Journal of Psychiatry, 155,* 976–978.

Kiraly, S. J., Ancill, R. J., & Dimitrova, G. (1997). The relationship of endogenous cortisol to psychiatric disorder: A review. *Canadian Journal of Psychiatry, 42,* 415–420.

Knoll, J. L., IV, Garver, D. L., Ramberg, J. E., Kingsbury, S. J., Croissant, D., & McDermott, B. (1998). Heterogeneity of the psychoses: Is there a neurodegenerative psychosis? *Schizophrenia Bulletin, 24*(3), 365–379.

Knutson, B., Wolkowitz, W. M., Cole, S. W., Chan, T., Moore, E. A., Johnson, R. C., Terpstra, J., Turner, R. A., & Reus, V. I. (1998). Selective alteration of personality and social behavior by serotonergic intervention. *American Journal of Psychiatry, 155,* 373–379.

Kobak, R. R., & Sceery, A. (1988). Attachment in late adolescence: Working models, affect regulation, and representations of self and others. *Child Development, 59,* 135–146.

Kolb, L. C. (1987). A neuropsychological hypothesis explaining posttraumatic stress disorders. *American Journal of Psychiatry, 144,* 989–995.

Kopp, C. B. (1989). Regulation of distress and negative emotions: A developmental view. *Developmental Psychology, 25,* 343–354.

Koreen, A. R., Siris, S. G., Chakos, M., Alvir, J., Mayerhoff, D., & Lieberman, J. (1993). Depression in first-episode schizophrenia. *American Journal of Psychiatry, 150,* 1643–1648.

Kovacs, M., & Devlin, B. (1998). Internalizing disorders in childhood. *Journal of Child Psychology and Psychiatry, 39,* 47–63.

Kraemer, G. W. (1992). A psychobiological theory of attachment. *Behavioral and Brain Sciences, 15,* 493–541.

Kraemer, G. W., Ebert, M. H., Schmidt, D. E., & McKinney, W. T. (1989). A longitudinal study of the effect of different social rearing conditions on cerebrospinal fluid norepinephrine and biogenic amine metabolites in rhesus monkeys. *Neuropsychopharmocology, 2,* 175–189.

Krueger, R. F., Caspi, A., Moffitt, T. E., Silva, P. A., & McGee, R. (1996). Personality traits are differentially linked to mental disorders: A multitrait–multidiagnosis study of an adolescent birth cohort. *Journal of Abnormal Psychology, 105,* 299–312.

Kugelmass, S., Faber, N., Ingraham, L. J., Frenkel, E., Nathan, M., Mirsky, A. F., & Shakhar, G. B. (1995). Reanalysis of SCOR and anxiety measures in the Israeli High-Risk Study. *Schizophrenia Bulletin, 21,* 205–217.

Kung, L., Conley, R., Chute, D. J., Smialek, J., & Roberts, R. C. (1998). Synaptic changes in the striatum of schizophrenic cases: A controlled postmortem ultrastructural study. *Synapse, 28,* 125–139.

LaGasse, L. L., Gruber, C. P., & Lipsitt, L. P. (1989). The infantile expression of avidity in relation to later assessments of inhibition and attachment. In J. S. Reznick (Ed.), *Perspectives on behavioral inhibition* (pp. 159–176). Chicago: University of Chicago Press.

Lambert, M. J. (1992). Psychotherapy outcome research: Implications for integrative and eclectic therapists. In J. C. Norcross & M. R. Goldfried (Eds.), *Handbook of psychotherapy integration* (pp. 94–129). New York: Basic Books.

Last, C. G., Hersen, M., Kazdin, A. E., Francis, G., & Grubb, H. J. (1987). Psychiatric illness in the mothers of anxious children. *American Journal of Psychiatry, 144,* 1580–1583.

Lazarus, R. S., & Folkman, S. (1984). *Stress, appraisal and coping.* New York: Springer.

LeDoux, J. E. (1992). Emotion as memory: Anatomical systems underlying indelible neural traces. In S. Christianson (Ed.), *The handbook of emotion and memory: Research and theory* (pp. 269–288). Hillsdale, NJ: Erlbaum.

LeDoux, J. E. (1993). Emotional networks in the brain. In M. Lewis & J. M. Haviland (Eds.), *Handbook of emotions* (pp. 109–118). New York: Guilford Press.

LeDoux, J. (1996). *The emotional brain.* New York: Simon & Schuster.

Lencz, T., Raine, A., Scerbo, A., Redmon, M., Brodish, S., Holt, L., & Bird, L. (1993). Impaired eye tracking in undergraduates with schizotypal personality disorder. *American Journal of Psychiatry, 150,* 152–154.

Lenzenweger, M. F., Dworkin, R. H., & Wethington, E. (1991). Examining the underlying structure of schizophrenic phenomenology: Evidence for a three-process model. *Schizophrenia Bulletin, 17*(3), 515–524.

Levenson, M. R., Aldwin, C. M., Bosse, R., & Spiro, A., III. (1988). Emotionality and mental health: Longitudinal findings from the normative aging study. *Journal of Abnormal Psychology, 97,* 94–96.

Levy, D. L., Holzman, P. S., Matthysse, S., & Mendell, N. R. (1993). Eye tracking dysfunction and schizophrenia: A critical perspective. *Schizophrenia Bulletin, 19,* 461–536.

Lewinsohn, P. M., Hoberman, H. M., & Rosenbaum, M. (1988). A prospective study of risk factors for unipolar depression. *Journal of Abnormal Psychology, 97,* 251–264.

Lewinsohn, P. M., Roberts, R. E., Rohde, P., Seeley, J. R., Gotlib, I. H., & Hops, H. (1994). Adolescent psychopathology: II. Psychosocial risk factors for depression. *Journal of Abnormal Psychology, 103,* 302–315.

Liddle, P. F., Friston, K. J., Frith, C. D., Hirsch, S. R., Jones, T., & Frackowiak, R. S. J. (1992). Patterns of cerebral blood flow in schizophrenia. *British Journal of Psychiatry, 160,* 179–186.

Lilenfeld, L., Kaye, W., & Strober, M. (1997). Genetics and family studies of anorexia nervosa and bulimia nervosa. *Balliere's Clinical Psychiatry: Eating Disorders, 3*(2), 177–199.

Linszen, D. H., Dingemans, P. M., Nugter, M. A., Van der Does, A. J. W., Scholte, W. F., & Lenior, M. A. (1997). Patient attributes and expressed emotion as risk factors for psychotic relapse. *Schizophrenia Bulletin, 23,* 119–130.

Liotti, G. (1995). Disorganized/disoriented attachment in the psychotherapy of the dissociative disorders. In S. Goldberg, R. Muir, & J. Kerr (Eds.), *Attachment theory: Social, developmental, and clinical perspectives* (pp. 343–363). Hillsdale, NJ: Analytic Press.

Loeber, R. (1991). Antisocial behavior: More enduring than changeable? *Journal of the American Academy of Child and Adolescent Psychiatry, 30,* 393–397.

Lyons, M. J., Eisen, S. A., Goldberg, J., True, W., Lin, N., Meyer, J. M., Toomey, R., Faraone, S., Merla-Ramos, M., & Tsuang, M. (1998). A registry-based twin study of depression in men. *Archives of General Psychiatry, 55,* 468–472.

Lyons, M. J., True, W. R., Eisen, S. A., Goldberg, J., Meyer, J. M., Farone, S. V., Eaves, L. J., & Tsuang, M. T. (1995). Differential heritability of adult and juvenile antisocial traits. *Archives of General Psychiatry, 52,* 906–915.

Lyons-Ruth, K. (1992). Maternal depressive symptoms, disorganized infant–mother attachment relationships and hostile–aggressive behavior in the preschool classroom: A prospective longitudinal view from infancy to age five. In D. Cicchetti & S. L. Toth (Eds.), *Developmental perspectives on depression* (pp. 131–171). Rochester, NY: University of Rochester Press.

Maccari, S., Piazza, P. V., Kabbaj, M., Barbazanges, A., Simon, H., & Le Moal, M. (1995). Adoption reverses the long-term impairment in glucocorticoid feedback induced by prenatal stress. *Journal of Neuroscience, 15,* 110–116.

MacLean, P. D. (1993). Cerebral evolution of emotion. In M. Lewis & J. M. Haviland (Eds.), *Handbook of emotions* (pp. 67–83). New York: Guilford Press.

Magai, C., & McFadden, S. (1995). *The role of emotions in social and personality development: History, theory, and research.* New York: Plenum Press.

Maher, B. A. (1996). Cognitive psychopathology in schizophrenia: Explorations in language, memory, associations, and movements. In S. Matthysse, D. L. Levy, J. Kagan, & F. M. Benes (Eds.), *Psychopathology: The evolving science of mental disorder* (pp. 433–454). New York: Cambridge University Press.

Maier, S. F., & Seligman, M. E. (1976). Learned helplessness: Theory and evidence. *Journal of Experimental Psychology, 105,* 3–46.

Main, M. (1995). Recent studies in attachment: Overview, with selected implications for clinical work. In S. Goldberg, R. Muir, & J. Kerr (Eds.), *Attachment theory: Social, developmental, and clinical perspectives* (pp. 407–474). Hillsdale, NJ: Analytic Press.

Main, M., & Goldwyn, R. (1984). Predicting rejection of her infant from mother's representation of her own experience: Implications for the abused–abusing intergenerational cycle. *International Journal of Child Abuse and Neglect, 8,* 203–217.

Main, M., Kaplan, N., & Cassidy, J. (1985). Security in infancy, childhood and adulthood: A move to the level of representation. In I. Bretherton & E. Waters (Eds.), Growing points of attachment theory and research. *Monographs of the Society for Research in Child Development, 50*(1–2, Serial No. 209), 66–104.

Main, M., & Solomon, J. (1990). Procedures for identifying infants as disorganized/disoriented during the Ainsworth Strange Situation. In M. T. Greenberg, D. Cicchetti, & E. M. Cummings (Eds.), *Attachment in the preschool years: Theory, research, and intervention* (pp. 121–160). Chicago: University of Chicago Press.

Malcarne, V. L., & Ingram, R. E. (1994). Cognition and negative affectivity. In R. H. Ollendick & R. J. Prinz (Eds.), *Advances in clinical child psychology* (Vol. 16, pp. 141–176). New York: Plenum Press.

Malloy, P., Bihrle, A., Duffy, J., & Cimino, C. (1993). The orbitomedial frontal syndrome. *Archives of Clinical Neuropsychology, 8,* 185–201.

Manassis, K., & Bradley, S. J. (1994). The development of childhood anxiety disorders: Toward an integrated model. *Journal of Applied Developmental Psychology, 15,* 345–366.

Manassis, K., Bradley, S. J., Goldberg, S., Hood, J., & Swinson, R. P. (1994). Attachment in mothers with anxiety disorders and their children. *Journal of the American Academy of Child and Adolescent Psychiatry, 33,* 1106–1113.

Mandal, M. K., Pandey, R., & Prasad, A. B. (1998). Facial expressions of emotions and schizophrenia: A review. *Schizophrenia Bulletin, 24*(1), 399–412.

Marcus, J., Hans, S. L., Auerbach, J. G., & Auerbach, A. G. (1993). Children at risk for schizophrenia: The Jerusalem Infant Development Study. II. Neurobehavioral deficits at school age. *Archives of General Psychiatry, 50,* 797–809.

Mathijssen, J. J. J. P., Koot, H. M., Verhulst, F. C., De Bruyn, E. E. J., & Oud, J. H. L. (1998). The relationship between mutual family relations and child psychopathology. *Journal of Child Psychology and Psychiatry, 39,* 477–487.

Max, J. E., Robin, D. A., Lindgren, S. D., Smith, W. J., Sato, Y., Mattheis, P. J., Stierwalt, J. A. G., & Castillo, C. S. (1997). Traumatic brain injury in children and adolescents: Psychiatric disorders at two years. *Journal of the American Academy of Child and Adolescent Psychiatry, 36,* 1278–1285.

Max, J. E., Smith, W. L., Sato, Y., Mattheis, P. J., Castillo, C. S., Lindgren, S. D., Robin, D. A., & Stierwalt, J. A. G. (1997). Traumatic brain injury in children and adolescents: Psychiatric disorders in the first three months. *Journal of the American Academy of Child and Adolescent Psychiatry, 36,* 94–102.

Mayberg, H. S., Liotti, M., Brannan, S. K., McGinnis, S., Mahurin, R. K., Jerabek, P. A., Silva, J. A., Tekell, J. L., Martin, C. C., Lancaster, J. L., & Fox, P. T. (1999). Reciprocal limbic–cortical function and negative mood: Converging

PET findings in depression and normal sadness. *American Journal of Psychiatry, 156,* 675–682.

McBurnett, K. (1992). Psychobiological approaches to personality and their applications to child psychopathology. In B. B. Lahey & A. E. Kazdin (Eds.), *Advances in clinical child psychology* (Vol. 14, pp. 107–164). New York: Plenum Press.

McCreadie, R. G., Williamson, D. J., Athawes, R. W. B., Connolly, M. A., & Tilak-Singh, D. (1994). The Nithsdale Schizophrenia Surveys: XIII. Parental rearing patterns, current symptomatology and relatives' expressed emotion. *British Journal of Psychiatry, 165,* 347–352.

McFarlane, A. C., & Yehuda, R. (1996). Resilience, vulnerability, and the course of posttraumatic reactions. In B. A. van der Kolk, A. C. McFarlane, & L. Weisaeth (Eds.), *Traumatic stress: The effects of overwhelming experience on mind, body, and society* (pp. 155–181). New York: Guilford Press.

McGaugh, J. L. (1992). Affect, neuromodulatory systems, and memory storage. In S. Christianson (Ed.), *The handbook of emotion and memory: Research and theory* (pp. 245–268). Hillsdale, NJ: Erlbaum.

McGlashan, T. H., & Fenton, W. S. (1992). The positive–negative distinction in schizophrenia: Review of natural history validators. *Archives of General Psychiatry, 49,* 63–72.

McGowan, S., Eastwood, S. L., Mead, A., Burnet, P. W. J., Smith, C., Flanigan,T. P., & Harrison, P. J. (1996). Hippocampal and cortical G protein (Gs alpha, Go alpha and Gi2 alpha) mRNA expression after electroconvulsive shock or lithium carbonate treatment. *European Journal of Pharmacology, 306,* 249–255.

McGuire, M. T., Raleigh, M. J., & Pollack, D. B. (1994). Personality features in vervet monkeys: The effects of sex, age, social status and group composition. *American Journal of Primatology, 33,* 1–13.

McGuire, P. K., Bench, C. J., Frith, C. D., Marks, I. M., Frackowiak, R. S. J., & Dolan, R. J. (1994). Functional anatomy of obsessive–compulsive phenomena. *British Journal of Psychiatry, 164,* 459–468.

Meaney, M. J., Diorio, J., Francis, D., Widdowson, J., LaPlante, P., Caldji, C., Sharma, S., Seckl, J. R., & Plotsky, P. M. (1996). Early environmental regulation of forebrain glucocorticoid receptor gene expression: Implications for adrenocorticalresponse to stress. *Developmental Neuroscience, 18,* 49–72.

Mednick, S. A., Parnas, J., & Schulsinger, F. (1987). The Copenhagen High Risk Project 1962–86. *Schizophrenia Bulletin, 13,* 485–495.

Meichenbaum, D. (1977). *Cognitive-behavior modification: An integrative approach.* New York: Plenum Press.

Messer, S. B., & Warren, C. S. (1995). *Models of brief psychodynamic therapy: A comparative approach.* New York: Guilford Press.

Messer, S. C., & Gross, A. M. (1995). Childhood depression and family interaction: A naturalistic observation study. *Journal of Clinical Child Psychology, 24,* 77–88.

Mesulam, M. M. (1985). *Principles of behavioral neurology.* Philadelphia: Davis.

Mezzacappa, E., Tremblay, R. E., Kindlon, D., Saul, J. P., Arseneault, L., Seguin, J., Pihl, R. O., & Earls, F. (1997). Anxiety, antisocial behavior, and heart rate regulation in adolescent males. *Journal of Child Psychology and Psychiatry, 38,* 457–469.

Miller, B. L., Darby, A., Benson, D. F., Cummings, J. L., & Miller, M. H. (1997). Aggressive, socially disruptive and antisocial behaviour associated with fronto-temporal dementia. *British Journal of Psychiatry, 170,* 150–155.

Mirsky, A. F. (1996). Familial factors in the impairment of attention in schizophrenia: Data from Ireland, Israel, and the District of Columbia. In S. Matthysse, D. L. Levy, J. Kagan, & F. M. Benes (Eds.), *Psychopathology: The evolving science of mental disorder* (pp. 364–406). New York: Cambridge University Press.

Mirsky, A. F., Ingraham, L. J., & Kugelmass, S. (1995). Neuropsychological assessment of attention and its pathology in the Israeli cohort. *Schizophrenia Bulletin, 21,* 193–204.

Mirsky, A. F., Kugelmass, S., Ingraham, L. J., Frenkel, E., & Nathan, M. (1995). Overview and summary: Twenty-five-year followup of high-risk children. *Schizophrenia Bulletin, 21,* 227–239.

Moffitt, T. E. (1993). The neuropsychology of conduct disorder. *Development and Psychopathology, 5,* 135–151.

Moffitt, T. E., Caspi, A., Dickson, N., Silva, P., & Stanton, W. (1996). Childhood-onset versus adolescent-onset antisocial conduct problems in males: Natural history from ages 3 to 18 years. *Development and Psychopathology, 8,* 399–424.

Monck, E., Graham, P., Richman, N., & Dobbs, R. (1994). Adolescent girls: II. Background factors in anxiety and depressive states. *British Journal of Psychiatry, 165,* 770–780.

Morgan, C. A., III, Grillon, C., Southwick, S. M., David, M., & Charney, D. S. (1996). Exaggerated acoustic startle reflex in Gulf war veterans with post-traumatic stress disorder. *American Journal of Psychiatry, 153,* 64–68.

Morice, R., & Delahunty, A. (1996). Frontal/executive impairments in schizophrenia. *Schizophrenia Bulletin, 22,* 125–137.

Moss, E., Rousseau, D., Parent, S., St.-Laurent, D., & Saintonge, J. (1998). Correlates of attachment at school age: Maternal reported stress, mother–child interaction, and behavior problems. *Child Development, 69,* 1390–1405.

Mueller, E., & Silverman, N. (1989). Peer relations in maltreated children. In D. Cicchetti & V. Carlson (Eds.), *Child maltreatment: Theory and research on the causes and consequences of child abuse and neglect* (pp. 529–578). New York: Cambridge University Press.

Murray, D., Cox, J. L., Chapman, G., & Jones, P. (1995). Childbirth: Life event or start of a long- term difficulty?: Further data from the Stoke-on-Trent Controlled Study of Postnatal Depression. *British Journal of Psychiatry, 166,* 595–600.

Nachmias, M., Gunnar, M., Mangelsdorf, S., Parritz, R. H., & Buss, K. (1996). Behavioral inhibition and stress reactivity: The moderating role of attachment security. *Child Development, 67,* 508–522.

Nelson, E. B., Sax, K. W., & Strakowski, S. M. (1998). Attentional performance in patients with psychotic and nonpsychotic major depression and schizophrenia. *American Journal of Psychiatry, 155,* 137–139.

Nelson, J. C., & Davis, J. M. (1997). DST studies in psychotic depression: A meta-analysis. *American Journal of Psychiatry, 154,* 1497–1503.

Nestor, P. G., Akdag, S. J., O'Donnell, B. F., Niznikiewicz, M., Law, S., Shenton, M. E., & McCarley, R. W. (1998). Word recall in schizophrenia: A connectionist model. *American Journal of Psychiatry, 155,* 1685–1690.

Neumann, C. S., & Walker, E. F. (1996). Childhood neuromotor soft signs, behavior problems, and adult psychopathology. In R. H. Ollendick & R. J. Prinz (Eds.), *Advances in clinical child psychology* (Vol. 18, pp. 173–203). New York: Plenum Press.

Newman, J. P., & Wallace, J. F. (1993). Diverse pathways to deficient self-regulation: Implications for disinhibitory psychopathology in children. *Clinical Psychology Review, 13,* 699–720.

Norman, R. M. G., Malla, A. K., Cortese, L., & Diaz, F. (1998). Aspects of dysphoria and symptoms of schizophrenia. *Psychological Medicine, 28,* 1433–1441.

Norman, R. M. G., Malla, A. K., Morrison-Stewart, S. L., Helmes, E., Williamson, P. C., Thomas, J., & Cortese, L. (1997). Neuropsychological correlates of syndromes in schizophrenia. *British Journal of Psychiatry, 170,* 134–139.

Nuechterlein, K. H., Snyder, K. S., & Mintz, J. (1992). Paths to relapse: Possible transactional processes connecting patient illness onset, expressed emotion, and psychotic relapse. *British Journal of Psychiatry, 161,* 88–96.

O'Brien, J. T. (1997). The 'glucocorticoid cascade' hypothesis: Prolonged stress may cause permanent brain damage. *British Journal of Psychiatry, 170,* 199–201.

O'Connor, T. G., Neiderhiser, J. M., Reiss, D., Hetherington, E. M., & Plomin, R. (1998). Genetic contributions to continuity, change, and co-occurrence of antisocial and depressive symptoms in adolescence. *Journal of Child Psychology and Psychiatry, 39,* 323–336.

O'Donnell, P., & Grace, A. A. (1998). Dysfunctions in multiple interrelated systems as the neurobiological bases of schizophrenic symptom clusters. *Schizophrenia Bulletin, 24*(2), 267–283.

Ogawa, J. R., Sroufe, L. A., Weinfeld, N. S., Carlson, E. A., & Egeland, B. (1997). Development and the fragmented self: Longitudinal study of dissociative symptomatology in a nonclinical sample. *Development and Psychopathology, 9,* 855–879.

Olin, S. S., & Mednick, S. A. (1996). Risk factors of psychosis: Identifying vulnerable populations premorbidly. *Schizophrenia Bulletin, 22*(2), 223–240.

Olney, J. W., & Farber, N. B. (1997). Discussion of Bogerts' temporolimbic system theory of paranoid schizophrenia. *Schizophrenia Bulletin, 23*(3), 533–536.

Olweus, D. (1979). Stability of aggressive reaction patterns in males: A review. *Psychological Bulletin, 86,* 852–875.

Oosterlaan, J., Logan, G. D., & Sergeant, J. A. (1998). Response inhibition in AD/HD, CD, comorbid AD/HD+CD, anxious, and control children: A meta-analysis of studies with the stop task. *Journal of Child Psychology and Psychiatry, 39,* 411–425.

Owens, M. J. (1996–1997). Molecular and cellular mechanisms of antidepressant drugs. *Depression and Anxiety, 4,* 153–159.

Ownby, R. L. (1998). Computational model of obsessive–compulsive disorder: Examination of etiologic hypothesis and treatment strategies. *Depression and Anxiety, 8,* 91–103.

Pakkenberg, B. (1990). Pronounced reduction of total neuron number in medio-dorsal thalamic nucleus and nucleus accumbens in schizophrenics. *Archives of General Psychiatry, 47,* 1023–1028.

Pakkenberg, B. (1993). Total nerve cell numbers in neocortex in chronic schizophrenics and controls estimated using optical dissectors. *Biological Psychiatry, 34,* 768–772.

Pallanti, S., Quercioli, L., & Pazzagli, A. (1997). Relapse in young paranoid schizophrenic patients: A prospective study of stressful life events, P300 measures, and coping. *American Journal of Psychiatry, 154,* 792–798.

Panksepp, J. (1993). Neurochemical control of moods and emotions: Amino acids to neuropeptides. In M. Lewis & J. M. Haviland (Eds.), *Handbook of emotions* (pp. 87–107). New York: Guilford Press.

Papez, J. W. (1937). A proposed mechanism of emotion. *Archives of Neurology and Psychiatry, 79,* 217–224.

Patterson, C. M., & Newman, J. P. (1993). Reflectivity and learning from aversive events: Toward a psychological mechanism for the syndromes of disinhibition. *Psychological Review, 100,* 716–736.

Patterson, G. R. (1982). *Coercive family process.* Eugene, OR: Castalia.

Patterson, G. R., Forgatch, M. S., Yoerger, K. L., & Stoolmiller, M. (1998). Variables that initiate and maintain an early-onset trajectory for juvenile offending. *Development and Psychopathology, 10,* 531–547.

Paul, S. M. (1988). Anxiety and depression: A common neurobiological substrate? *Journal of Clinical Psychiatry, 49,* 13–16.

Perls, F., Hefferline, R., & Goodman, P. (1951). *Gestalt therapy.* New York: Dell.

Persson-Blennow, I., Binett, B., & McNeil, T. F. (1988). Offspring of women with nonorganic psychosis: Antecedents of anxious attachment to the mother at one year of age. *Acta Psychiatrica Scandinavica, 78,* 66–71.

Pettem, O., West, M., Mahoney, A., & Keller, A. (1993). Depression and attachment problems. *Journal of Psychiatry and Neuroscience, 18,* 78–81.

Pfefferbaum, A., Ford, J. M., White, P. M., & Roth, W. T. (1989). P3 in schizophrenia is affected by stimulus modality, response requirements, medication status, and negative symptoms. *Archives of General Psychiatry, 46,* 1035–1044.

Pianta, R., Egeland, B., & Erickson, M. F. (1989). The antecedents of maltreatment: Results of the Mother–Child Interaction Research Project. In D. Cicchetti & V. Carlson (Eds.), *Child maltreatment: Theory and research on the causes and consequences of child abuse and neglect* (pp. 203–253). New York: Cambridge University Press.

Pine, D. S., Coplan, J. D., Wasserman, G. A., Miller, L. S., Fried, J. E., Davies, M., Cooper, T. B., Greenhill, L., Shaffer, D., & Parsons, B. (1997). Neuroendocrine response to fenfluramine challenge in boys: Associations with aggressive behavior and adverse rearing. *Archives of General Psychiatry, 54,* 839–846.

Pine, D. S., Wasserman, G. A., Fried, J. E., Parides, M., & Shaffer, D. (1997). Neurological soft signs: One-year stability and relationship to psychiatric symptoms in boys. *Journal of the American Academy of Child and Adolescent Psychiatry, 36,* 1579–1586.

Plomin, R., & Stocker, C. (1989). Behavioral genetics and emotionality. In J. S. Reznick (Ed.), *Perspectives on behavioral inhibition* (pp. 219–240). Chicago: University of Chicago Press.

Posner, M. I., & Rothbart, M. K. (1992). Attentional mechanisms and conscious experience. In D. Milner & M. Rugg (Eds.), *The neuropsychology of consciousness* (pp. 91–111). San Diego, CA: Academic Press.

Post, R. M. (1992). Transduction of psychosocial stress into the neurobiology of recurrent affective disorder. *American Journal of Psychiatry, 149,* 999–1010.

Post, R. M., Weiss, S. B., Leverich, G. S., George, M. S., Frye, M., & Ketter, T. A. (1996). Developmental psychobiology of cyclic affactive illness: Implications for early therapeutic intervention. *Development and Psychopathology, 8,* 273–305.

Post, R. M., Weiss, S. R. B., & Smith, M. (1995). Sensitization and kindling: Implications for the evolving neural substrates of post-traumatic stress disorder. In M. J. Friedman, D. S. Charney, & A. Y. Deutch (Eds.), *Neurobiology and clinical consequences of stress: From normal adaptation to PTSD* (pp. 203–224). Philadelphia: Lippincott–Raven.

Prescott, C. A., & Gottesman, I. I. (1993). Genetically mediated vulnerability to schizophrenia. *Psychiatric Clinics of North America, 16*(2), 245–267.

Prochaska, J. O., DiClemente, C. C., & Norcross, J. C. (1992, September). In search of how people change: Application to addictive behaviors. *American Psychologist,* 1102–1114.

Purcell, R., Maruff, P., Kyrios, M., & Pantelis, C. (1998). Neuropsychological deficits in obsessive–compulsive disorder: A comparison with unipolar depression, panic disorder, and normal controls. *Archives of General Psychiatry, 55,* 415–423.

Pynoos, R. S. (1993). Traumatic stress and developmental psychopathology in children and adolescents. In J. Oldham, M. Riba, & A. Tasman (Eds.), *American Psychiatric Press review of psychiatry* (Vol. 12, pp. 205–238). Washington, DC: American Psychiatric Press.

Radke-Yarrow, M., McCann, K., DeMulder, E., Belmont, B., Martinez, P., & Richardson, D. T. (1995). Attachment in the context of high-risk conditions. *Development and Psychopathology, 7,* 247–265.

Raine, A. (1997). Autonomic nervous system factors underlying disinhibited, antisocial, and violent behavior. *Annals of the New York Academy of Sciences, 794,* 46–59.

Raine, A., Benishay, D., Lencz, T., & Scarpa, A. (1997). Abnormal orienting in schizotypal personality disorder. *Schizophrenia Bulletin, 23*(1), 75–82.

Raine, A., Brennan, P., Mednick, B., & Mednick, S. A. (1996). High rates of violence, crime, academic problems, and behavioral problems in males with both early neuromotor deficits and unstable family environments. *Archives of General Psychiatry, 53,* 544–549.

Raine, A., Brennan, P., & Mednick, S. A. (1994). Birth complications combined with early maternal rejection at age 1 year predispose to violent crime at age 18 years. *Archives of General Psychiatry, 51,* 984–988.

Raine, A., Reynolds, C., Venables, P. H., Mednick, S. A., & Farrington, D. P. (1998). Fearlessness, stimulation-seeking, and large body size at age 3 years as early predispositions to childhood aggression at age 11 years. *Archives of General Psychiatry, 55,* 745–751.

Raine, A., Venables, P. H., & Mednick, S. A. (1997). Low resting heart rate at age 3 years predisposes to aggression at age 11 years: Evidence from the Mauritius Child Health Project. *Journal of the American Academy of Child and Adolescent Psychiatry, 36,* 1457–1464.

Raine, A., Venables, P. H., & Williams, M. (1995). High autonomic arousal and electrodermal orienting at age 15 years as protective factors against criminal behavior at age 29 years. *American Journal of Psychiatry, 152,* 1595–1600.

Rapee, R. M., Mattick, R., & Murrell, E. (1986). Cognitive mediation in the affective component of spontaneous panic attacks. *Journal of Behavior Therapy and Experimental Psychiatry, 17,* 245–253.

Rapoport, J. L., & Wise, S. P. (1989). Obsessive–compulsive disorder: Evidence for basal gangia dysfunction. *Psychopharmacology Bulletin, 24,* 380–384.

Rauch, S. L., Jenike, M. A., Alpert, N. M., Baer, L., Breiter, H. C. R., Savage, C. R., & Fischman, A. J. (1994). Regional cerebral blood flow measured during symptom provocation in obsessive–compulsive disorder using oxygen 15-labeled carbon dioxide and positron emission tomography. *Archives of General Psychiatry, 51,* 62–70.

Reznick, J. S. (Ed.). (1989). *Perspectives on behavioral inhibition.* Chicago: University of Chicago Press.

Reznick, J. S., Gibbons, J. L., Johnson, M. O., & McDonough, P. M. (1989). Behavioral inhibition in a normative sample. In J. S. Reznick (Ed.), *Perspectives on behavioral inhibition* (pp. 25–49). Chicago: University of Chicago Press.

Rogeness, G. A., & McClure, E. B. (1996). Development and neurotransmitter–environmental interactions. *Development and Psychopathology, 8,* 183–199.

Rogers, C. R. (1951). *Client-centered therapy.* Boston: Houghton Mifflin.

Rogosch, F. A., Cicchetti, D., & Aber, J. L. (1995). The role of child maltreatment in early deviations in cognitive and affective processing abilities and later peer relationship problems. *Development and Psychopathology, 7,* 591–609.

Rolls, E. T. (1992). Neurophysiology and functions of the primate amygdala. In J. P. Aggleton (Ed.), *The amygdala: Neurobiological aspects of emotion, memory, and mental dysfunction* (pp. 143–165). New York: Wiley–Liss.

Rosenbaum, J. F., Biederman, J., Bolduc, E. A., Hirshfeld, D. R., Faraone, S. V., & Kagan, J. (1992). Comorbidity of parental anxiety disorders as risk for childhood-onset anxiety in inhibited children. *American Journal of Psychiatry, 149,* 475–481.

Rosenbaum, J. F., Biederman, J., Gersten, M., Hirshfield, D. R., Meminger, S. R., Herman, J. B., Kagan, J., Reznick, J. S., & Snidman, N. (1988). Behavioral inhibition in children of parents with panic disorder and agoraphobia: A controlled study. *Archives of General Psychiatry, 45,* 463–470.

Rosenbaum, J. F., Biederman, J., Hirshfeld, D. R., Bolduc, E. A., & Chaloff, J. (1991). Behavioral inhibition in children: A possible precursor to panic disorder or social phobia. *Journal of Clinical Psychiatry, 52*(Suppl.), 5–9.

Rosenberg, D. R., Auerbach, D. H., O'Hearn, K. M., Seymour, A. B., Birmaher, B., & Sweeney, J. A. (1997). Oculomotor response inhibition abnormalities in pediatric obsessive–compulsive disorder. *Archives of General Psychiatry, 54,* 831–838.

Rosenberg, D. R., Keshavan, M. S., O'Hearn, K. M., Dick, E. L., Bagwell, W. W., Seymour, A. B., Montrose, D. M., Pierri, J. N., & Birmaher, B. (1997). Frontostriatal measurement in treatment-naive children with obsessive–compulsive disorder. *Archives of General Psychiatry, 54,* 824–830.

Rosenblum, L. A., Coplan, J. D., Friedman, S., Bassoff, T., Gorman, J. M., & Andrews, M. W. (1994). Adverse early experiences affect noradrenergic and serotenergic functioning in adult primates. *Biological Psychiatry, 35*(4), 221–227.

Ross, D. E., Buchanan, R. W., Medoff, D., Lahti, A. C., & Thaker, G. K. (1998). Association between eye tracking disorder in schizophrenia and poor sensory integration. *American Journal of Psychiatry, 155,* 1352–1357.

Roth, A., & Fonagy, P. (1996). *What works for whom?: A critical review of psychotherapy research.* New York: Guilford Press.

Rothbart, M. K. (1981). Measuement of temperament in infancy. *Child Development, 52,* 569–578.

Rothbart, M. K., & Bates J. E. (1998). Temperament. In. W. Damon (Series Ed.) & N. Eisenberg (Vol. Ed.), *Handbook of child psychology: Vol. 3. Social, emotional, and personality development* (5th ed., pp. 105–176). New York: Wiley.

Rothbart, M. K., Derryberry, D., & Posner, M. I. (1994). A psychological approach to the development of temperament. In J. E. Bates & T. D. Wachs (Eds.), *Temperament: Individual differences at the interface of biology and behavior* (pp. 83–116). Washington, DC: American Psychological Association.

Rubin, K. H., Coplan, R. J., Fox, N. A., & Calkins, S. D. (1995). Emotionality, emotion regulation, and preschoolers' social adaptation. *Development and Psychopathology, 7,* 49–62.

Rubin, K. H., Stewart, S. L., & Coplan, R. J. (1995). Social withdrawal in childhood: Conceptual and empirical perspectives. In R. H. Ollendick & R. J. Prinz (Eds.), *Advances in clinical child psychology* (Vol. 17, pp. 157–196). New York: Plenum Press.

Rund, B. R. (1998). A review of longitudinal studies of cognitive functions in schizophrenia patients. *Schizophrenia Bulletin, 24*(3), 425–435.

Rund, B. R., Orbeck, A. L., & Landro, N. I. (1992). Vigilance deficits in schizophrenics and affectively disturbed patients. *Acta Psychiatrica Scandinavica, 86,* 207–212.

Russek, L. G., King, S. H., Russek, S. J., & Russek, H. I. (1990). The Harvard Mastery of Stress Study 35-year follow-up: Prognostic significance of patterns of psychological arousal and adaptation. *Psychosomatic Medicine, 52,* 271–285.

Rutter, M. (1989). Pathways from childhood to adult life. *Journal of Child Psychology and Psychiatry, 30,* 23–51.

Rutter, M., Graham, P., & Yule, W. (1970). *A neuropsychiatric study in childhood* (Clinics in Developmental Medicine Nos. 35–36). London: Heinemann.

Ryan, R. M., Kuhl, J., & Deci, E. L. (1997). Nature and autonomy: An organizational view of social and neurobiological aspects of self-regulation in behavior and development. *Development and Psychopathology, 9,* 701–728.

Sackheim, H. A., Devanand, D. P., & Nobler, M. S. (1995). Electroconvulsive therapy. In F. E. Bloom & D. J. Kupfer (Eds.), *Psychopharmacology: The fourth generation of progress* (pp. 1123–1141). New York: Raven Press.

Safran, J. D., & Segal, Z. V. (1990). *Interpersonal process in cognitive therapy*. New York: Basic Books.

Sameroff, A. J. (1989). Models of developmental regulation: The envirotype. In D. Cicchetti (Ed.), *Rochester Symposium on Developmental Psychopathology: Vol. 1. The emergence of a discipline* (pp. 41–68). Hillsdale, NJ: Erlbaum.

Sanders, M. R. (1996). New directions in behavioral family intervention with children. In T. H. Ollendick & R. J. Prinz (Eds.), *Advances in clinical child psychology* (Vol. 18, pp. 283–330). New York: Plenum Press.

Sanders, M. R., & Markie-Dadds, C. (1992). Toward a technology of prevention of disruptive behaviour disorders: The role of behavioural family intervention. *Behavior Change, 9,* 186–200.

Sanderson, R. S., Rapee, R. M., & Barlow, D. H. (1989). The influence of an illusion of control on panic attacks induced via inhalation of 5.5% carbon dioxide-enriched air. *Archives of General Psychiatry, 46,* 157–162.

Sapolsky, R. M. (1994). *Why zebras don't get ulcers: A guide to stress, stress-related diseases, and coping*. New York: Freeman.

Saykin, A. J., Gur, R. C., Gur, R. E., Mozley, P. D., Mozley, L. H., Resnick, S. M., Kester, B., & Stafiniak, P. (1991). Neuropsychological function in schizophrenia: Selective impairment in memory and listening. *Archives of General Psychiatry, 48,* 618–624.

Schachar, R., & Logan, G. D. (1990). Implusivity and inhibitory control in normal development and childhood psychopathology. *Developmental Psychology, 26,* 710–720.

Schmitz, S., Fulker, D. W., & Mrazek, D. A. (1995). Problem behavior in early and middle childhood: An initial behavior genetic analysis. *Journal of Child Psychology and Psychiatry, 36*(8), 1443–1458.

Schneider, M. L., Clarke, A. S., Kraemer, G. W., Roughton, E. C., Lubach, G. R., Rimm-Kaufman, S., Schmidt, D., & Ebert, M. (1998). Prenatal stress alters brain biogenic amine levels in primates. *Development and Psychopathology, 10,* 427–440.

Schneider, M. L., & Coe, C. L. (1993). Repeated social stress during pregnancy impairs neuromotor development of the primate infant. *Journal of Developmental and Behavioral Pediatrics, 14,* 81–87.

Schneider, M. L., Coe, C. L., & Lubach, G. R. (1992). Endocrine activation mimics the adverse effects of prenatal stress on the neuromotor development of the infant primate. *Developmental Psychobiology, 25,* 427–439.

Schore, A. N. (1994). *Affect regulation and the origins of the self*. Hillsdale, NJ: Erlbaum.

Schore, A. N. (1996). The experience-dependent maturation of a regulatory system in the orbital prefrontal cortex and the origin of developmental psychopathology. *Development and Psychopathology, 8,* 59–87.

Schothorst, P., & van Engeland, H. (1996). Long-term behavioral sequelae of prematurity. *Journal of the American Academy of Child and Adolescent Psychiatry, 35,* 175–183.

Schraeder, B. D., Heverly, M. A., & O'Brien, C. M. (1996). Home and classroom behavioral adjustment in very low birthweight children: The influence of caregiver stress and goodness of fit. *Children's Health Care, 25*(2), 117–131.

Schulkin, J., McEwen, B. S., & Gold, P. W. (1994). Allostasis, amygdala, and anticipatory angst. *Neuroscience and Biobehavioral Reviews, 18*, 385–396.

Schwartz, C., Snidman, N., & Kagan, J. (1996). Early childhood temperament as a determinant of externalizing behavior in adolescence. *Development and Psychopathology, 8*, 527–537.

Schwartz, D., Dodge, K. A., Pettit, G. S., & Bates, J. E. (1997). The early socialization of aggressive victims of bullying. *Child Development, 68*, 665–675.

Schwartz, D., McFadyen-Ketchum, S. A., Dodge, K. A., Pettit, G. S., & Bates, J. E. (1998). Peer group victimization as a predictor of children's behavior problems at home and in school. *Development and Psychopathology, 10*, 87–99.

Scott, J. P., & Fuller, J. L. (1965). *Genetics and the social behavior of the dog.* Chicago: University of Chicago Press.

Seeman, M. V. (1997). Psychopathology in women and men: Focus on female hormones. *American Journal of Psychiatry, 154*, 1641–1647.

Seeman, P., Bzowej, N. H., Guan, H. C., Bergeron, C., Reynolds, G. P., Bird, E. D., Riederer, P., Jellinger, K., Watanabe, S., & Tourtellote, W. (1987). Human brain dopamine receptors in children and aging adults. *Synapse, 1*, 399–405.

Segal, M. (1985). Mechanisms of action of noradrenaline in the brain. *Physiological Psychology, 13*, 172–178.

Segal, Z. V., Williams, J. M., Teasdale, J. D., & Gemar, M. (1996). A cognitive science perspective on kindling and episode sensitization in recurrent affective disorder. *Psychological Medicine, 26*, 371–380.

Selemon, L. D., Rajkowska, G., & Goldman-Rakic, P. S. (1995). Abnormally high neuronal density in the schizophrenic cortex: A morphometric analysis of prefrontal area 9 and occipital area 17. *Archives of General Psychiatry, 52*, 805–818.

Shalev, A. Y. (1996). Stress versus traumatic stress: From acute homeostatic reactions to chronic psychopathology. In B. A. van der Kolk, A. C. McFarlane, & L. Weisaeth (Eds.), *Traumatic stress: The effects of overwhelming experience on mind, body, and society* (pp. 77–101). New York: Guilford Press.

Shapiro, F., & Forrest, M. S. (1997). *EMDR: The breakthrough therapy for overcoming anxiety, stress, and trauma.* New York: Basic Books.

Sharma, R., Lancaster, E., Lee, D., Lewis, S., Sigmundsson, R., Takei, N., Gurling, H., Barta, P., Pearlson, G., & Murray, R. (1998). Brain changes in schizophrenia: Volumetric MRI study of families multiply affected with schizophrenia—The Maudsley Family Study 5. *British Journal of Psychiatry, 173*, 132–138.

Shaw, D. S., & Bell, R. Q. (1993). Developmental theories of parental contributors to antisocial behavior. *Journal of Abnormal Child Psychology, 21*, 493–518.

Shaw, D. S., Keenan, K., Vondra, J. I., Delliquadri, E., & Giovanelli, J. (1997). Antecedents of preschool children's internalizing problems: A longitudinal study of low-income families. *Journal of the American Academy of Child and Adolescent Psychiatry, 36*, 1760–1767.

Shaw, D. S., Owens, E. B., Vondra, J. I., Keenan, K., & Winslow, E. B. (1996). Early risk factors and pathways in the development of early disruptive behavior problems. *Development and Psychopathology, 8,* 679–699.

Shirk, S. R., Boergers, J., Eason, A., & Van Horn, M. (1998). Dysphoric interpersonal schemata and preadolescents' sensitization to negative events. *Journal of Clinical Child Psychology, 27,* 54–68.

Sifneos, P. E. (1973). The prevalence of "alexithymic" characteristics in psychosomatic patients. *Psychotherapy and Psychosomatics, 22,* 255–262.

Sigvardsson, S., Bohman, M., & Cloninger, C. R. (1987). Structure and stability of childhood personality: Prediction of later social adjustment. *Journal of Child Psychology and Psychiatry, 28,* 929–946.

Silberg, J. L., Heath, A. C., Kessler, R., Neale, M. C., Meyer, J. M., Eaves, L. J., & Kendler, K. S. (1990). Genetic and environmental effects on self-reported depressive symptoms in a general population twin sample. *Journal of Psychiatric Research, 24,* 197–212.

Silberg, J., Meyer, J., Pickles, A., Simonoff, E., Eaves, L., Hewitt, J., Maes, H., & Rutter, M. (1995). Heterogeneity among juvenile antisocial behaviours: Findings from the Virginia Twin Study of Adolescent Behavioural Development. In G. R. Bock & J. A. Goode (Eds.), *Genetics of criminal and antisocial behaviour* (Ciba Foundation Symposium No. 194, pp. 76–92). Chichester, England: Wiley.

Silberg, J., Rutter, M., Meyer, J., Maes, H., Hewitt, J., Simonoff, E., Pickles, A., Loeber, R., & Eaves, L. (1996). Genetic and environmental influences on the covariation between hyperactivity and conduct disturbance in juvenile twins. *Journal of Child Psychology and Psychiatry, 37,* 803–816.

Smith, O. A., & DeVito, J. L. (1984). Central neural integration for the control of automatic responses associated with emotion. *Annual Review of Neuroscience, 7,* 43–65.

Solomon, Z., Laor, N., & McFarlane, A. C. (1996). Acute posttraumatic reactions in soldiers and civilians. In B. A. van der Kolk, A. C. McFarlane, & L. Weisaeth (Eds.), *Traumatic stress: The effects of overwhelming experience on mind, body, and society* (pp. 102–114). New York: Guilford Press.

Sonuga-Barke, E. J. S., Thompson, M., Stevenson, J., & Viney, D. (1997). Patterns of behaviour problems among pre-school childeren. *Psychological Medicine, 27,* 909–918.

Spangler, G., & Grossmann, K. E. (1993). Biobehavioral organization in securely and insecurely attached infants. *Child Development, 64,* 1439–1450.

Spohn, H. E. (1996). Neuroleptic treatment effects in relation to psychotherapy, social skills training, and social withdrawal in schizophrenics. In S. Matthysse, D. L. Levy, J. Kagan, & F. M. Benes (Eds.), *Psychopathology: The evolving science of mental disorder* (pp. 353–361). New York: Cambridge University Press.

Spoont, M. R. (1992). Modulatory role of serotonin in neural information processing: Implications for human psychopathology. *Psychological Bulletin, 112,* 330–350.

Squires-Wheeler, E., Friedman, D., Skodol, A. E., & Erlenmeyer-Kimling, L. (1993). A longitudinal study relating P3 amplitude to schizophrenia spectrum disorders and to global personality functioning. *Biological Psychiatry, 33,* 774–785.

Sroufe, L. A. (1989a). Pathways to adaptation and maladaptation: Psychopathology as developmental deviation. In D. Cicchetti (Ed.), *Rochester Symposium on Developmental Psychopathology: Vol. 1. The emergence of a discipline* (pp. 13–40). Hillsdale, NJ: Erlbaum.

Sroufe, L. A. (1989b). Relationships, self, and individual adaptation. In A. J. Sameroff & R. N. Emde (Eds.), *Relationship disturbances in early childhood: A developmental approach* (pp. 70–94). New York: Basic Books.

Sroufe, L. A. (1991). Considering normal and the abnormal together: The essence of developmental psychopathology. *Development and Psychopathology, 2,* 335–347.

Staal, W. G., Hulshoff Pol, H. E., Schnack, H., van der Schot, A. C., & Kahn, R. S. (1998). Partial volume decrease of the thalamus in relatives of patients with schizophrenia. *American Journal of Psychiatry, 155,* 1784–1786.

Stansbury, K., & Gunnar, M. R. (1994). Adrenocortical activity and emotion regulation. In N. A. Fox (Ed.), The development of emotion regulation: Biological and behavioral considerations. *Monographs of the Society for Research in Child Development 59*(2–3, Serial No. 240), 108–134.

Stearns, C. Z. (1993). Sadness. In M. Lewis & J. M. Haviland (Eds.), *Handbook of emotions* (pp. 547–561). New York: Guilford Press.

Stein, M. B., Koverola, C., Hanna, C., Torchia, M. G., & McClarty, B. (1997). Hippocampal volume in women victimized by childhood sexual abuse. *Psychological Medicine, 21,* 951–959.

Stern, D. N. (1985). *The interpersonal world of the infant.* New York: Basic Books.

Stevens, J. R. (1997). Anatomy of schizophrenia revisited. *Schizophrenia Bulletin, 23*(3), 373–383.

Stevenson, J. (1996). Developmental changes in the mechanisms linking language disabilities and behavior disorder. In J. H. Beitchman, N. J. Cohen, M. M. Konstantareas, & R. Tannock (Eds.), *Language, learning, and behavior disorders* (pp. 78–99). New York: Cambridge University Press.

Stevenson-Hinde, J. (1989). Behavioral inhibition: Issues of context. In J. S. Reznick (Ed.), *Perspectives on behavioral inhibition* (pp. 125–138). Chicago: University of Chicago Press.

Stevenson-Hinde, J., & Glover, A. (1996). Shy girls and boys: A new look. *Journal of Child Psychology and Psychiatry, 37,* 181–187.

Stevenson-Hinde, J., Stillwell-Barnes, R., & Zunz, M. (1980). Subjective assessment of rhesus monkeys over four successive years. *Primates, 21,* 66–82.

Stewart, S. L., & Rubin, K. H. (1995). The social problem-solving skills of anxious-withdrawn children. *Development and Psychopathology, 7,* 323–336.

Stiefel, G. S., Plunkett, J. W., & Meisels, S. J. (1987). Affective expression among preterm infants of varying levels of biological risk. *Infant Behavior and Development, 10,* 151–164.

Stiles, W. B., Elliott, R., LLewelyn, S. P., Firth-Cozens, J. A., Margison, F. R., Shapiro, D. A., & Hardy, G. (1990). Assimilation of problematic experiences by clients in psychotherapy. *Psychotherapy, 27,* 411–420.

Stocker, C. M. (1995). Differences in mothers' and fathers' relationships with siblings: Links with children's behavior problems. *Development and Psychopathology, 7,* 499–513.

Stormshak, E. A., Bierman, K. L., & the Conduct Problems Prevention Research Group. (1998). The implications of different developmental patterns of disruptive behavior problems for school adjustment. *Development and Psychopathology, 10,* 451–467.

Strelau, J. (1994). The concepts of arousal and arousability as used in temperament studies. In J. E. Bates & T. D. Wachs (Eds.), *Temperament: Individual differences at the interface of biology and behavior* (pp. 117–141). Washington, DC: American Psychological Association Press.

Stubbe, D. E., Zahner, G. E. P., Goldstein, M. J., & Leckman, J. F. (1993). Diagnostic specificity of a brief measure of expressed emotion: A community study of children. *Journal of Child Psychology and Psychiatry, 34,* 139–154.

Sturgeon, D., Turpin, G., Kuipers, L., Berkowitz, R., & Leff, J. (1984). Psychophysiological responses of schizophrenic patients to high and low expressed emotion relatives: A follow-up study. *British Journal of Psychiatry, 145,* 62–69.

Suess, G. J., Grossmann, K. E., & Sroufe, L. A. (1992). Effects of infant attachment to mother and father on quality of adaptation in preschool: From dyadic to individual organisation of self. *International Journal of Behavioral Development, 15,* 43–65.

Suomi, S. J. (1991a). Adolescent depression and depressive symptoms: Insights from longitudinal studies with rhesus monkeys. *Journal of Youth and Adolescence, 20,* 273–287.

Suomi, S. J. (1991b). Primate separation models of affective disorders. In J. Madden IV (Ed.), *Neurobiology of learning, emotion and affect* (pp. 195–214). New York: Raven Press.

Suomi, S. J. (1995). Influence of attachment theory on ethological studies of biobehavioral development in nonhuman primates. In S. Goldberg, R. Muir, & J. Kerr (Eds.), *Attachment theory: Social, developmental, and clinical perspectives* (pp. 185–201). Hillsdale, NJ: Analytic Press.

Swedo, S., Leonard, H. L., Mittelman, B. B., Allen, A. J., Rapoport, J. L., Dow, S. P., Kanter, M. E., Chapman, F., & Zabriskie, J. (1997). Identification of children with pediatric autoimmune neuropsychiatric disorders associated with streptococcal infections by a marker associated with rheumatic fever. *American Journal of Psychiatry, 154,* 110–112.

Sykes, D. H., Hoy, E. A., Bill, J. M., McClure, B. G., Halliday, H. L., & Reid, M. M. (1997). Behavioural adjustment in school of very low birthweight children. *Journal of Child Psychology and Psychiatry, 38,* 315–325.

Szatmari, P., Offord, D. R., Siegel, L. S., Finlayson, M. A. J., & Tuff, L. (1990). The clinical significance of neurocognitive impairments among children with psychiatric disorders: Diagnosis and situational specificity. *Journal of Child Psychology and Psychiatry, 31,* 287–299.

Tannock, R., & Schachar, R. (1996). Executive dysfunction as an underlying mechanism of behavior and language problems in attention deficit hyperactivity disorder. In J. H. Beitchman, N. J. Cohen, M. M. Konstantareas, & R. Tannock (Eds.), *Language, learning and behavior disorders: Developmental, biological, and clinical perspectives* (pp. 128–155). New York: Cambridge University Press.

Tarrant, C. J., & Jones, P. B. (1999). Precursors to schizophrenia: Do biological markers have any specificity? *Canadian Journal of Psychiatry, 44,* 335–349.

Tarrier, N. (1989). Electrodermal activity, expressed emotion and outcome in schizophrenia. *British Journal of Psychiatry, 155*(Suppl.), 51–56.

Tarrier, N., Barrowclough, C., Porceddu, K., & Watts, S. (1988). The assessment of psychophysiological reactivity to the expressed emotion of the relatives of schizophrenic patients. *British Journal of Psychiatry, 152,* 618–624.

Taylor, G. J., Bagby, R. M., & Parker, J. D. A. (1997). *Disorders of affect regulation: Alexithymia in medical and psychiatric illness.* Cambridge, England: Cambridge University Press.

Teicher, M. H., Ito, Y., Glod, C. A., Andersen, S. L., Dumont, N., & Ackerman, E. (1997). Preliminary evidence for abnormal cortical development in physically and sexually abused children using EEG coherence and MRI. *Annals of the New York Academy of Sciences, 821,* 160–175.

Thapar, A., Hervas, A., & McGuffin, P. (1995). Childhood hyperactivity scores are highly heritable and show sibling competition effects: Twin study evidence. *Behavior Genetics, 25,* 537–544.

Thapar, A., & McGuffin, P. (1994). A twin study of depressive symptoms in childhood. *British Journal of Psychiatry, 165,* 259–269.

Thapar, A., & McGuffin, P. (1997). Anxiety and depressive symptoms in childhood: A genetic study of comorbidity. *Journal of Child Psychology and Psychiatry, 38,* 651–656.

Thomas, A., Chess, S., & Birch, H. G. (1968). *Temperament and behavior disorders in children.* New York: New York University Press.

Thompson, R. A. (1994). Emotion regulation: A theme in search of definition. In N. A. Fox (Ed.), The development of emotion regulation: Biological and behavioral considerations. *Monographs of the Society for Research in Child Development, 59*(2–3, Serial No. 240), 53–72.

Thompson, R. A., & Calkins, S. D. (1996). The double-edged sword: Emotional regulation for children at risk. *Development and Psychopathology, 8,* 163–182.

Tibbo, P., & Warneke, L. (1999). Obsessive–complusive disorder in schizophrenia: Epidemiologic and biologic overlap. *Journal of Psychiatry and Neuroscience, 24*(1), 15–24.

Tienari, P. (1991). Interaction between genetic vulnerability and family environment: The Finnish adoptive family study of schizophrenia. *Acta Psychiatrica Scandinavica, 84,* 460–465.

Todd, R. D., Swarzenski, B., Rossi, P. G., & Visconti, P. (1995). Structural and functional development of the human brain. In D. Cicchetti & D. J. Cohen (Eds.), *Developmental psychopathology: Vol. 1. Theory and methods* (pp. 161–194). New York: Wiley.

Tomkins, S. S. (1962). *Affect, imagery, consciousness: Vol. 1. The positive affects.* New York: Springer.

Tomkins, S. S. (1963). *Affect, imagery, consciousness: Vol 2. The negative affects.* New York: Springer.

Tompson, M., Asarnow, J. R., Goldstein, M. J., & Miklowitz, D. J. (1990). Thought disorder and communication problems in children with schizophrenia spectrum and depressive disorders and their parents. *Journal of Clinical Child Psychiatry, 19,* 159–168.

Torgersen, S., & Alnaes, R. (1992). Differential perception of parental bonding in schizotypal and borderline personality disorder patients. *Comprehensive Psychiatry, 33,* 34–38.

Torgersen, S., Onstad, S., Skre, I., Edvardsen, J., & Kringlen, E. (1993). "True" schizotypal personality disorder: A study of co-twins and relatives of schizophrenic probands. *American Journal of Psychiatry, 150,* 1661–1667.

Tremblay, R. E., Masse, L. C., Vitaro, F., & Dobkin, P. L. (1995). The impact of friends' deviant behavior on early onset of delinquency: Longitudinal data from 6 to 13 years of age. *Development and Psychopathology, 7,* 649–667.

Trevarthen, C., & Aitken, K. J. (1994). Brain development, infant communication, and empathy disorders: Intrinsic factors in child mental health. *Development and Psychopathology, 6,* 597–633.

Tronick, E. Z., & Gianino, A. F. (1986). The transmission of maternal disturbance to the infant. In E. Z. Tronick & T. Field (Monograph Eds.), *Maternal depression and infant disturbance.* W. Damon (Ed.), *New directions for child development* (Vol. 34, pp. 5–11). San Francisco: Jossey-Bass.

Truax, C. B., & Carkhuff, R. R. (1967). *Toward an effective counselling and psychotherapy: Training and practice.* Chicago: Aldine.

Tubman, J. G., & Lerner, R. M. (1994). Continuity and discontinuity in the affective experiences of parents and children: Evidence from the New York Longitudinal Study. *American Journal of Orthopsychiatry, 64,* 112–125.

Tucker, D. M., & Williamson, P. A. (1984). Asymmetric neural control systems in human self-regulation. *Psychological Review, 91,* 185–215.

Tyrer, P., Seivewright, N., Murphy, S., Ferguson, B., Kingdon, D., Barczak, P., Brothwell, J., Darling, C., Gregory, S., & Johnson, A. L. (1988, July). The Nottingham Study of Neurotic Disorder: Comparison of drug and psychological treatments. *Lancet,* 235–240.

van den Boom, D. C. (1994). The influence of temperament and mothering on attachment and exploration: An experimental manipulation of sensitive responsiveness among lower-class mothers with irritable infants. *Child Development, 65,* 1457–1477.

van der Kolk, B. A. (1994). The body keeps the score: Memory and the evolving psychobiology of posttraumatic stress. *Harvard Review of Psychiatry, 1,* 253–265.

van der Kolk, B. A. (1996). The body keeps the score: Approaches to the psychobiology of posttraumatic stress disorder. In B. A. van der Kolk, A. C. McFarlane, & L. Weisaeth (Eds.), *Traumatic stress: The effects of overwhelming experience on mind, body, and society* (pp. 214–241). New York: Guilford Press.

van der Kolk, B. A., & McFarlane, A. C. (1996). The black hole of trauma. In B. A. van der Kolk, A. C. McFarlane, & L. Weisaeth (Eds.), *Traumatic stress: The effects of overwhelming experience on mind, body, and society* (pp. 3–23). New York: Guilford Press.

van der Kolk, B. A., McFarlane, A. C., & Weisaeth, L. (Eds.). (1996). *Traumatic stress: The effects of overwhelming experience on mind, body, and society.* New York: Guilford Press.

van IJzendoorn, M. H., & Bakermans-Kranenburg, M. J. (1996). Attachment representations in mothers, fathers, adolescents, and clinical groups: A meta-analytic search for normative data. *Journal of Consulting and Clinical Psychology, 64,* 8–21.

van IJzendoorn, M. H., Goldberg, S., Kroonenberg, P. M., & Frenkel, O. (1992). The relative effects of maternal and child problems on the quality of attachment: A meta-analysis of attachment in clinical samples. *Child Development, 63,* 840–858.

van IJzendoorn, M. H., Schuengel, C., & Bakermans-Kranenburg, M. J. (1999). Disorganized attachment in early childhood: Meta-analysis of precursors, concomitants and sequelae. *Development and Psychopathology, 11,* 225–249.

Vaughan, C. E., & Leff, J. (1976). The influence of family and social factors on the course of psychiatric illness. *British Journal of Psychiatry, 129,* 125–137.

Vollema, M. G., & van den Bosch, R. J. (1995). The multidimensionality of schizotypy. *Schizophrenia Bulletin, 21,* 19–31.

Vostanis, P., & Nicholls, J. (1995). Nine-month changes of maternal expressed emotion in conduct and emotional disorders of childhood: A follow-up study. *Journal of Child Psychology and Psychiatry, 36,* 833–846.

Vostanis, P., Nicholls, J., & Harrington, R. (1994). Maternal expressed emotion in conduct and emotional disorders of childhood. *Journal of Child Psychology and Psychiatry, 35,* 365–376.

Wahlberg, K.-E., Wynne, L. C., Oja, H., Keskitalo, P., Pykalainen, L., Lahti, I., Moring, J., Naarala, M., Sorri, A., Seitamaa, M., Läksy, K., Kolassa, J., & Tienari, P. (1997). Gene–environment interaction in vulnerability to schizophrenia: Findings from the Finnish Adoptive Family Study of Schizophrenia. *American Journal of Psychiatry, 154,* 355–362.

Walker, E. F., & Lewine, R. J. (1990). Prediction of adult-onset schizophrenia from childhood home movies of the patients. *American Journal of Psychiatry, 147,* 1052–1056.

Walker, E., Lewis, N., Loewy, R., & Palyo, S. (1999). Motor dysfunction and risk for schizophrenia. *Development and Psychopathology, 11,* 509–523.

Walker, E. F., Neumann, C. G., Baum, K., Davis, D. M., DiForio, D., & Bergman, A. (1996). The developmental pathways to schizophrenia: Potential moderating effects of stress. *Development and Psychopathology, 8,* 647–665.

Warner, R. (1995). Time trends in schizophrenia: Changes in obstetric risk factors with industrialization. *Schizophrenia Bulletin, 21,* 483–500.

Warren, S. L., Huston, L., Egeland, B., & Sroufe, L. A. (1997). Child and adolescent anxiety disorders and early attachment. *Journal of the American Academy of Child and Adolescent Psychiatry, 36,* 637–644.

Watson, D., & Clark, L. A. (1994). Emotions, moods, traits and temperaments: Conceptual distinctions and empirical findings. In P. Ekman & R. J. Davidson (Eds.), *The nature of emotion: Fundamental questions* (pp. 89–93). New York: Oxford University Press.

Webster-Stratton, C., & Spitzer, A. (1996). Parenting a young child with conduct problems: new insights using qualitative methods. In R. H. Ollendick & R. J.

Prinz (Eds.), *Advances in clinical child psychology* (Vol. 18, pp. 1–62). New York: Plenum Press.

Webster-Stratton, C., & Hammond, M. (1997). Treating children with early-onset conduct problems: A comparison of child and parent training interventions. *Journal of Consulting and Clinical Psychology, 65,* 93–109.

Weiger, W. A., & Bear, D. M. (1988). An approach to the neurology of aggression. *Journal of Psychiatric Research, 22,* 85–98.

Weinberger, D. R., Berman, K. F., & Zec, R. F. (1986). Physiologic dysfunction of dorsolateral prefrontal cortex in schizophrenics: I. Regional cerebral blood flow evidence. *Archives of General Psychiatry, 43,* 114–124.

Weinberger, J. (1993). Common factors in psychotherapy. In G. Stickler & J. R. Gold (Eds.), *Comprehensive handbook of psychotherapy integration* (pp. 43–56). New York: Plenum Press.

Weiskrantz, L. (1956). Behavioral changes associated with ablation of the amygdaloid complex in monkeys. *Journal of Comparative and Physiological Psychology, 49,* 381–391.

Weiss, E. L., Longhurst, J. G., & Mazure, C. M. (1999). Childhood sexual abuse as a risk factor for depression in women: Psychosocial and neurobiological correlates. *American Journal of Psychiatry, 156,* 816–828.

Weiss, J. (1990, March). Unconscious mental functioning. *Scientific American,* pp. 103–109.

Werry, J. S., & McClellan, J. M. (1992). Predicting outcome in child and adolescent (early onset) schizophrenia and bipolar disorder. *Journal of the American Academy of Child and Adolescent Psychiatry, 31,* 147–150.

Whitaker, A. H., Van Rossem, R., Feldman, J. F., Schonfeld, I. S., Pinto-Martin, J. A., Torre, C., Shaffer, D., & Paneth, N. (1997). Psychiatric outcomes in low-birth-weight children at age 6 years: Relation to neonatal cranial ultrasound abnormalities. *Archives of General Psychiatry, 54,* 847–856.

Wickramaratne, P. J., & Weissman, M. M. (1998). Onset of psychopathology in offspring by developmental phase and parental depression. *Journal of the American Academy of Child and Adolescent Psychiatry, 37,* 933–942.

Wiedl, K. H., & Schottner, B. (1991). Coping with symptoms related to schizophrenia. *Schizophrenia Bulletin, 17*(3), 525–538.

Williams, L. M. (1996). Cognitive inhibition and schizophrenic symptom subgroups. *Schizophrenia Bulletin, 22,* 139–151.

Winnicott, D. (1965). *The maturational process and the facilitating environment.* London: Hogarth Press.

Wolfe, D. A., Wekerle, C., Reitzel-Jaffe, D., & Lefebvre, L. (1998). Factors associated with abusive relationships among maltreated and nonmaltreated youth. *Development and Psychopathology, 10,* 61–85.

Woods, B. T. (1998). Is schizophrenia a progressive neurodevelopmental disorder?: Toward a unitary pathogenetic mechanism. *American Journal of Psychiatry, 155,* 1661–1670.

Wootton, J. M., Frick, P. J., Shelton, K. K., & Silverthorn, P. (1997). Ineffective parenting and childhood conduct problems: The moderating role of callous–unemotional traits. *Journal of Consulting and Clinical Psychology, 65,* 301–308.

Wuerker, A. M. (1996). Communication patterns and expressed emotion in families of persons with mental disorders. *Schizophrenia Bulletin, 22*(4), 671–690.

Yehuda, R., & McFarlane, A. C. (1995). Conflict between current knowledge about posttraumatic stress disorder and its original conceptual basis. *American Journal of Psychiatry, 152,* 1705–1713.

Young, E. A., Abelson, J. L., Curtis, G. C., & Nesse, R. M. (1997). Childhood adversity and vulnerability to mood and anxiety disorders. *Depression and Anxiety, 5,* 66–72.

Zahn-Waxler, C., Cole, P. M., & Barrett, K. C. (1991). Guilt and empathy: Sex differences and implications for the development of depression. In J. Garber & K. A. Dodge (Eds.), *The development of emotion regulation and dysregulation* (pp. 243–272). Cambridge, England: Cambridge University Press.

Zahn-Waxler, C., Iannotti, R. J., Cummings, E. M., & Denham, S. (1990). Antecedents of problem behaviors in children of depressed mothers. *Development and Psychopathology, 2,* 271–291.

Zahn-Waxler, C., Schmitz, S., Fulker, D., Robinson, J., & Emde, R. (1996). Behavior problems in 5-year-old monozygotic and dizygotic twins: Genetic and environmental influences, patterns of regulation, and internalization of control. *Development and Psychopathology, 8,* 103–122.

Zaidel, D. W., Esiri, M. M., & Harrison, P. J. (1997). Size, shape, and orientation of neurons in the left and right hippocampus: Investigation of normal asymmetries and alterations in schizophrenia. *American Journal of Psychiatry, 154,* 812–818.

Zametkin, A. J., & Rapoport, J. L. (1987). Noradrenergic hypothesis of attention deficit disorder with hyperactivity: A critical review. In H. Y. Meltzer (Ed.), *Psychopharmacology: The third generation of progress* (pp. 837–842). New York: Raven Press.

Zeanah, C. H., Benoit, D., Barton, M., Regan, C., Hirshberg, L. M., & Lipsitt, L. P. (1993). Representations of attachment in mothers and their one-year-old infants. *Journal of the American Academy of Child and Adolescent Psychiatry, 32,* 278–286.

Zobel, A. W., Yassouridis, A., Frieboes, R.-M., & Holsboer, F. (1999). Prediction of medium-term outcome by cortisol response to the combined dexamethasone-CRH test in patients with remitted depression. *American Journal of Psychiatry, 156,* 949–951.

Zoccolillo, M. (1992). Concurrence of conduct disorder and its adult outcomes with depressive and anxiety disorders: A review. *Journal of the American Academy of Child and Adolescent Psychiatry, 31,* 547–556.

Zucker, K. J., & Bradley, S. J. (1995). *Gender identity disorder and psychosexual problems in children and adolescents.* New York: Guilford Press.

Zuckerman, M. (1994). Impulsive unsocialized sensation seeking: The biological foundations of a basic dimension of personality. In J. E. Bates & T. D. Wachs (Eds.), *Temperament: Individual differences at the interface of biology and behavior* (pp. 219–258). Washington, DC: American Psychological Association.

Index

Abuse
  defined, 82
  in development of internalizing
      disorders, 19, 180
  developmental outcomes, 94
  intergenerational transmission, 95–96
  neurobiological response, 95
  psychopathology and, 5, 36, 94–95
  risk of externalizing disorder, 217–218
Acetylcholine, 12, 121, 226
Adrenocorticotropic hormone, 85, 86, 124,
      162, 189
  stress response, 191
Affective functioning
  amygdalar system in, 123–125, 148–149
  attachment and, 65–71, 72–73, 80, 105
  attentional processes in, 33, 99–100, 101
  brain factors in, 10–12, 28, 127–128
  brain hemisphere differences, 117–118,
      127–128
  clinical significance, 3–4
  developmental process, 29–32, 67
  in disruptive behavior disorders, 211,
      218–222, 227–228
  effects of dysfunctional parenting, 75–76
  emotional feeling and, 4, 27–28
  family psychosocial factors, 173–184
  long-term outcomes of dysregulation,
      38–39
  model of psychopathology, 3, 23, 29,
      30, 35–37, 267–268

neurobiological basis, 112–113, 114–115,
      133–138
positive and negative states, 3–4, 11–12,
      28, 158
psychotic disorders as disorders of,
      230–231
regulatory structure and process, 28–29,
      97–99
schemata and, 33–35
social competence and, 32–33
therapeutic goals, 146–149
unconscious processes in, 147, 148
Aggressive behavior, 22
  brain function in, 226–227
  defensive behavior and, 125–126
  heritability, 52–53
  information-processing patterns, 222
  maladaptive coping, 102–103
  neurobiological model of affect
      dysregulation, 137–138
  parental conflict and, 107, 215–216
  physiological correlates, 210
  predisposing family factors, 175
  serotonergic system and, 224, 225–226
  See also Disruptive behavior disorders
Alcoholism, 201
Alexithymia, 109, 149–150
Ambivalent attachments, 7–8, 30, 57–58,
      105
Amino acid neurophysiology, 121–122
  See also specific acid

317